Methods in Molecular Biology

Series Editor
John M. Walker
School of Life and Medical Sciences
University of Hertfordshire
Hatfield, Hertfordshire, AL10 9AB, UK

For further volumes:
http://www.springer.com/series/7651

Hypertension

Methods and Protocols

Edited by

Rhian M. Touyz

Institute of Cardiovascular and Medical Sciences, University of Glasgow, Glasgow, Scotland, United Kingdom

Ernesto L. Schiffrin

Lady Davis Institute for Medical Research and Department of Medicine, Jewish General Hospital, McGill University, Montreal, QC, Canada

Humana Press

Editors
Rhian M. Touyz
Institute of Cardiovascular and Medical Sciences
University of Glasgow
Glasgow, Scotland
United Kingdom

Ernesto L. Schiffrin
Lady Davis Institute for Medical Research
and Department of Medicine
Jewish General Hospital
McGill University
Montreal, QC, Canada

ISSN 1064-3745 ISSN 1940-6029 (electronic)
Methods in Molecular Biology
ISBN 978-1-4939-6623-3 ISBN 978-1-4939-6625-7 (eBook)
DOI 10.1007/978-1-4939-6625-7

Library of Congress Control Number: 2016956249

Printed on acid-free paper

This Humana Press imprint is published by Springer Nature
The registered company is Springer Science+Business Media LLC
The registered company address is: 233 Spring Street, New York, NY 10013, U.S.A.

Preface

Despite the availability of a plethora of very effective antihypertensive drugs, the treatment of hypertension remains suboptimal and the prevalence of hypertension is increasing, contributing to the major cause of morbidity and mortality worldwide. Reasons for this relate, in part, to a lack of understanding of the exact mechanisms underlying the pathogenesis of hypertension, which is complex involving interactions between genes, physiological processes, and environmental factors. To gain insights into this complexity, studies at the molecular, subcellular, and cellular levels are needed to better understand mechanisms responsible for arterial hypertension and associated target organ damage of the vascular system, brain, heart, and kidneys.

This book provides a comprehensive compendium of protocols that the hypertension researcher can use to dissect out fundamental principles and molecular mechanisms of hypertension, extending from genetics of experimental hypertension to biomarkers in clinical hypertension.

The book is written in a user-friendly way and has been organized into seven sections, comprising (1) Genetics and omics of hypertension; (2) The renin-angiotensin-aldosterone system; (3) Vasoactive agents and hypertension; (4) Signal transduction and reactive oxygen species; (5) Novel cell models and approaches to study molecular mechanisms of hypertension; (6) Vascular physiology; and (7) New approaches to manipulate mouse models to study molecular mechanisms of hypertension.

The chapters follow the format of the book series on Molecular Methods. Each chapter has a general overview followed by well-described and detailed protocols and includes step-by-step protocols, lists of materials and reagents needed to complete the experiments, and a helpful notes section offering tips and tricks of the trade as well as troubleshooting advice.

Many protocol-based books and reviews related to hypertension research are available. Here we have carefully selected some new topics that are evolving in the field of molecular biology of hypertension. We hope these will be useful in advancing the understanding of hypertension at the molecular, subcellular, and cellular levels.

Glasgow, Scotland, UK — *Rhian M. Touyz*
Montreal, QC, Canada — *Ernesto L. Schiffrin*

Contents

Contributors

AMAYA ALBALAT • *School of Natural Sciences, University of Stirling, Stirling, UK*
NATALIA ALENINA • *Max-Delbrück-Center for Molecular Medicine (MDC), Berlin, Germany*
JOHNY AL-KHOURY • *Department of Anatomy and Cell Biology, Faculty of Medicine, University of Sherbrooke, Sherbrooke, QC, Canada*
SAMANTHA ALVAREZ-MADRAZO • *Institute of Cardiovascular and Medical Sciences, BHF Glasgow Cardiovascular Research Centre, University of Glasgow, Glasgow, UK*
ANGELICA AMANSO • *Division of Cardiology, Department of Medicine, Emory University, Atlanta, GA, USA*
MICHAEL BADER • *Max-Delbrück-Center for Molecular Medicine (MDC), Berlin, Germany*
TLILI BARHOUMI • *Lady Davis Institute for Medical Research, Jewish General Hospital, McGill University, Montreal, QC, Canada*
GHASSAN BKAILY • *Department of Anatomy and Cell Biology, Faculty of Medicine, University of Sherbrooke, Sherbrooke, QC, Canada*
THIAGO BRUDER-NASCIMENTO • *Kidney Research Centre, Department of Medicine, Ottawa Hospital Research Institute, University of Ottawa, Ottawa, ON, Canada; Department of Pharmacology, Medical School of Ribeirao Preto, University of Sao Paulo, Sao Paulo, Brazil*
MERCEDES L. DE BOLD • *Department of Pathology and Laboratory Medicine, Faculty of Medicine, Ottawa Heart Institute, University of Ottawa and the Cardiovascular Endocrinology Laboratory, Ottawa, ON, Canada*
ADOLFO J. DE BOLD • *Department of Pathology and Laboratory Medicine, Faculty of Medicine, Ottawa Heart Institute, University of Ottawa and the Cardiovascular Endocrinology Laboratory, Ottawa, ON, Canada*
ANA M. BRIONES • *Department of Pharmacology, School of Medicine, Instituto de Investigación Hospital Universitario La Paz (IdiPAZ), Universidad Autónoma de Madrid, Madrid, Spain*
K. BRIDGET BROSNIHAN • *Department of Surgery, Hypertension & Vascular Research, Cardiovascular Sciences Center, Wake Forest School of Medicine, Winston-Salem, NC, USA*
DYLAN BURGER • *Kidney Research Centre, Ottawa Hospital Research Institute, University of Ottawa, Ottawa, ON, Canada*
KEVIN D. BURNS • *Division of Nephrology, Department of Medicine, Kidney Research Centre, Ottawa Hospital Research Institute, University of Ottawa, Ottawa, ON, Canada*
G.E. CALLERA • *Kidney Research Centre, Department of Medicine, Ottawa Hospital Research Institute, University of Ottawa, Ottawa, ON, Canada*
R.M. CAREY • *University of Virgina, School of Medicine, Fontaine Research Park, Charlottesville, VA, USA*
AURELIE NGUYEN DINH CAT • *Institute of Cardiovascular and Medical Sciences, BHF Glasgow Cardiovascular Research Centre, University of Glasgow, Glasgow, Scotland, UK*

Mark C. Chappell • *Department of Surgery, Hypertension & Vascular Research, Cardiovascular Sciences Center, Wake Forest University School of Medicine, Winston-Salem, NC, USA*
Allen W. Cowley Jr • *Department of Physiology, Medical College of Wisconsin, Milwaukee, WI, USA*
Eleanor Davies • *Institute of Cardiovascular and Medical Sciences, BHF Glasgow Cardiovascular Research Centre, University of Glasgow, Glasgow, UK*
Christian Delles • *Institute of Cardiovascular and Medical Sciences, BHF Glasgow Cardiovascular, Research Centre, Medical Sciences University of Glasgow, Glasgow, UK*
Satoru Eguchi • *Department of Physiology, Cardiovascular Research Centre, Lewis Katz School of Medicine, Temple University, Philadelphia, PA, USA*
Katherine Elliott • *Department of Physiology, Cardiovascular Research Centre, Lewis Katz School of Medicine at Temple University, Philadelphia, PA, USA*
R.A. Felder • *University of Virgina, School of Medicine, Charlottesville, VA, USA*
Denise C. Fernandes • *Vascular Biology Laboratory, Heart Institute (InCor), University of São Paulo School of Medicine, São Paulo, Brazil*
Anderson J. Ferreira • *National Institute of Science and Technology in Nanobiopharmaceutics, Federal University of Minas, Gerais, Brazil; Department of Morphology, Biological Science Institute, Federal University of Minas, Gerais, Brazil*
Rodrigo A. Fraga-Silva • *National Institute of Science and Technology in Nanobiopharmaceutics, Federal University of Minas, Gerais, Brazil; Institute of Bioengineering, Elcole Polytechnique Federale De Lausanne, Lausanne, Switzerland*
Yamil Gerena • *School of Pharmacy, Medical Sciences Campus UPR, San Juan, PR, USA*
J.J. Gildea • *Department of Pathology, University of Virginia, Charlottesville, VA, USA*
Renata C. Gonçalves • *Vascular Biology Laboratory, Heart Institute (InCor), University of São Paulo School of Medicine, São Paulo, Brazil*
Kathirvel Gopalakrishnan • *Center for Hypertension and Personalized Medicine, Department of Physiology and Pharmacology, University of Toledo College of Medicine, Toledo, OH, USA; Program in Physiological Genomics, Center for Hypertension and Personalized Medicine, Department of Physiology and Pharmacology, University of Toledo College of Medicine and Life Sciences, Toledo, OH, USA*
Kathy K. Griendling • *Division of Cardiology, Department of Medicine, Emory University, Atlanta, GA, USA*
Caryl E. Hill • *Department of Neuroscience, John Curtin School of Medical Research, Australian National University, Canberra, ACT, Australia*
Holger Husi • *School of Natural Sciences, University of Stirling, Stirling, UK*
Danielle Jacques • *Department of Anatomy and Cell Biology, Faculty of Medicine, University of Sherbrooke, Sherbrooke, QC, Canada*
Bina Joe • *Center for Hypertension and Personalized Medicine, Bioinformatics, Proteomics and Genomics Program, Department of Surgery, University of Toledo College of Medicine, Toledo, OH, USA; Center for Hypertension and Personalized Medicine, Department of Physiology and Pharmacology, University of Toledo College of Medicine, Toledo, OH, USA; Program in Physiological Genomics, Center for Hypertension and Personalized Medicine, Department of Physiology and Pharmacology, University of Toledo College of Medicine and Life Sciences, Toledo, OH, USA*

P.A. JOSE • *Department of Medicine and Physiology, University of Maryland School of Medicine, Baltimore, MD, USA*

HENRY L. KEEN • *Department of Pharmacology, Roy J. and Lucille A. Carver College of Medicine, University of Iowa, Iowa City, IA, USA*

B.A. KEMP • *Division of Endocrinology and Metabolism, University of Virginia, Charlottesville, VA, USA*

ALISON J. KRIEGEL • *Department of Physiology, Medical College of Wisconsin, Milwaukee, WI, USA*

IVANA Y. KUO • *Department of Pharmacology, School of Medicine, Yale University, New Haven, CT, USA*

TERRY KURTH • *Department of Physiology, Medical College of Wisconsin, Milwaukee, WI, USA*

FRANCISCO R.M. LAURINDO • *Vascular Biology Laboratory, Heart Institute (InCor), University of São Paulo School of Medicine, São Paulo, Brazil*

ROBERTO Q. LAUTNER • *National Institute of Science and Technology in Nanobiopharmaceutics, Federal University of Minas, Gerais, Brazil*

Department of Physiology and Biophysics, Biological Science Institute, Federal University of Minas, Gerais, Brazil

ERIC LAZARTIGUES • *Department of Pharmacology and Experimental Therapeutics and Cardiovascular Center of Excellence, Louisiana State University Health Sciences Center, New Orleans, LA, USA*

MINGYU LIANG • *Center of Systems Molecular Medicine, Department of Physiology, Medical College of Wisconsin, Milwaukee, WI, USA*

YONG LIU • *Department of Physiology, Medical College of Wisconsin, Milwaukee, WI, USA*

GERVAISE LOIRAND • *INSERM, UMR_S1087-CNRS UMR_C6291, Nantes, France; CHU de Nantes, Nantes, France; CHU de Nantes, l'institut du thorax, Nantes, France*

RHEURE A.M. LOPES • *British Heart Foundation Glasgow Cardiovascular Research Centre, Institute of Cardiovascular and Medical Sciences, University of Glasgow, Glasgow, UK*

ALICIA N. LYLE • *Division of Cardiology, Department of Medicine, Emory University, Atlanta, GA, USA*

SCOTT M. MACKENZIE • *BHF Glasgow Cardiovascular Research Centre, Institute of Cardiovascular and Medical Sciences, University of Glasgow, Glasgow, UK*

KOREN K. MANN • *Lady Davis Institute for Medical Research and Department of Oncology Jewish General Hospital, McGill University, Montreal, QC, Canada*

DAVID L. MATTSON • *Center of Systems Molecular Medicine, Department of Physiology, Medical College of Wisconsin, Milwaukee, WI, USA*

MARTIN MCBRIDE • *Institute of Cardiovascular and Medical Sciences, BHF Glasgow Cardiovascular Research Centre, University of Glasgow, Glasgow, UK*

H.E. MCGRATH • *Department of Pathology, Univeristy of Virginia, Charlottesville, VA, USA*

WALMOR C. DE MELLO • *School of Medicine, Medical Sciences Campus UPR, San Juan, PR, USA*

HARALD MISCHAK • *School of Natural Sciences, University of Stirling, Stirling, UK; Mosaiques Diagnostics GmbH, Hannover, Germany; Institute of Cardiovascular and Medical Sciences, BHF Glasgow Cardiovascular Research Centre, University of Glasgow, Glasgow, UK*

AUGUSTO C. MONTEZANO • *British Heart Foundation Glasgow Cardiovascular Research Centre, Institute of Cardiovascular and Medical Sciences, University of Glasgow, Glasgow, UK*
WILLIAM MULLEN • *School of Natural Sciences, University of Stirling, Stirling, UK*
KARLA B. NEVES • *British Heart Foundation Glasgow Cardiovascular Research Centre, Institute of Cardiovascular and Medical Sciences, University of Glasgow, Glasgow, UK*
PAUL OLEYNIK • *Ottawa Hospital Research Institute, University of Ottawa, Ottawa, ON, Canada*
SANDOSH PADMANABHAN • *BHF Glasgow Cardiovascular Research Centre, Institute of Cardiovascular and Medical Sciences, University of Glasgow, Glasgow, UK*
PIERRE PARADIS • *Lady Davis Institute for Medical Research, Jewish General Hospital, McGill University, Montreal, QC, Canada*
KIM BRINT PEDERSEN • *Department of Pharmacology and Experimental Therapeutics and Cardiovascular Center of Excellence, Louisiana State University Health Sciences Center, New Orleans, LA, USA*
YOHANN RAUTUREAU • *Lady Davis Institute for Medical Research, Jewish General Hospital, McGill University, Montreal, QC, Canada*
FRANCISCO J. RIOS • *British Heart Foundation Glasgow Cardiovascular Research Centre, Institute of Cardiovascular and Medical Sciences, University of Glasgow, Glasgow, UK*
ROBSON A.S. SANTOS • *National Institute of Science and Technology in Nanobiopharmaceutics, Federal University of Minas, Gerais, Brazil*
Department of Physiology and Biophysics, Biological Science Institute, Federal University of Minas, Gerais, Brazil
VINCENT SAUZEAU • *INSERM, UMR_S1087-CNRS UMR_C6291, Nantes, France; Université de Nantes, Nantes, France; CHU de Nantes, l'institut du thorax, Nantes, France*
ERNESTO L. SCHIFFRIN • *Lady Davis Institute for Medical Research and Department of Medicine, Jewish General Hospital, McGill University, Montreal, QC, Canada*
CHRISTIN SCHULZ • *BHF Glasgow Cardiovascular Research Centre, Institute of Cardiovascular and Medical Sciences, University of Glasgow, Glasgow, UK*
R.E. VAN SCIVER • *Department of Mircobiology and Molecular Cell Biology, Eastern Virginia Medical School, Norfolk, Virginia*
SIMON YANICK • *Department of Anatomy and Cell Biology, Faculty of Medicine, University of Sherbrooke, Sherbrooke, QC, Canada*
CURT D. SIGMUND • *Department of Pharmacology, Roy J. and Lucille A. Carver College of Medicine, University of Iowa, Iowa City, IA, USA*
SRINIVAS SRIRAMULA • *Department of Pharmacology and Experimental Therapeutics and Cardiovascular Center of Excellence, Louisiana State University Health Sciences Center, New Orleans, LA, USA*
MIHAIL TODIRAS • *Max-Delbrück-Center for Molecular Medicine (MDC), Berlin, Germany*
RHIAN. M. TOUYZ • *Kidney Research Centre, Department of Medicine, Ottawa Hospital Research Institute, University of Ottawa, Ottawa, ON, Canada*
BHF Glasgow Cardiovascular Research Centre, Canada and Institute of Cardiovascular and Medical Sciences, University of Glasgow, Glasgow, Scotland, UK
SOFIA TSIROPOULOU • *Institute of Cardiovascular and Medical Sciences, BHF Glasgow Cardiovascular Research Centre, University of Glasgow, Glasgow, UK*

Kristie S. Usa • *Department of Physiology, Medical College of Wisconsin, Milwaukee, WI, USA*
David Weaver • *Center for Hypertension and Personalized Medicine, Bioinformatics, Proteomics and Genomics Program, Department of Surgery, University of Toledo College of Medicine, Toledo, OH, USA; Center for Hypertension and Personalized Medicine, Department of Physiology and Pharmacology, University of Toledo College of Medicine, Toledo, OH, USA*
Huijing Xia • *Department of Pharmacology and Experimental Therapeutics and Cardiovascular Center of Excellence, Louisiana State University Health Sciences Center, New Orleans, LA, USA*
Fengxia Xiao • *Division of Nephrology, Department of Medicine, Ottawa Hospital Research Institute, University of Ottawa, Ottawa, ON, Canada*

Chapter 1

Large-Scale Transcriptome Analysis

David Weaver, Kathirvel Gopalakrishnan, and Bina Joe

Abstract

Genomic variants identified to be linked with complex traits such as blood pressure are fewer in coding sequences compared to noncoding sequences. This being the case, there is an increasing need to query the expression of genes at a genome scale to then correlate the cause of alteration in expression to the function of variants regardless of where they are located. To do so, quering transcriptomes using microarray technology serves as a good experimental tool. This Chapter presents the basic methods needed to conduct a microarray experiment and points to resources avaiable online to complete the analysis and generate data regarding the transcriptomic status of a tissue sample relevant to hypertension.

Key words Microarray, mRNA, lncRNA, array, Chip, blood pressure

1 Introduction

Various genetic studies provide clear and compelling evidence for at least 20–30% of all the factors that contribute to the development of hypertension can be attributed to genetics. Despite a number of classical approaches applied to both human and model organism research, the precise identities of the underlying genetic elements that control blood pressure remain largely unknown. Thus, the quest for genes/genetic elements controlling blood pressure continues to be a daunting task.

The conventional methods for locating genetic elements that control blood pressure include linkage analysis and substitution mapping. These techniques are reviewed elsewhere. The results of such mapping studies point to discrete regions of the genome, within the limits of which, genetic elements can be expected to reside and influence blood pressure. To further the investigations on these prioritized regions, technological advances in large-scale hybridization technologies have become invaluable tools. In the early 2000s, when microarray technologies were being developed for determining the extent of differential gene expression between

Rhian M. Touyz and Ernesto L. Schiffrin (eds.), *Hypertension: Methods and Protocols*, Methods in Molecular Biology, vol. 1527, DOI 10.1007/978-1-4939-6625-7_1, © Springer Science+Business Media LLC 2017

two samples, we [1–3] and others [2–6] used these technologies to assess the mRNA expression status of candidate genes within the genomic segments prioritized by mapping studies for hypertension and metabolism-related phenotypes [7]. Some of these mapping studies led to the detection of differentially expressed genes as potentially novel candidate genes for blood pressure regulation in rats. A good example is the prioritization of the gene coding for the nuclear receptor 2, factor 2 [1]. This gene located on rat chromosome 1 was prioritized through a rat microarray experiment [1] and many years later also prioritized in human hypertension through a reanalysis of a genome-wide association study [8].

During the decade since the microarray platform came into existence, this technology has not only expanded in terms of its ability to detect and analyze transcriptomes comprising of mRNAs, but has grown dynamically to encompass the analysis of noncoding RNAs such as microRNAs and long noncoding RNAs (LncRNAs), and PiwiRNAs. Given that very little is known regarding the role of these new classes of noncoding RNAs in the genetics of hypertension and that the basic principles and methodologies associated with a microarray experiment for either mRNAs or noncoding RNAs remains essentially unchanged, the microarray technology can be predicted to be a mainstay in the quest for genetic elements controlling blood pressure.

Therefore, in this chapter, we chose to describe the methods to conduct and analyze a microarray experiment. The chapter also catalogs information on pertinent websites that we have accessed during our studies for analyzing our datasets.

2 Sample Preparation for Microarray

2.1 Total RNA Isolation

The quality of the RNA is essential to the overall success of the analysis. Since the most appropriate protocol for the isolation of RNA can be source dependent, we recommend using one of the commercially available kits designed for RNA isolation such as TRIZOL (Life technologies) or QIAzol (QIAGEN). RNA thus obtained is of poor quality for hybridization experiments. A cleanup procedure using an RNA cleanup kit such as RNeasy Kit (Ambion) is important.

2.2 Reagents and Materials Required

1. TRIZOL Reagent: Invitrogen Life Technologies, P/N 15596-018, or QIAzol™ Lysis Reagent: QIAGEN, P/N 79306.
2. RNeasy Mini Kit: QIAGEN, P/N 74104.
3. 10× TBE: Cambrex, P/N 50843.
4. Absolute ethanol (stored at −20 °C for RNA precipitation; store ethanol at room temperature for use with the GeneChip Sample Cleanup Module and IVT cRNA Kit).
5. 80% ethanol (in DEPC-treated water) (stored at −20 °C for RNA precipitation; store ethanol at room temperature for use with the GeneChip Sample Cleanup Module).

6. 3 M sodium acetate (NaOAc): Sigma-Aldrich, P/NS7899.
7. Chloroform.
8. Isopropyl alcohol.
9. 75 % ethanol (in DEPC-treated water).
10. RNase-free water.
11. Ethidium bromide: Sigma-Aldrich, P/N E8751.
12. 1 N NaOH.
13. 1 N HCl.
14. Sterile, RNase-free, microcentrifuge vials, 1.5 mL: USA Scientific, P/N 1415-2600 (or equivalent).
15. Micropipettors, (P-2, P-20, P-200, P-1000): Rainin Pipetman or equivalent.
16. Sterile barrier, RNase-free pipette tips. (Tips must be pointed, not rounded, for efficient use with the probe arrays.) Beveled pipette tips may cause damage to the array septa and cause leakage.
17. Mini agarose gel electrophoresis unit with appropriate buffers.
18. UV spectrophotometer or Nanodrop or Bioanalyzer.
19. Nonstick RNase-free microcentrifuge tubes, 0.5 mL and 1.5 mL: Ambion, P/N12350 and P/N 12450, respectively.

2.3 Isolation of RNA from Mammalian Cells or Tissues Using TRIZOL Reagent

TRIZOL Reagent is a ready-to-use reagent for the isolation of total RNA from cells and tissues (rat kidney or heart). This technique performs well with small quantities of tissue (50–100 mg) and cells (5×10^6), and large quantities of tissue (≥1 g) and cells (>10^7), of animal origin. The simplicity of the TRIZOL Reagent method allows simultaneous processing of a large number of samples. The entire procedure can be completed in 1 h.

2.4 Precautions for Preventing RNase Contamination

RNases can be introduced accidentally into the RNA preparation at any point in the isolation procedure through improper technique. Because RNase activity is difficult to inhibit, it is essential to prevent its introduction. The following guidelines should be observed when working with RNA.

1. Always wear disposable gloves. Skin often contains bacteria and molds that can contaminate an RNA preparation and be a source of RNases. Practice good microbiological technique to prevent microbial contamination.
2. Use sterile, disposable plasticware and automatic pipettes reserved for RNA work to prevent cross-contamination with RNases from shared equipment. For example, a laboratory that is using RNA probes will likely be using RNase A or T1 to reduce background on filters, and any nondisposable items (such as automatic pipettes) can be rich sources of RNases.
3. In the presence of TRIZOL Reagent, RNA is protected from RNase contamination. Downstream sample handling requires

that nondisposable glassware or plasticware be RNase-free. Glass items can be baked at 150 °C for 4 h, and plastic items can be soaked for 10 min in 0.5 M NaOH, rinsed thoroughly with water, and autoclaved.

2.5 Homogenization

2.5.1 Tissues

Homogenize tissue samples in 1 mL of TRIZOL Reagent per 50–100 mg of tissue (rat kidney or heart) using a glass-Teflon® or power homogenizer (Polytron, or Tekmar's TISSUMIZER® or equivalent). The sample volume should not exceed 10% of the volume of TRIZOL Reagent used for homogenization. As a rule, *make sure that the solution remains pink in color and does not turn brown*.

Following homogenization, remove insoluble material from the homogenate by centrifugation at 12,000 × *g* for 10 min at 2–8 °C. The resulting pellet contains extracellular membranes, polysaccharides, and high molecular weight DNA, while the supernate contains RNA.

2.6 Phase Separation

Incubate the homogenized samples for 5 min at 15–30 °C to permit the complete dissociation of nucleoprotein complexes. Add 0.2 mL of chloroform per 1 mL of TRIZOL Reagent. Cap sample tubes securely. Shake tubes vigorously by hand for 15 s and incubate them at 15–30 °C for 2–3 min. Centrifuge the samples at no more than 12,000 × *g* for 15 min at 2–8 °C. Following centrifugation, the mixture separates into a lower red, phenol-chloroform phase, an interphase, and a colorless upper aqueous phase. RNA remains exclusively in the aqueous phase. The volume of the aqueous phase is about 60% of the volume of TRIZOL Reagent used for homogenization.

2.7 RNA Precipitation

Transfer the aqueous phase to a fresh tube and precipitate the RNA from the aqueous phase by mixing with isopropyl alcohol. Use 0.5 mL of isopropyl alcohol per 1 mL of TRIZOL Reagent used for the initial homogenization. Incubate samples at 15–30 °C for 10 min and centrifuge at no more than 12,000 × *g* for 10 min at 2–8 °C. The RNA precipitate, often invisible before centrifugation, forms a gel-like pellet on the side and bottom of the tube.

2.8 RNA Wash

Remove the supernate. Wash the RNA pellet once with 75% ethanol, adding at least 1 mL of 75% ethanol per 1 mL of TRIZOL Reagent used for the initial homogenization. Mix the sample by vortexing and centrifuge at no more than 7500 × *g* for 5 min at 2–8 °C.

2.9 Redissolving the RNA

At the end of the procedure, briefly dry the RNA pellet (air-dry or vacuum-dry for 5–10 min). Do not dry the RNA by centrifugation under vacuum. It is important not to let the RNA pellet dry completely as this will greatly decrease its solubility. Partially dissolved RNA samples have an A260/280 ratio < 1.6. Dissolve RNA in RNase-free water incubating for 10 min at 55–60 °C.

2.10 Precipitation of RNA

It is not necessary to precipitate total RNA following isolation or cleanup with the RNeasy Mini Kit. Adjust elution volumes from the RNeasy column to prepare for cDNA synthesis based upon expected RNA yields from your experiment. Ethanol precipitation is required following TRIZOL or QIAzol reagent isolation and hot phenol extraction methods.

2.11 Precipitation Procedure

1. Add 1/10 volume 3 M NaOAc, pH 5.2, and 2.5 volumes ethanol.
2. Mix and incubate at −20 °C for at least 1 h.
3. Centrifuge at ≥ 12,000 × *g* in a microcentrifuge for 20 min at 4 °C.
4. Wash pellet twice with 80 % ethanol.
5. Air-dry pellet. Check for dryness before proceeding.
6. Resuspend pellet in DEPC-treated H_2O.

The appropriate volume for resuspension depends on the expected yield and the amount of RNA required for the cDNA synthesis. Please read ahead to the cDNA synthesis protocol in order to determine the appropriate resuspension volume at this step.

Important: If going directly from TRIZOL-isolated total RNA to cDNA synthesis, it is beneficial to perform a second cleanup on the total RNA before starting. After the ethanol precipitation step in the TRIZOL extraction procedure, perform a cleanup using the QIAGEN RNeasy Mini Kit. Much better yields of labeled cRNA are obtained from the in vitro transcription-labeling reaction when this second cleanup is performed.

2.12 Quantification of RNA

Quantify the RNA yield by a spectrophotometric method using the convention that one absorbance unit at 260 nm equals 40 μg/mL RNA.

1. The absorbance should be checked at 260 and 280 nm for determination of sample concentration and purity.
2. The A260/A280 ratio should be close to 2.0 for pure RNA (ratios between 1.9 and 2.1 are acceptable; refer to Fig. 1 for an example).

Using the RNA isolated, there are several choices for proceeding with the microarray experiment. The choices are:

1. Submit the isolated RNA for conversion to cDNA and hybridization by a commercial vendor or core facility for microarrays.

   To do so, document the spectrophotometric quality check information and ship the RNA on dry ice.
2. Convert the RNA to cDNA in the laboratory for hybridization experiments.

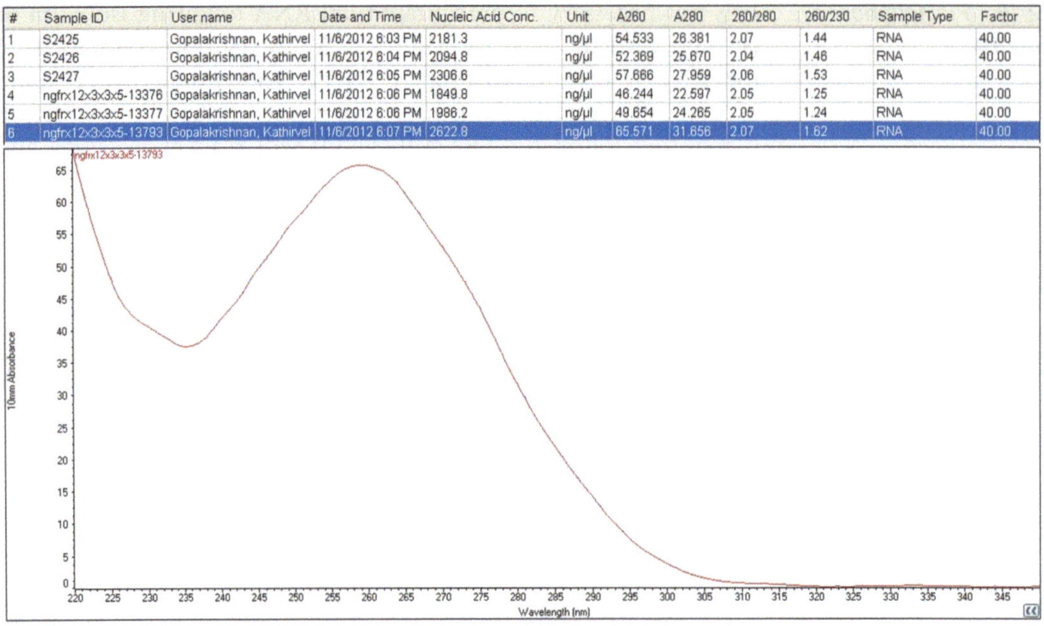

#	Sample ID	User name	Date and Time	Nucleic Acid Conc.	Unit	A260	A280	260/280	260/230	Sample Type	Factor
1	S2425	Gopalakrishnan, Kathirvel	11/6/2012 6:03 PM	2181.3	ng/µl	54.533	26.381	2.07	1.44	RNA	40.00
2	S2426	Gopalakrishnan, Kathirvel	11/6/2012 6:04 PM	2094.8	ng/µl	52.369	25.670	2.04	1.46	RNA	40.00
3	S2427	Gopalakrishnan, Kathirvel	11/6/2012 6:05 PM	2306.6	ng/µl	57.666	27.959	2.06	1.53	RNA	40.00
4	ngfrx12x3x3x5-13376	Gopalakrishnan, Kathirvel	11/6/2012 6:06 PM	1849.8	ng/µl	46.244	22.597	2.05	1.25	RNA	40.00
5	ngfrx12x3x3x5-13377	Gopalakrishnan, Kathirvel	11/6/2012 6:06 PM	1986.2	ng/µl	49.654	24.265	2.05	1.24	RNA	40.00
6	ngfrx12x3x3x5-13793	Gopalakrishnan, Kathirvel	11/6/2012 6:07 PM	2622.8	ng/µl	65.571	31.656	2.07	1.62	RNA	40.00

Fig. 1 Representative absorption spectrum of a good-quality RNA sample

Several cDNA preparation kits are available from commercial vendors such as Bio-Rad, Life Technologies, and QIAGEN.

3. Use the RNA for preparation for Affymetrix arrays: In this case, Affymetrix has a unique procedure for one-cycle cDNA synthesis, target labeling, and cRNA preparations. Follow the Affymetrix manual, which is quite detailed and self-explanatory for the most part.

   Please note that besides Affymetrix, there are a number of additional commercial microarray service providers for your hybridization experiments (Table 1).

2.13 Microarray Hybridization, Washing and Staining of Sample Targets

For experiments described in our work [9], we used the Affymetrix GeneChip® microarrays (http://www.affymetrix.com/estore/). The Affymetrix system used consisted of the Affymetrix GeneChip® Hybridization Oven 640, the Affymetrix GeneChip® Fluidics Station 450, and the Affymetrix GeneChip® Scanner 3000 6G. The software utilized was the Affymetrix GeneChip® Operating Software (GCOS), version 1.4. Manuals used for protocols were the GeneChip® Expression Analysis Technical Manual (catalog number 702232, Revision 3) (http://media.affymetrix.com/support/downloads/manuals/expression_analysis_manual.pdf) and the GeneChip® Expression, Wash, Stain and Scan User Manual (catalog number 702731, Revision 3) (http://media.affymetrix.com/support/downloads/manuals/wash_stain_scan_cartridge_arrays_manual.pdf). For user-prepared protocols, in the Analysis

Table 1
Details of some of the microarray service providers in the United States

Microarray service provider	Website	
Affymetrix 3420 Central Expressway Santa Clara, CA 95051 USA	http://www.affymetrix.com/estore/	Affymetrix® platform
Illumina, Inc. 5200 Illumina Way San Diego, CA 92122 USA	http://www.illumina.com/	Illumina® platform
Star Array Unit 223, Innovation Center BLK 2, 18 Nanyang Drive, Singapore 637723	http://www.star-array.com/technology.html	Illumina® platform
QIAGEN Inc. 27220 Turnberry Lane Valencia, CA 91355 USA	http://www.sabiosciences.com/RTPCR.php	RT^2 ProfilerTM PCR Array platform
Agilent 5301 Stevens Creek Blvd Santa Clara, CA 95051 USA	http://www.genomics.agilent.com/CollectionOverview.aspx?PageType=Application&SubPageType=ApplicationOverview&PageID=103	Agilent gene expression microarray platform
Roche NimbleGen, Inc. 500 South Rosa Road Madison, WI 53719 USA	http://www.nimblegen.com/products/expression/index.html	NimbleGen platform
Arraystar	http://www.arraystar.com/index.asp	Illumina® platform
Otogenetics	http://www.otogenetics.com/rnaseq_page_010812.htm	

Technical manual, refer to Appendix B, and in the Wash, Stain and Scan manual, refer to Chapter 2.

In recent years, Affymetrix has updated both the sample preparation protocols and the system equipment. For example, Affymetrix has since discontinued the GCOS software and now uses the Affymetrix GeneChip® Command Console (AGCC) (http://www.affymetrix.com/esearch/search.jsp?pd=131429&N=4294967292) with the GeneChip® Expression Console (http://www.affymetrix.com/esearch/search.jsp?pd=131414&N=4294967292) to generate similar data. All experimental procedures performed in this manuscript utilized the GCOS software (*see* **Note 1**). The Affymetrix scanner has been upgraded to a 3000 7G model which scans with an increased resolution of 7 μm and allows for different types of Affymetrix microarrays to be utilized in research. It is highly recommended that the researcher refer to Affymetrix for the most updated expression analysis methodology (http://www.affymetrix.com/estore/).

Important aspects for designing a microarray study: Most microarray experiments are run with a minimum of six samples (three control and three experimental) to achieve data that can be mined with statistical programs. The longest step of the process is the overnight (16 h) hybridization. For washing and staining following hybridization, the fluidics station can process four arrays at a time, and normally, eight arrays can be run in 1 day with subsequent scanning of the arrays. If the user is running more than eight samples, it is recommended that all samples be processed at one time to create all of the sample hybridization cocktails. Once created, they can be stored at −20 °C until ready for hybridization to the arrays.

For example, assume an experiment consists of 24 arrays for processing: 12 control samples (sample #'s 1–12) and 12 experimental samples (sample #'s 13–24). As eight samples can be run per day, the overall work should be planned as outlined in the following timeline. It is highly recommended that the user does not process only samples from the same group on the same day. In our example, on day 1, control sample #'s 1–4 and experimental sample #'s 13–16 are processed.

Experimental timeline example for 24 samples

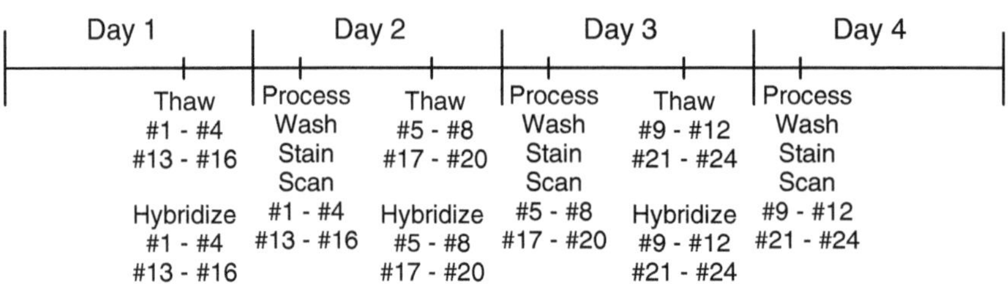

Day 1 afternoon	Thaw "control" or normotensive strain samples 1–4 and "experimental" or hypertensive strain samples 13–16. Apply the hybridization cocktails to microarrays and hybridize overnight
Day 2 morning	Prepare solutions for washing and staining. Process "control" or normotensive strain samples 1–4 and "experimental" or hypertensive strain samples 13–16 with the fluidics station. Scan these eight arrays
Day 2 afternoon	Thaw "control" or normotensive samples 5–8 and "experimental" or hypertensive strain samples 17–20. Apply the hybridization cocktails to microarrays and hybridize overnight
Day 3 morning	Prepare solutions for washing and staining. Process "control" or normotensive strain samples 5–8 and "experimental" or hypertensive strain samples 17–20 with the fluidics station. Scan these eight arrays
Day 3 afternoon	Thaw "control" or normotensive strain samples 9–12 and "experimental" or hypertensive strain samples 21–24. Apply the hybridization cocktails to microarrays and hybridize overnight
Day 4 morning	Prepare solutions for washing and staining. Process controls 9–12 and experimentals 21–24 with the fluidics station. Scan these eight arrays to complete the generation of experimental data

2.14 Materials

Affymetrix manuals are available online and are very user-friendly. The protocols listed by Affymetrix should be strictly followed (http://www.affymetrix.com/support/technical/manuals.affx).

All solutions should be prepared using ultrapure water (purified deionized water with a sensitivity of 18 MW at 25 °C), unless otherwise specified, and analytical grade reagents. Prepare all stock solutions at room temperature and store at the proper temperatures listed.

2.14.1 Hybridization Components, Stock Solutions and Buffers

1. Water, Molecular Biology Grade (Fisher Scientific, Pittsburgh, PA).
2. Acetylated Bovine Serum Albumin (BSA) solution (50 mg/mL) (catalog number 15561-020) (Life Technologies).
3. Herring Sperm DNA (catalog number D1811) (Promega Corporation).
4. GeneChip® Hybridization Control Kit (catalog number 900454) (Affymetrix, Santa Clara, CA) Contains the 20× Eukaryotic Hybridization Control Stock composed of premixed biotin-labeled bioB, bioC, bioD and cre, in staggered amounts, which is added directly in the preparation of the hybridization cocktail. These controls allow for monitoring of the hybridization process for troubleshooting. The kit also contains the Control Oligonucleotide B2 (3 nM) which is used for alignment of array probe cell features for image analysis.

5. 5 M NaCl, RNase-free, DNase-free (Life Technologies, Grand Island, NY).
6. MES hydrate SigmaUltra (catalog number M5287) (Sigma-Aldrich).
7. MES Sodium Salt (catalog number M5057 or M3058) (Sigma-Aldrich).
8. EDTA Disodium Salt, 0.5 M solution (catalog number E7889) (Sigma-Aldrich).
9. Dimethyl sulfoxide (DMSO) (catalog number D5879) (Sigma-Aldrich).
10. Sufact-Amps 20 (Tween-20), 10% (catalog number 28320) (Pierce Chemical).
11. GeneChip® Rat Genome 230 2.0 Arrays (Affymetrix).
12. 12× MES stock solution: 1.22 M MES, 0.89 M [Na+]. Molecular Biology Grade water should be used in creating this solution. Add about 500 mL Molecular Biology Grade water to a 1-L graduated cylinder. Weigh 64.61 g MES hydrate and transfer to the cylinder. Weigh 193.3 g MES Sodium Salt and transfer to the cylinder. Mix and adjust the volume to 1000 mL with Molecular Biology Grade water. (A magnetic stirring bar helps to dissolve the materials into solution.) The pH should be between 6.5 to 6.7 (*see* **Note 2**). Filter the solution through a 0.2 mm filter. The solution should be shielded from light and stored at 2–8 °C. (*see* **Note 3**).
13. 2× Hybridization buffer: 100 mM MES, 1 M [Na+], 20 mM EDTA, 0.01% Tween-20. In a 100 mL beaker, combine 8.3 mL of 12× MES stock solution, 17.7 mL of 5 M NaCl (RNase-free, DNase-free), 4.0 mL of 0.5 M EDTA, 0.1 mL of 10% Tween-20 and 19.9 mL ultrapure water. Mix and filter the 50 mL of solution through a 0.2 mm filter. The solution should be shielded from light and stored at 2–8 °C.

2.14.2 Washing and Staining Components, Stock Solutions and Buffers

1. Streptavidin, R-Phycoerythrin Conjugate (SAPE), 1 mg/mL (catalog number S-866) (Life Technologies).
2. PBS, pH 7.2 (catalog number 20012-027) (Life Technologies).
3. UltrapureTM 20× SSPE (3 M NaCl, 0.2 M NaH_2PO_4, 0.02 M EDTA) (catalog number 15591043) (Life Technologies).
4. IgG from goat serum, reagent grade (catalog number I5256-10MG) (Sigma-Aldrich). For 10 mg/mL Goat IgG stock, resuspend 10 mg in 1 mL of PBS, pH 7.2 (or 150 mM NaCl) and store at 4 °C. Larger volume stocks can be stored at −20 °C until use.
5. Biotinylated anti-streptavidin antibody from goat (catalog number BA-0500) (Vector Laboratories).

6. Stringent wash buffer: 100 mM MES, 0.1 M [Na+], 0.01% Tween-20. In a 1-L graduated cylinder, combine 83.3 mL of 12× MES stock solution, 5.2 mL of 5 M NaCl (RNase-free, DNase-free), 1.0 mL of 10% Tween-20 and 910.5 mL ultrapure water. Mix and filter the solution through a 0.2 mm filter. The solution should be shielded from light and stored at 2–8 °C.
7. Non-stringent wash buffer: 6× SSPE, 0.01% Tween-20. In a 1-L graduated cylinder, combine 300 mL of 20× SSPE, 1.0 mL of 10% Tween-20 and 699 mL ultrapure water. Mix and filter the solution through a 0.2 mm filter. The solution can be stored at room temperature.
8. 2× Stain buffer: 100 mM MES, 1 M [Na+], 0.05% Tween-20. In a 500 mL graduated cylinder, combine 41.7 mL 12× MES stock solution, 92.5 mL 5 M NaCl (RNase-free, DNase-free), 2.5 mL 10% Tween-20 and 113.3 mL of ultrapure water. Mix and filter the solution through a 0.2 mm filter. The solution should be shielded from light and stored at 2–8 °C.

3 Methods

3.1 Eukaryotic Target Hybridization

The methods presented in this manuscript are based on our experience conducting experiments using the Affymetrix GeneChip® Rat Genome 230 2.0 Arrays. The preparation of the hybridization cocktails is for use with the Affymetrix GeneChip® Rat Genome 230 2.0 Arrays, which are the standard (49 Format/64 Format) arrays (*see* **Note 4**) from Affymetrix. The samples were processed according to the Affymetrix GeneChip® Expression Analysis Technical Manual (catalog number 702232, Revision 3) (http://media.affymetrix.com/support/downloads/manuals/expression_analysis_manual.pdf).

Use sterile, RNase-free microcentrifuge vials and sterile barrier pipette tips for all procedures.

1. In a 1.5 mL microcentrifuge vial, mix the following to create the hybridization cocktail for each sample: 15 μg of prepared fragmented and labeled cRNA, 5 μL control oligonucleotide B2 (3 nM), 15 μL 20× eukaryotic hybridization controls (*see* **Note 5**), 3 μL herring sperm DNA (10 mg/mL), 3 μL acetylated bovine serum albumin (BSA) solution (50 mg/mL), 150 μL 2× hybridization buffer, 30 μL DMSO. Bring the final volume to 300 μL with nuclease-free water.
2. Allow the arrays to equilibrate to room temperature immediately before use (*see* **Note 6**).
3. Heat the hybridization cocktail to 99 °C for 5 min in a heat block (*see* **Note 7**).

4. While the sample is heating, the microarray cartridge needs to be filled with 200 μL of 1× hybridization buffer (*see* **Note 8**). On the back of the GeneChip® cartridge, there are two rubber septa. To fill the array, first insert a clean, unused pipette tip into the upper septa for venting. Using a micropipetter, insert the tip into the remaining septa to fill with the 1× hybridization buffer for pre-hybridization wetting. Remove all tips and incubate the array filled with 1× hybridization buffer in the GeneChip® Hybridization Oven at 45 °C for 10 min with rotation at 60 rpm.
5. Transfer the hybridization cocktail (that has been heated to 99 °C) to a 45 °C heat block for 5 min.
6. Following the 5 min incubation, spin the hybridization cocktail in a microcentrifuge for 5 min to collect any insoluble material from the hybridization mixture.
7. Remove the array from the hybridization oven. Vent the array, as above when loading, and then extract the 1× hybridization buffer. Leave the venting pipette tip in place and fill the GeneChip® with 200 μL of the hybridization cocktail. Be sure to avoid any insoluble matter at the bottom of the microcentrifuge tube.
8. Place the sample-filled array in the hybridization oven. Rotate at 60 rpm for 16 h at 45 °C.
9. During the latter part of the overnight 16 h incubation, proceed to the following section to prepare reagents required at the end of the hybridization.

3.2 Microarray Washing and Staining

The washing and staining of the Affymetrix GeneChip® Rat Genome 230 2.0 Arrays are automated using the Affymetrix GeneChip® Fluidics Station 450. To wash, stain, and scan an array, a sample file must be created using the GCOS software (or the updated AGCC software http://www.affymetrix.com/esearch/search.jsp?pd=131429&N=4294967292). Registering the sample file (EXP file in GCOS, ARR file in AGCC) is the beginning of the Affymetrix data flow. The created sample file will be referred to for the washing, staining, and subsequent scanning of the array by the automated instrument protocols. Samples should be processed according to the Affymetrix GeneChip® Expression, Wash, Stain and Scan User Manual (catalog number 702731, Revision 3) (http://media.affymetrix.com/support/downloads/manuals/wash_stain_scan_cartridge_arrays_manual.pdf).

The manual provides step-by-step directions for using the Affymetrix GeneChip® Fluidics Station 450. Once samples are registered, they can be automatically processed using the manufacturer's protocol. The manual lists materials for staining solutions based on an individual array. It is recommended that the researcher mix up the solutions for the number of samples being processed that day and aliquot them appropriately. It is highly recommended that the user prepare for one additional solution "set" to the number being processed. If the user is processing six arrays, enough of both, the Streptavidin, R-Phycoerythrin (SAPE) solution mix and the antibody solution should be created to allow for processing of seven arrays as seen in the following example. It is important to make fresh solutions on the day of the washing and staining of the array.

1. Mix the following for the SAPE solution mix (Streptavidin, R-Phycoerythrin stain):

Component	Volume/reaction	# of samples	Volume for 7 reactions
2× Stain buffer	600.0 µL	7	4200.0 µL
BSA (50 mg/mL)	48.0 µL	7	336.0 µL
Streptavidin Phycoerythrin (SAPE)	12.0 µL	7	84.0 µL
DI H_2O	540.0 µL	7	3780.0 µL
Total	1200.0 µL	7	8400.0 µL

Aliquot 600.0 µL of the SAPE solution mix into 1.5 mL microcentrifuge tubes. For the seven samples example, the user would have fourteen microcentrifuge tubes each containing 600.0 µL volume of SAPE solution mix.

2.

Component	Volume/reaction	# of samples	Volume for 7 reactions
2× Stain Buffer	300.0 µL	7	2100.0 µL
BSA (50 mg/mL)	24.0 µL	7	168.0 µL
Goat Ig G stock (10 mg/mL)	6.0 µL	7	42.0 µL
Biotinylated antibody (0.5 mg/mL)	3.6 µL	7	25.2 µL
DI H_2O	266.4 µL	7	1864.8 µL
Total	1200 µL	7	4200.0 µL

Aliquot 600.0 µL of the antibody solution mix into 1.5 mL microcentrifuge tubes. For the samples example, the user would have seven microcentrifuge tubes each containing 600.0 µL volume of antibody solution mix.

3. Once the above solutions have been freshly prepared, remove the arrays from the hybridization oven.
4. Using venting, similar to when filling the arrays, remove the hybridization cocktail and place it in a clean microcentrifuge tube. (The hybridization cocktails can be stored at −80 °C and can be reused up to three times on other arrays.) Fill the array

cartridge with 250 μL of the non-stringent wash buffer. The array is now ready for washing and staining in the fluidics station. As the station can only process four arrays at a time, other arrays to be processed can be stored temporarily at 4 °C for up to 3 h.

5. The fluidics station needs to be primed to ensure the lines are filled with the appropriate buffers and is ready for running protocols. The non-stringent wash buffer should be filled in the Wash A buffer reservoir on the machine. The stringent wash buffer should be filled in the Wash B buffer reservoir. Run the Prime_450 maintenance protocol with empty microcentrifuge tubes in the stain holder positions 1, 2, and 3.
6. After priming, the fluidics station is ready to accept arrays for washing and staining. Using the proper protocol enter the sample file name, the array name, and the probe array type. Select the fluidics protocol script for processing the arrays. For our experiments, the fluidics script used was the EukGE-WS2v5_450. Follow instructions on the LCD window on the fluidics station for loading the array into the machine and for loading of the sample holders. There are three sample holders on the machine module. Place one vial containing 600.0 μL SAPE stain solution in sample holder 1. Place one vial containing 600.0 μL antibody solution in sample holder 2. Place one vial containing 600.0 μL SAPE stain solution in sample holder 3. Press down on the needle lever to snap needles into position which will start the run.
7. When the protocol is complete, the LCD window will display the message EJECT & INSPECT CARTRIDGE. Press down on the cartridge lever to the eject position and remove the array. *Do not* engage the washblock until the array has been inspected for the presence of bubbles or air pockets. If the array has no bubbles, it is ready for scanning. If there are bubbles present, reinsert the array back into the washblock probe array holder and engage the washblock. The array will be drained and refilled. Recheck the array for any bubbles and when none are present, continue on scanning the array. Engage all washblocks for the fluidics station to continue to complete the protocol and prime for the next wash protocol.
8. If the arrays are not scanned immediately following washing and staining, they can be stored at 4 °C, in the dark, until ready for scanning for a maximum of 24 h.
9. A shutdown protocol should be run on the fluidics station at the end of the daily session.

3.3 Microarray Scanning

The scanning of the Affymetrix GeneChip® Rat Genome 230 2.0 Arrays are automated using the Affymetrix GeneChip® Scanner 3000. The sample file created using the GCOS software (or the updated AGCC software) will be referenced for scanning of the array. After washing and staining of the array, the sample file will be available in the scanner software. Samples were scanned according to the Affymetrix GeneChip® Expression, Wash, Stain and Scan User Manual (catalog number 702731, Revision 3) (http://media.affymetrix.com/support/downloads/manuals/wash_stain_scan_cartridge_arrays_manual.pdf).

The manual provides step-by-step directions for using the AGGC software to operate the Affymetrix GeneChip® Scanner 3000. Once samples are washed and stained, they can be scanned using the manufacturer's protocol (*see* **Note 9**).

The output of the scanning creates two files for each array. The first file created during scanning is the raw pixelated image of the array and is referred to as a .DAT file. The Affymetrix software saves this file and aligns a grid onto the image to locate and identify the probe cell features. The control oligonucleotide B2 included in the hybridization cocktail allows for this alignment. The software takes each pixelated probe feature from the .DAT file and automatically calculates a single intensity value for each probe feature (non-pixelated) to create a second image file. This file contains all of the probe cell intensity data that is referred to as the .CEL file. *It is the most important file that is generated* and is used by Affymetrix or other third-party software to determine single gene intensity values based on their respective probe intensities.

3.4 Scanned Image Analysis

The Affymetrix expression software, either GCOS or the Affymetrix Expression Console, can be used to visualize the .CEL files for verification of a problem-free array and can be used to analyze the data to generate reports to ensure the microarrays in an experiment are suitable for subsequent data analysis.

Affymetrix created their gene expression arrays utilizing sets of 25-mer oligonucleotide probes designed specifically for each individual gene. An individual gene probe set is composed of 11 perfect match primers (PM) and 11 mismatch primers (MM) (the middle base of the 25-mer perfect match is changed). In other words, each gene has a set of 22 individual probes whose intensities are available to be used for analysis in determining a single intensity of the specified gene using Affymetrix software or other third-party software.

A visual inspection of the array should be done to determine all areas of the array suitable for analysis.

1. The array image should be clear of "bubbles" (areas where there was no hybridization due to air bubbles trapped in the array during hybridization), scratches, or other problematic areas. If these areas are present, they need to be masked and not used in subsequent analysis.

2. The image should have an overall "equal" image intensity without large areas of extreme intensity.
3. When the grid is applied on the array, the border of the array should be examined for a checkerboard appearance in each corner of the array and an alternating pattern on the border edges of the entire array that are aligned within the grid boxes. This alignment uses the hybridization of the control oligonucleotide B2 at these specific probe cells on the array.
4. In the center section of the array image, a small cross should be present which is also a result of the control oligonucleotide B2 hybridization and should be aligned within the grid boxes.
5. If alignment does not automatically occur directly, manual adjustment can be made to the grid using an Affymetrix manual protocol. In our experience over 10 years, we have never had to adjust any grid alignments, nor have we had to use any masking of problematic areas of the microarrays.

Prior to data analysis, the arrays to be included in an experiment must be evaluated to ensure they are within certain parameters to be considered comparable and suitable for data analysis. To do this, the user will rely on a report file (.RPT) that can be generated with GCOS or the Affymetrix Expression Console software (*see* **Note 10**). In either GCOS or the Expression Console, the researcher will use the MAS 5.0 algorithm to analyze each array independently in order to obtain a report regarding the performance of the array. It is important to identify any obvious problems at this point before submitting data from the experimental set of arrays to a multichip analysis method, either in the Expression Console or with third-party software. For the generation of a MAS 5.0 algorithm .RPT file, the researcher should use the GCOS software to create a tabular formatted analysis results file or .CHP file. The software allows for scaling and normalization of each array as it is analyzed by the MAS 5.0 algorithm to create the .CHP file. Our experiments used a scaling setting for all probe sets (set at 150) to achieve a scale factor for each array which will be referred to below. No normalization adjustments were made to the data and Affymetrix default settings were used for all other limits. Once a .CHP file is created, the software can then be used to create a report (.RPT) file.

The report file contains information to evaluate performance of the array. Various laboratories may use different limit settings for deciding which arrays can be compared with confidence. The top heading of each report file lists the file name, probe array type, and the algorithm used. The following list contains those parameters, which in our hands provide confident assurance to continue on with the arrays for multichip analysis.

1. Scaling factor (SF): In creating our .CHP file, we used an all-probes scaling setting of 150 on each array. The SF for each array should be compared and should be approximately equivalent. For example, if the SF of one array is 1.215 and the second array has a SF of 1.561, these arrays overall are of approximately equal intensity. If one array's SF is 1.335 and the second is 26.321, they can't be compared with any confidence.
2. Background: The average background on the array should be less than 100. All arrays in an experimental set should have similar values.
3. Noise (RawQ): The noise is a reflection of the normal operation of the machine and should be less than 10.
4. Total probe sets: The percentages of number present should be in a range of 5–10 % of each other. Depending on the experimental conditions, the set of control samples and the set of experimental samples should each be similar among like samples.
5. Housekeeping controls: The housekeeping controls are representative of successful processing of the sample as the source of these genes are naturally occurring genes present in the sample. The housekeeping genes have intensity readings for probes from both the 3′ and 5′ ends and can be used to generate a 3′ to 5′ ratio value. If full mRNA templates were present in the sample, the ratio representing both ends of the gene that was processed through the amplification steps in the preparation of the sample should theoretically be equal to 1. If the starting mRNA was degraded and processed, this ratio would vary as the 3′ end of the mRNA would not be present for amplification. In our experiments, GAPDH (rat) was used as the housekeeping gene, and the acceptance value for the 3′/5′ ratio was 3 or less. Other common housekeeping genes on the Affymetrix rat genome array include beta-actin and hexokinase.
6. Spike controls: These controls are the Affymetrix Eukaryotic Hybridization Controls (mixed biotin-labeled bioB, bioC, bioD, and cre, in staggered amounts) incorporated as part of the hybridization cocktail. The bioC, bioD, and cre should all have present calls for both the 3′ and 5′ regions. The bioB is the control that is spiked in the least amount to test the lower limit of the readability by the scanner and has three regions that are investigated (3′, 5′, and middle). It is recommended that at least two of the three regions have present calls.

Once the above visual evaluations and report standards have been met, the arrays are ready for analysis of the entire data set. The .CEL files for each array can be transferred out of either the GCOS or AGCC software and uploaded into various third-party statistical packages for the mining of significant results.

4 Notes

1. Affymetrix has discontinued support of the GCOS software, and the only available operating system is the AGCC software (http://www.affymetrix.com/esearch/search.jsp?pd=131429&N=4294967292). The researcher will have to use the AGCC software to do experiments with the Affymetrix system.
2. Following preparation of the solution, the pH normally does not need much adjustment. To avoid a sudden pH change, use either 1 N HCl to lower the pH or 1 N NaOH to increase the pH.
3. Do not autoclave the solution. If the solution turns yellow with time, discard the solution.
4. Affymetrix sells premade Hybridization, Wash and Stain kits (catalog number 900720) (Affymetrix) with all of the necessary components for the hybridization, array post-hybridization washing, and staining.
5. Frozen stocks of 20× Eukaryotic Hybridization Controls are heated to 65 °C for 5 min to completely resuspend the cRNA before dispensing.
6. It is important to allow the arrays to be at room temperature prior to use. The rubber septa (on the back of the array for loading) need to be equilibrated to room temperature; otherwise, they may be prone to cracking which can result in leaks.
7. It is recommended that lock caps be used on the microcentrifuge tubes during the high heat incubation to ensure the lids do not open as a result of the increased temperature.
8. Make up a small volume of 1× hybridization buffer by making a 1:1 dilution of the 2× hybridization buffer. The 200 μL volume will not completely fill the array. Move the array, while looking in the array window, to ensure the array is completely wetted. The solution should be shielded from light and stored at 2–8 °C. Another option is to make a 1× array holding buffer: 100 mM MES, 1 M [Na+], 0.01 % Tween-20. For 100 mL, combine 8.3 mL of 12× MES stock solution, 18.5 mL of 5 M NaCl (RNase-free, DNase-free), 0.1 mL of 10% Tween-20, and 73.1 mL ultrapure water. Mix and filter the solution through a 0.2 μm filter. The solution should be shielded from light and stored at 2–8 °C.
9. The scanner uses a laser and has a safety interlock system; however, users should always be aware of the hazardous nature of laser light. It is important to let the scanner laser warm up for at least 10 min prior to scanning for the laser to stabilize.
10. As mentioned previously, our experiments were carried out with the GCOS operating system. This software had the capa-

bility to generate tabular results files (.CHP files) directly, but is no longer supported by Affymetrix. One should refer to the Affymetrix Expression Console software operating manual (http://media.affymetrix.com/support/downloads/manuals/expression_console_userguide.pdf) to create .CHP files and subsequent report files. Both GCOS and the Expression Console software use the MAS 5.0 algorithm to calculate a significance or *p*-value for each probe set on an individual array in creating the .CHP file. Report files (.RPT) can be generated from .CHP files. The Expression Console provides more in-depth information in its .RPT file than the GCOS software. The Expression Console also has available multichip analysis methods: Robust Multichip Analysis (RMA) algorithm or Probe Logarithmic Intensity Error Estimation (PLIER) algorithm. Reports can be generated for .CHP files created with either multichip analysis and should be evaluated by Affymetrix protocols.

5 Data Analysis

Many computer programs are available from both commercial and educational sources to analyze the large amounts of data generated in a microarray experiment. It is highly recommended that the researcher consult with a biostatistician to assist in the appropriate analysis of the data set.

Our experimental data was analyzed with the R statistical program (http:cran.r-project.org/), a freely downloadable statistical package. The R program is a high-level statistical package which requires an in-depth knowledge for writing program scripts to properly analyze the data. With the guidance of our on-site statistician, we used an available Affymetrix limma GUI (user guidance interface) within the R program to perform comparison analysis between the control and experimental groups. This format has drop-down menus of choices in the setup of the analysis criteria and requires the creation of a small identification file of the samples to reference the Affymetrix .CEL files that will be analyzed.

6 Downloading and Installing R Statistical Program

1. Search on the Internet using the keyword "Cran R."
2. Go to the The Comprehensive **R** Archive Network link.
3. Click on Windows in Download and Install R.
4. Click on base.
5. Click on Download R 2.8.1 for Windows.
6. Save on Desktop.

7. Run R-2.8.1-win32.exe file on your computer.
8. Once loaded, open R program.
9. Under Packages pull-down menu, choose select repositories.
10. Highlight (select) all BioC components and press OK.
11. Under Packages pull-down menu, choose Install package(s).
12. From the menu choose the affylmGUI package and press OK. (A number of required components will be installed.)
13. Under Packages pull-down menu, choose Load package.
14. From the menu choose the affylmGUI and press OK.
15. After first-time loading, you will only need to do **steps 14** and **15** when using the affylmGUI.

R statistical program with the affylmGUI (for Affymetrix .CEL files) does the evaluation of your data set.

In this analysis, importation of the raw data in the Affymetrix .CEL file format is accomplished by directing the affylmGUI to the folder containing the Renamed files. The remaining is done to remove # notations that cause the R program errors. As part of the import, a Target file is created from the information categorizing the data as to the type of a .CEL file (treated or control file). This Target file is referenced in the affylmGUI for parameter descriptions and type. Once loaded, the data is normalized using Robust Multiarray Averaging (RMA). After normalization, a linear model fit is completed. Contrast parameters are then input (treated versus control), and a Table of Genes Ranked in order of Differential Expression can be created.

Mining of the data for meaningful genes of interest involves using different adjustments and cutoffs determined by the user. The *p*-values are adjusted using the Benjamini-Hochberg method (BH). We normally employ a cutoff of p-value <0.05 and delete those with p values greater than 0.05. Further reduction can be obtained by using the B-statistic, which is the log odds that the gene is differentially expressed. A cutoff of $B=1.386$ would correspond to the probability of 80% that a gene is differentially expressed. For this example, the edited table would be entitled "adjusted p value less than 0.05 & B greater than 1.386 genes with fold change."

The *M*-value (*M*) is the value of the contrast (treated versus control), and this represents a log2 fold change between two or more experimental conditions. Positive *M*-values indicate an increase in the treated compared to the control. Negative *M*-values indicate a decrease in the treated compared to the control. Use the absolute values of the *M*-values and create a fold change column by raising 2 to the power of *M*-value. The sign of the *M*-value determines whether the fold change listed is an increase or decrease and was used to create the Increase/Decrease column.

7 Pathway Analysis

To query gene product networks that may be affected in your experimental system, we input our data [1, 9, 10] into Ingenuity Systems Pathway Analysis (http://ingenuity.com/). Other websites with similar pathway analyses capabilities are as follows:

1. EADGENE http://www.eadgene.info/ToolsResources/ASGPathwaysAnalysisSoftware/tabid/226/Default.aspx
2. DAVID Bioinformatics Resources 6.7 http://david.abcc.ncifcrf.gov/
3. FunNet: Functional analysis of Transcriptional networks http://www.funnet.info/
4. GFINDer: Genome Function INtegrated Discoverer http://www.medinfopoli.polimi.it/GFINDer/
5. Rat Genome Database http://rgd.mcw.edu

8 Microarray Data Submission to the Gene Expression Omnibus (GEO) Database

The Gene Expression Omnibus (GEO) is a public repository of the National Center for Biotechnology Information (NCBI) of the National Institutes of Health (NIH), USA, which archives and freely distributes microarray, next-generation sequencing, and other forms of high-throughput functional genomic data submitted by the scientific community. Most reputed journals require that microarray data should be deposited into a MIAME (minimum information about microarray experiments)-compliant public repository like GEO. To submit data, you first need to establish your identity by setting up your own GEO account, with a username and password (Fig. 2).

After the successful creation of the account, go to the main page (http://www.ncbi.nlm.nih.gov/geo/) and log in with your username and password and follow the steps below.

1. Click on the new submission to reach the data submission page.
2. Under the Data types select the array platform which you used for your experiment. Example input "Affymetrix." This will take you to the page with details specific for submission of data collected using the Affymetrix platform.

The GEO archive spreadsheet-based submission method is recommended for Affymetrix data deposits. With this submission option, you should provide the following components.

1 A Microsoft Excel metadata worksheet containing descriptive information and protocols for the overall experiment and individual samples. (You can use the Affymetrix GEO archive

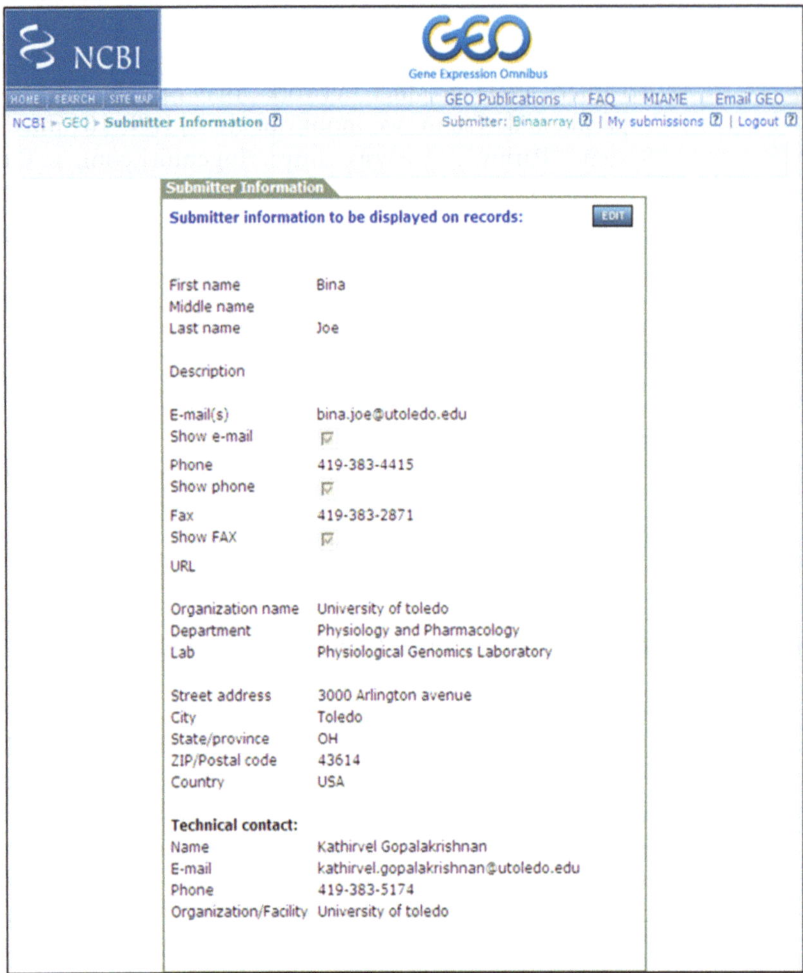

Fig. 2 Screenshot as it appears on your computer after you input your username and password at the NCBI GEO database

templates and examples provided in the same web page to create your metadata worksheet. Please refer to Fig. 3.)

2 CEL files.

3 Processed data. This is the probe set summary data generated by the primary analysis software (e.g., Expression Console, MicroArray Suite 5.0, Genotyping Console, GTYPE/CNAT, GTGS, Tiling Array Software, or GeneChip-compatible/other third-party software). These data may be submitted either as CHP files or a matrix table (*see* examples in templates below). Please submit the data used to draw the conclusions of your

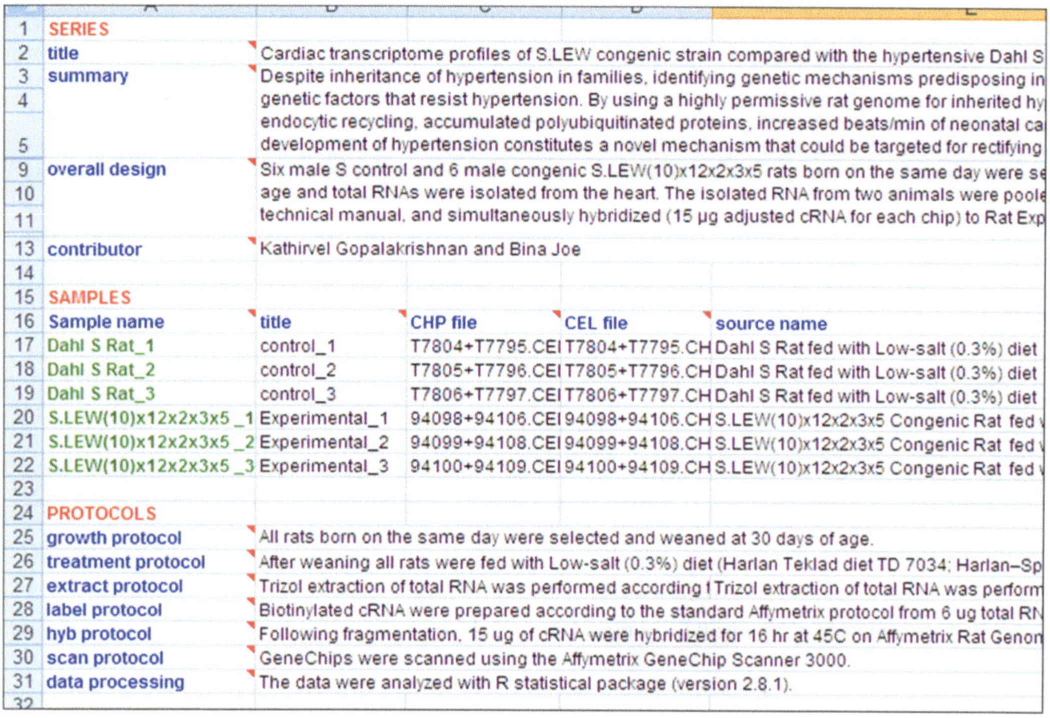

	A	B	C	D	E
1	SERIES				
2	title	Cardiac transcriptome profiles of S.LEW congenic strain compared with the hypertensive Dahl S			
3	summary	Despite inheritance of hypertension in families, identifying genetic mechanisms predisposing in			
4		genetic factors that resist hypertension. By using a highly permissive rat genome for inherited hy			
5		endocytic recycling, accumulated polyubiquitinated proteins, increased beats/min of neonatal ca development of hypertension constitutes a novel mechanism that could be targeted for rectifying			
9	overall design	Six male S control and 6 male congenic S.LEW(10)x12x2x3x5 rats born on the same day were se			
10		age and total RNAs were isolated from the heart. The isolated RNA from two animals were poole			
11		technical manual, and simultaneously hybridized (15 µg adjusted cRNA for each chip) to Rat Exp			
13	contributor	Kathirvel Gopalakrishnan and Bina Joe			
14					
15	SAMPLES				
16	Sample name	title	CHP file	CEL file	source name
17	Dahl S Rat_1	control_1	T7804+T7795.CEI	T7804+T7795.CH	Dahl S Rat fed with Low-salt (0.3%) diet
18	Dahl S Rat_2	control_2	T7805+T7796.CEI	T7805+T7796.CH	Dahl S Rat fed with Low-salt (0.3%) diet
19	Dahl S Rat_3	control_3	T7806+T7797.CEI	T7806+T7797.CH	Dahl S Rat fed with Low-salt (0.3%) diet
20	S.LEW(10)x12x2x3x5 _1	Experimental_1	94098+94106.CEI	94098+94106.CH	S.LEW(10)x12x2x3x5 Congenic Rat fed
21	S.LEW(10)x12x2x3x5 _2	Experimental_2	94099+94108.CEI	94099+94108.CH	S.LEW(10)x12x2x3x5 Congenic Rat fed
22	S.LEW(10)x12x2x3x5 _3	Experimental_3	94100+94109.CEI	94100+94109.CH	S.LEW(10)x12x2x3x5 Congenic Rat fed
23					
24	PROTOCOLS				
25	growth protocol	All rats born on the same day were selected and weaned at 30 days of age.			
26	treatment protocol	After weaning all rats were fed with Low-salt (0.3%) diet (Harlan Teklad diet TD 7034; Harlan–Sp			
27	extract protocol	Trizol extraction of total RNA was performed according t	Trizol extraction of total RNA was perform		
28	label protocol	Biotinylated cRNA were prepared according to the standard Affymetrix protocol from 6 ug total RN			
29	hyb protocol	Following fragmentation, 15 ug of cRNA were hybridized for 16 hr at 45C on Affymetrix Rat Genon			
30	scan protocol	GeneChips were scanned using the Affymetrix GeneChip Scanner 3000.			
31	data processing	The data were analyzed with R statistical package (version 2.8.1).			

Fig. 3 Screenshot of a sample Microsoft Excel metadata worksheet

study. For instance, do not submit CHP files analyzed with MAS5.0 if your submission is related to a publication based on GC-RMA data. In this case, you should submit the GC-RMA probe set summary data instead of MAS5.0 CHP files.

The two datasheets needed for submission are the raw data worksheet and the processed (normalized) data with BH adjustment. Screenshots of these two worksheets are shown in Figs. 4 and 5.

Before the upload, bundle all parts (Excel file containing the metadata spreadsheet and matrix spreadsheet, raw data files, CEL files, and CHP files if relevant) together into a .zip, .rar, or .tar archive using a program like WinZip and transfer to GEO by selecting the "GEOarchive" option on the Direct Deposit page. There you can select data release date and data type: new or update.

After the successful data upload you will receive an email from the GEO database confirming your data submission. Behind the scenes, the GEO database personnel will check and validate your data before public release. Upon final release your data will appear as shown in Fig. 6.

1	Probe ID	T7804+T7795.CEL	T7805+T7796.CEL	T7806+T7797.CEL	94098+94106.CEL	94099+94108.CEL	94100+94109.CEL
2	1367452_at	11.60185737	11.6836487	11.65157286	11.65794414	11.61693749	11.64622207
3	1367453_at	11.11586901	11.08175567	11.00202891	11.02417604	11.08262624	11.09996724
4	1367454_at	10.73274599	10.78493981	10.65688252	10.77067547	10.76756024	10.73277215
5	1367455_at	11.92588861	11.98583422	12.03625662	11.9687957	12.01043526	11.95896224
6	1367456_at	11.53814097	11.60545428	11.69666797	11.60033161	11.58964213	11.56833991
7	1367457_at	9.977584092	10.07854827	10.21113841	10.1149985	10.05736258	9.98459235
8	1367458_at	8.660594613	8.682944197	8.600055003	8.684416396	8.722105831	8.643189069
9	1367459_at	12.58573832	12.59421034	12.56530074	12.5817246	12.58335267	12.5989734
10	1367460_at	11.62653356	11.63305156	11.75266674	11.59534212	11.7175601	11.65344018
11	1367461_at	9.895064719	9.941391674	10.03106135	10.0199525	9.944447324	9.985345967
12	1367462_at	11.20973934	11.37727823	11.45987887	11.34693247	11.34276172	11.39965095
13	1367463_at	11.7110346	11.69100325	11.6474258	11.60913308	11.64058062	11.66034666
14	1367464_at	9.631304508	9.661621769	9.694579088	9.659657449	9.735347961	9.650575134
15	1367465_at	10.07035309	10.18312538	10.32065146	10.10566135	10.17226253	10.22791879
16	1367466_at	10.35985773	10.34905561	10.49371961	10.44607564	10.27687047	10.40313956
17	1367467_at	11.38510805	11.4803838	11.47266101	11.50930049	11.42254426	11.44494064
18	1367468_at	10.43947111	10.34362277	10.46680176	10.35725354	10.22629312	10.4277691
19	1367469_at	12.92389713	12.86566969	12.90717869	12.87476207	12.9061872	12.90907868
20	1367470_at	10.66357274	10.6577666	10.68217447	10.72667087	10.63356593	10.69288019

Fig. 4 Partial screenshot of Microsoft Excel metadata worksheet

1	probe ID	log2-fold change	Fold change	P.Value	Gene Symbol
2	1379740_at	1.8458	3.5944	0.0010	LOC361346
3	1380293_at	1.5387	2.9054	0.0006	LOC361346
4	1388630_at	1.4840	2.7972	0.0007	---
5	1388774_at	1.4043	2.6468	0.0004	Mbd2
6	1383505_at	1.3737	2.5913	0.0167	---
7	1393094_at	1.3052	2.4712	0.0006	---
8	1384247_at	-0.5931	1.5085	0.0438	---
9	1377563_at	-0.6459	1.5647	0.0374	Lmod3
10	1377112_at	-0.7038	1.6288	0.0374	Cda
11	1369983_at	-0.7090	1.6346	0.0374	Ccl5
12	1378848_at	-0.7359	1.6655	0.0374	LOC361187

Fig. 5 Partial screenshot of processed (normalized) data with BH adjustment

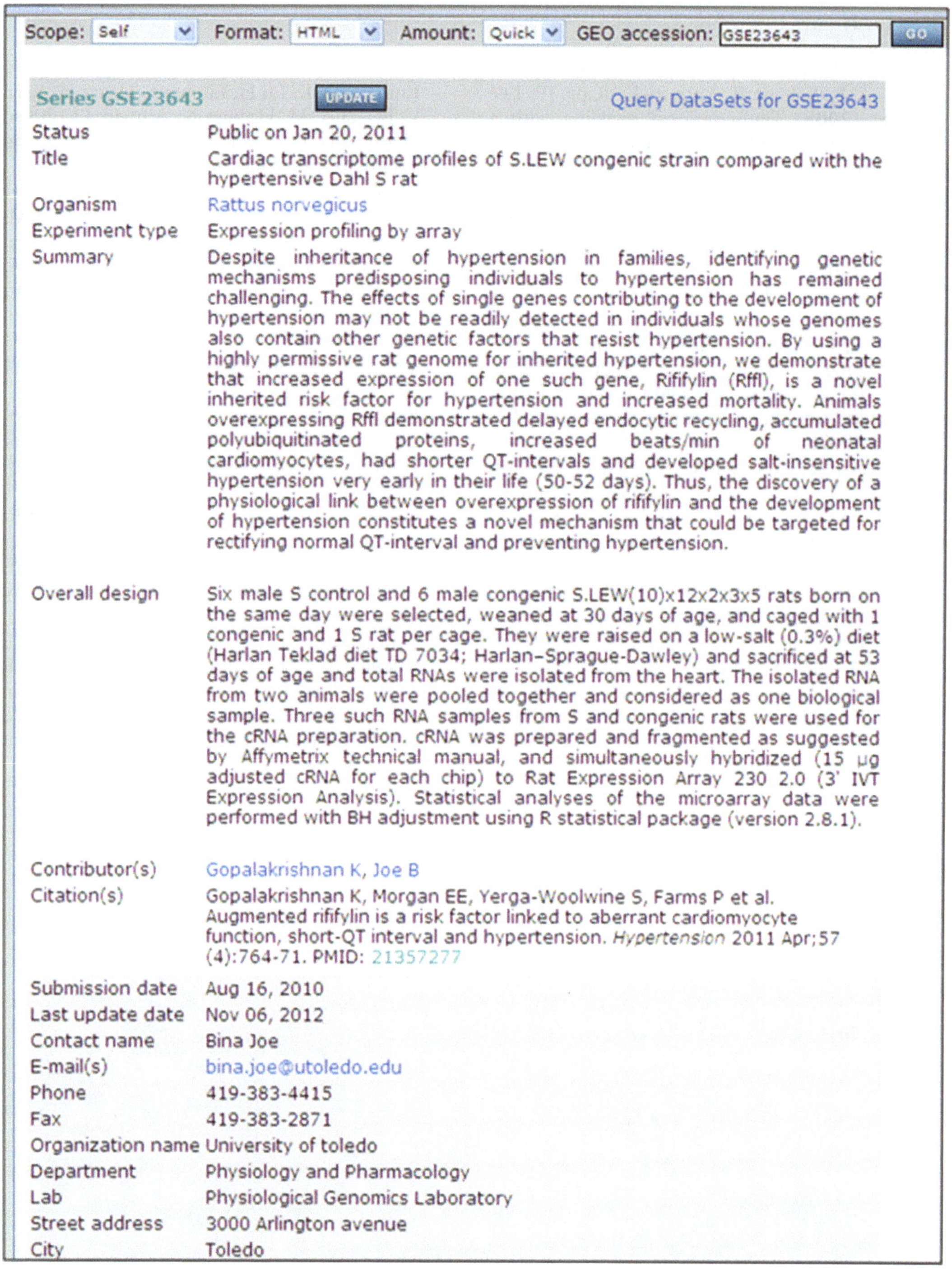

Scope: Self Format: HTML Amount: Quick GEO accession: GSE23643 GO

Series GSE23643 UPDATE Query DataSets for GSE23643

Status	Public on Jan 20, 2011
Title	Cardiac transcriptome profiles of S.LEW congenic strain compared with the hypertensive Dahl S rat
Organism	Rattus norvegicus
Experiment type	Expression profiling by array
Summary	Despite inheritance of hypertension in families, identifying genetic mechanisms predisposing individuals to hypertension has remained challenging. The effects of single genes contributing to the development of hypertension may not be readily detected in individuals whose genomes also contain other genetic factors that resist hypertension. By using a highly permissive rat genome for inherited hypertension, we demonstrate that increased expression of one such gene, Rififylin (Rffl), is a novel inherited risk factor for hypertension and increased mortality. Animals overexpressing Rffl demonstrated delayed endocytic recycling, accumulated polyubiquitinated proteins, increased beats/min of neonatal cardiomyocytes, had shorter QT-intervals and developed salt-insensitive hypertension very early in their life (50-52 days). Thus, the discovery of a physiological link between overexpression of rififylin and the development of hypertension constitutes a novel mechanism that could be targeted for rectifying normal QT-interval and preventing hypertension.
Overall design	Six male S control and 6 male congenic S.LEW(10)x12x2x3x5 rats born on the same day were selected, weaned at 30 days of age, and caged with 1 congenic and 1 S rat per cage. They were raised on a low-salt (0.3%) diet (Harlan Teklad diet TD 7034; Harlan-Sprague-Dawley) and sacrificed at 53 days of age and total RNAs were isolated from the heart. The isolated RNA from two animals were pooled together and considered as one biological sample. Three such RNA samples from S and congenic rats were used for the cRNA preparation. cRNA was prepared and fragmented as suggested by Affymetrix technical manual, and simultaneously hybridized (15 μg adjusted cRNA for each chip) to Rat Expression Array 230 2.0 (3' IVT Expression Analysis). Statistical analyses of the microarray data were performed with BH adjustment using R statistical package (version 2.8.1).
Contributor(s)	Gopalakrishnan K, Joe B
Citation(s)	Gopalakrishnan K, Morgan EE, Yerga-Woolwine S, Farms P et al. Augmented rififylin is a risk factor linked to aberrant cardiomyocyte function, short-QT interval and hypertension. *Hypertension* 2011 Apr;57 (4):764-71. PMID: 21357277
Submission date	Aug 16, 2010
Last update date	Nov 06, 2012
Contact name	Bina Joe
E-mail(s)	bina.joe@utoledo.edu
Phone	419-383-4415
Fax	419-383-2871
Organization name	University of toledo
Department	Physiology and Pharmacology
Lab	Physiological Genomics Laboratory
Street address	3000 Arlington avenue
City	Toledo

Fig. 6 Final appearance of data after complete input of all required data into the NCBI GEO database

References

1. Joe B, Letwin NE, Garrett MR, Dhindaw S, Frank B, Sultana R, Verratti K, Rapp JP, Lee NH (2005) Transcriptional profiling with a blood pressure QTL interval-specific oligonucleotide array. Physiol Genomics 23:318–326
2. Okuda T, Sumiya T, Iwai N, Miyata T (2002) Difference of gene expression profiles in spontaneous hypertensive rats and Wistar-Kyoto rats from two sources. Biochem Biophys Res Commun 296:537–543
3. Okuda T, Sumiya T, Mizutani K, Tago N, Miyata T, Tanabe T, Kato H, Katsuya T, Higaki J, Ogihara T, Tsujita Y, Iwai N (2002) Analyses of differential gene expression in genetic hypertensive rats by microarray. Hypertens Res 25:249–255
4. Hubner N, Wallace CA, Zimdahl H, Petretto E, Schulz H, Maciver F, Mueller M, Hummel O, Monti J, Zidek V, Musilova A, Kren V, Causton H, Game L, Born G, Schmidt S, Muller A, Cook SA, Kurtz TW, Whittaker J, Pravenec M, Aitman TJ (2005) Integrated transcriptional profiling and linkage analysis for identification of genes underlying disease. Nat Genet 37:243–253
5. Pravenec M, Wallace C, Aitman TJ, Kurtz TW (2003) Gene expression profiling in hypertension research: a critical perspective. Hypertension 41:3–8
6. Petretto E, Mangion J, Dickens NJ, Cook SA, Kumaran MK, Lu H, Fischer J, Maatz H, Kren V, Pravenec M, Hubner N, Aitman TJ (2006) Heritability and tissue specificity of expression quantitative trait loci. PLoS Genet 2, e172
7. Aitman TJ, Glazier AM, Wallace CA, Cooper LD, Norsworthy PJ, Wahid FN, Al-Majali KM, Trembling PM, Mann CJ, Shoulders CC, Graf D, St Lezin E, Kurtz TW, Kren V, Pravenec M, Ibrahimi A, Abumrad NA, Stanton LW, Scott J (1999) Identification of Cd36 (Fat) as an insulin-resistance gene causing defective fatty acid and glucose metabolism in hypertensive rats. Nat Genet 21:76–83
8. Browning BL, Browning SR (2008) Haplotypic analysis of Wellcome Trust Case Control Consortium data. Hum Genet 123: 273–280
9. Garrett MR, Meng H, Rapp JP, Joe B (2005) Locating a blood pressure quantitative trait locus within 117 kb on the rat genome: substitution mapping and renal expression analysis. Hypertension 45:451–459
10. Gopalakrishnan K, Kumarasamy S, Yan Y, Liu J, Kalinoski A, Kothandapani A, Farms P, Joe B (2012) Increased expression of rififylin in A<330 Kb congenic strain is linked to impaired endosomal recycling in proximal tubules. Front Genet 3:138

Chapter 2

Methods to Assess Genetic Risk Prediction

Christin Schulz and Sandosh Padmanabhan

Abstract

It is recognized that traditional risk factors do not identify everyone who will develop cardiovascular disease. There is a growing interest in the discovery of novel biomarkers that will augment the predictive potential of traditional cardiovascular risk factors. The era of genome-wide association studies (GWAS) has resulted in the discovery of common genetic polymorphisms associated with a multitude of cardiovascular traits and raises the possibility that these variants can be used in clinical risk prediction. Assessing and evaluating the new genetic risk markers and quantification of the improvement in risk prediction models that incorporate this information is a major challenge. In this paper we discuss the key metrics that are used to assess prediction models—discrimination, calibration, reclassification, and demonstration on how to calculate and interpret these metrics.

Key words Genome-wide association, Genetic risk score, ROC, AUC, Reclassification, Prediction

1 Introduction

Cardiovascular disease (CVD) risk prediction has a central role in cardiovascular prevention strategies, and there are ongoing large-scale efforts to refine and improve risk assessment methods [1]. Risk estimates are commonly used in clinical practice to identify individuals at high risk of developing CVD and select those individuals for intensive preventive measures, but they can also motivate individuals to adhere to recommended lifestyle advice or therapies. The major cardiovascular risk factors, namely, male sex, hypertension, cholesterol, smoking, and diabetes mellitus, have been known for over 30 years and have been used in various risk prediction algorithm scores (Framingham Risk Score [2, 3], QRISK [4], SCORE [5]). It is estimated that around 15–20% of myocardial infarction (MI) patients have none of the traditional risk factors and would be considered low risk by current prediction algorithms [6]. Several studies have evaluated the predictive power of the addition of single SNPs and combinations of risk SNPs to genetic risk scores for MI risk. Additions of single SNPs at 9p21 to the Framingham Risk Score did

Rhian M. Touyz and Ernesto L. Schiffrin (eds.), *Hypertension: Methods and Protocols*, Methods in Molecular Biology, vol. 1527, DOI 10.1007/978-1-4939-6625-7_2, © Springer Science+Business Media LLC 2017

not improve risk prediction consistently [7, 8]. A genetic risk score comprising 101 validated SNPs from large-scale GWAS of MI and other cardiovascular risk factors was evaluated for cardiovascular risk prediction in 19,313 women. After adjustment for traditional risk factors, the genetic risk score was not associated with CVD events, and the addition of the genetic risk score to a standard risk prediction model did not significantly improve discrimination or reclassification [9]. Despite the incorporation of multiple CAD-associated SNPs, genetic risk scores to date have explained less than 5% of the interindividual variance in risk [10] and have not led to clinically meaningful improvements in risk prediction. However, the modest improvements in risk reclassification seen in some of these studies [11] highlight the future potential for the use of genetic markers for risk prediction as additional genetic variants are discovered.

1.1 Genetic Variants and as Novel Biomarkers

There is a major drive to discover novel biomarkers that can enhance the current conventional risk scores. Genetic variants have attracted a lot of interest as markers that may enhance risk prediction models. There are various reasons—measurement of genetic variants is now accurate and cheap, and variants would only need to be measured once as they are fixed at conception and therefore may be relevant for younger individuals before the conventional risk factors, such as hyperlipidemia, hypertension, and diabetes mellitus, become apparent. The case for risk prediction with genetic polymorphisms must be held to the same standards as used for other biomarkers. Significant improvement to well-validated risk scores by the addition of a genetic biomarker must be demonstrated by the use of standard metrics, to evaluate their clinical performance. More importantly, any genetic marker should also provide incremental risk information over and above a model that incorporates family history [12, 13].

1.2 Assessment of Risk Prediction Equations

The first step in assessing a new risk score incorporating genetic information should show a significant statistical association with the outcome of interest. However, this significant association has no relationship to its clinical utility. A number of metrics are used in the assessment of a new risk score to determine their ability to discriminate future cases from non-cases, the calibration of the model, the model fit, the informativeness of the model for the outcome of interest, risk reclassification, and clinical utility [1, 14, 15]. A minimum of three criteria other than statistical significance have been proposed in the evaluation of new biomarkers: discrimination, calibration, and reclassification [16]. Recently recommendations on how to report evaluations of risk prediction models that include genetic variants have been published [17].

1.3 Discrimination

Discrimination is a measure of how well a model is able to distinguish between subjects who will have an event from those who will not (the ability of a risk model to rank order individuals' risks). A test's discriminatory ability is measured by its C statistic, which represents the area under the receiver operating characteristic curve (visualised by plotting "sensitivity" in relation to "1-specificity"). The numeric value of the C statistic represents the probability of a randomly selected patient who develops the disease (a "case") having a higher risk score than a randomly selected non-case. The C statistic can vary from 1.0 (perfect discrimination) to 0.5 (random chance, indicating that the score being applied is no better than flipping a coin). C statistics <0.70 are thought to indicate inadequate discrimination by current convention; those between 0.70 and 0.80 are considered acceptable and those between 0.80 and 0.90 excellent. The Framingham Risk Score, which is based on traditional cardiovascular risk factors, yields a C statistic of 0.63–0.78 [18].

1.4 Calibration

Calibration compares the predicted risk with the observed risk in groups of individuals with varying baseline risk (assess the ability of a risk prediction model to predict accurately the absolute level of risk that is subsequently observed) [19]. Calibration is often assessed visually by dividing the population at risk into quantiles of predicted risk and plotting the predicted risk versus the observed event rate for each quantile. The Hosmer-Lemeshow goodness-of-fit test is used to test the calibration of a risk model, and a P-value < 0.05 for such a test would indicate poor calibration of the model for the population. Treatment decisions are dependent on estimates of predicted risk, and thus well-calibrated models will have a major impact on clinical management.

1.5 Reclassification

The Hosmer-Lemeshow statistic is a global measure of calibration giving equal weight to all combinations of predicted and observed risk. This may not be very useful for the most common treatment decision scenario involving individuals who fall into an "intermediate" risk category. Reclassification tests whether the addition of a new risk marker results in a substantial proportion of individuals being moved ("reclassified") across a predefined treatment threshold [14]. Simply quantifying the proportion of individuals reclassified across a given threshold ignores whether that reclassification was correct. To quantify the appropriateness and amount of overall reclassification, Pencina et al. [15] have proposed two indices, the net reclassification improvement (NRI) and the integrative discrimination index (IDI). The NRI is calculated by splitting the sample into those who develop events and those who do not and tallying the number who are correctly classified (up-classified in the event group and down-classified in the nonevent group) or incorrectly classified (down-classified in the event group and up-classified in the nonevent group). NRI is the net number of correct reclassifications in both groups. The integrative discrimination index (IDI) indicates how far individuals are moving on average along the continuum of predicted risk [15]. If the IDI is small, even in the presence of significant NRI, then the change in predicted risk will be small on average (those at higher baseline risk will likely change more than those at lower baseline risk) [1].

2 Materials

Genetic risk prediction requires high quality data which includes all relevant covariates and genotypic information with no missing information. For prospective analysis, a high event rate is essential for an adequately powered study.

2.1 Prior Knowledge

Familiarity with standard statistical methods including linear and logistic regression, survival analysis, and Cox proportional hazard model is essential. Any standard statistical package like SPSS or STATA can be used to do regression or survival analyses, and the results of these can be imported into R for risk prediction analyses. For specific risk prediction assessment, the following section demonstrates calculating measures of discrimination, calibration, and reclassification using the R statistical package. A detailed knowledge of R is not essential.

2.2 Installing R

R (www.r-project.org) is a commonly used, free statistics software. R allows you to carry out statistical analyses in an interactive mode, as well as allowing simple programming. Installation versions for Windows, Mac, and Linux are available on the R website—http://cran.r-project.org/. A basic introduction to R is available online, and a lot of information is available either on www.r-project.org or by simply doing an online search.

http://en.wikibooks.org/wiki/Statistical_Analysis:_an_Introduction_using_R/R_basics

http://en.wikibooks.org/wiki/R_Programming

The highlighted text below indicates the actual command that needs to be typed at the R command prompt (*see* **Note 1**).

2.3 Installing and Using R Packages

To perform risk prediction analysis in R, there are programs available that can be loaded in R and will generate the metrics easily. The following packages need to be installed on the local machine and invoked for analyses.

1. Required R packages—The R packages required can be downloaded manually from the R website or installed directly from R. The required packages are:

   Hmisc (http://biostat.mc.vanderbilt.edu/wiki/Main/Hmisc)

   Rms (http://biostat.mc.vanderbilt.edu/rms/)

   PredictABEL (http://www.genabel.org/packages/PredictABEL)

2. Installing an R package
   (a) Start R by double-clicking on the R icon.
   (b) Install packages from the menu: Packages → Install package(s). The first time you do this, R will ask for a mirror; choose the nearest one to you from the pop-up list

that appears. After this another pop-up list appears with a list of R packages. Select the package you want to install from the list. For risk prediction analyses, install three R packages—Hmisc, rms, and PredictABEL.

(c) Installing packages from the command line is performed by typing (*see* **Note 2**)

install.packages("rms").

3. To access the function of the installed package, you must load the package using the command—library(packagename).

library(rms)

3 Methods

3.1 Preparing Data for Analysis

Prepare a data table for analysis. R can import tables generated as Excel files, text files, or even SPSS files. The Hmisc R package is one of the many packages that can facilitate the import of these file formats. Create two tables as shown below—one for survival analysis (Table 1) and one for binary outcome analysis (Table 2). The columns and the data definitions are shown (*see* **Note 3**).

1. Importing files into R and quality check

Load the Hmisc package

```
library(Hmisc)
```

Table 1
Survival table

Column name	Type of data	Value
ID	Individual ID	Unique id
Survival	Time to event	Days, months, or years
Status	Censored	1 = event; 0 = no event
Age	Continuous	
Sex	Binary	1 = male; 2 = female
BMI	Continuous	
Smoking	Factor	0 = nonsmoker; 1 = ex-smoker; 3 = current smoker
Diabetes	Binary	0 = no; 1 = yes
Cholesterol	Continuous	
HDL	Continuous	
Systolic BP	Continuous	
GRS	Continuous	Genetic risk score

Table 2
Binary outcome

Column name	Type of data	Value
ID	Individual ID	Unique id
Outcome	Binary	0 = no; 1 = yes
Age	Continuous	
Sex	Binary	1 = male; 2 = female
BMI	Continuous	
Smoking	Factor	0 = nonsmoker; 1 = ex-smoker; 3 = current smoker
Diabetes	Binary	0 = no; 1 = yes
Cholesterol	Continuous	
HDL	Continuous	
SystolicBP	Continuous	
GRS	Continuous	Genetic risk score

#Read the survival data file into a data frame called "surv_tbl" (*see* **Note 4**)

#if tab-limited file

```
surv_tbl<-read.table("datafile.txt",
header=True, sep="\t")
```

#check the number of rows and columns in the table

```
dim(surv_tbl)
```

2. Missing values (*see* **Note 5**)

#remove any rows with missing data

```
surv_tbl <- na.omit(surv_tbl)
```

#check again the number of rows available for analysis

```
dim(surv_tbl)
```

3. Check for multicollinearity (*see* **Note 6**)

   Multicollinearity occurs when two or more predictors in the model are correlated and provide redundant information about the response. This leads to increased standard error of estimates of the beta coefficients (decreased reliability). An easy method is to compute correlations between all pairs of predictors. If some are close to 1 or −1, remove one of the two correlated predictors from the model.

4. Remove outliers

   The data table may contain variables with extreme values which may either be true or spurious due to transcription errors.

A careful review of the data is required with review of the distributions and obvious spurious outliers need to be removed. Sometimes a threshold of >4 SD is used to remove outliers.

3.2 Calculation of Genetic Risk Score (GRS) (See Note 7)

1. GRS is calculated as a weighted mean using reported effect sizes from reference studies as weights per copy of the coded allele.
2. Select the set of *n* SNPs (S1…S*n*) that will be used for the calculation of GRS. This can be SNPs that have been validated in large GWAS meta-analyses. If using SNPs discovered in a new study, then it is appropriate to test risk prediction in an independent population and not in the population from which SNPs and effect sizes were obtained from.
3. Check that the SNPs are independent of each other by reviewing pair-wise r^2. Pair-wise LD between SNPs can be checked using the SNP Annotation and Proxy Search website http://www.broadinstitute.org/mpg/snap/ldsearchpw.php
4. Recode the genotype for each SNP as 0/1/2 based on the number of risk alleles for each individual. The recoded genotype is denoted by *gi* for the *i*th SNP. If using imputed genotypes, then use the expected allele dosage (which takes real values between 0.0 and 2.0 for imputed SNPs).
5. If more than 60% of SNP genotypes are missing for an individual, then set GRS as missing for that individual.
6. Obtain the beta coefficients of the risk allele from published GWAS meta-analyses. The beta coefficients are denoted by *bi* for the *i*th SNP.
7. Calculate the weighted risk score for *n* SNPs as follows:

$$\text{GRS} = g_1 b_1 + g_2 b_2 + \ldots g_n b_n$$

3.3 Association of GRS with Quantitative or Binary Traits or Incident Events

1. For testing association between GRS and a quantitative phenotype like systolic BP or cholesterol, a linear regression model with the trait as a dependent variable and GRS along with other relevant covariates as independent variables is used.
2. For a qualitative phenotype like HTN or MI, binary logistic regression models adjusted for covariates as above are used.
3. For incident events, a Cox proportional hazard model is used with GRS as a covariate. For incident outcome associations, for example, CV events, Cox model should be adjusted for known risk predictors like total cholesterol, HDL cholesterol, current smoking, and baseline diabetes, to form the baseline model. To form the second model, add GRS to the baseline list of covariates.

3.4 Generating Predicted Risks for Each Individual

The two outcomes of interest are binary outcomes (disease present or absent) or a survival event consisting of time to event and a censor variable. The former is analyzed using logistic regression and the latter using Cox proportional hazard model.

To assess predictive potential of a genetic risk score, two models are built: one using traditional risk factors and the second which includes traditional risk factors plus the genetic risk score.

For logistic regression analysis and risk prediction, the PredictABEL package is the easiest to use to perform both the regression analysis followed by discrimination and reclassification analyses. To assess the predictive potential of Cox regression models, the predicted risks for Cox models need to be generated separately and then used in PredictABEL.

1. Predicted risks using logistic regression—from PredictABEL. The following protocol is annotated example from the PredictABEL manual.

   # specify dataset with outcome and predictor variables. Here Table 2 is read into the data frame object outc_tbl.

   ```
   outc_tbl<-read.table("datafile.txt",
   header=True)
   ```

   # specify column number of the outcome variable. This is the column number of the outc_tbl which has the binary outcome info.

   ```
   cOutcome <- 2
   ```

   # specify column numbers of nongenetic predictors—age, sex, BMI, smoking, diabetes, cholesterol, HDL, systolic BP

   ```
   cNonGenPred1 <- c(3:10)

   cNonGenPred2 <- c(3:10)
   ```

   # specify column numbers of nongenetic predictors that are categorical—none in current table, so coded as 0.

   ```
   cNonGenPredCat1 <- c(0)

   cNonGenPredCat2 <- c(0)
   ```

   # specify column numbers of genetic predictors—the GRS column is specified in model 2 and not in model 1.

   ```
   cGenPred1 <- c(0)

   cGenPred2 <- c(11)
   ```

   # specify column numbers of genetic predictors that are categorical—none in current table, so coded as 0. If the GRS is recoded into binary or categorical data like quartiles, then specify this column here.

   ```
   cGenPredsCat1 <- c(0)

   cGenPredsCat2 <- c(0)
   ```

   # fit logistic regression models

   ```
   riskmodel1 <- fitLogRegModel(data= outc_tbl,
   cOutcome=cOutcome,
   ```

```
cNonGenPreds=cNonGenPred1, cNonGenPredsCat=cNo
nGenPredCat1,

cGenPreds=cGenPred1, cGenPredsCat=cGenPredsCat1)

riskmodel2 <- fitLogRegModel(data= outc_tbl,
cOutcome=cOutcome,

cNonGenPreds=cNonGenPred2, cNonGenPredsCat=cNo
nGenPredCat2,

cGenPreds=cGenPred2, cGenPredsCat=cGenPredsCat2)
```

#Calculate predicted risk for each model. The results, namely, predRisk1 and predRisk2, will be used in all subsequent analyses.

```
predRisk1 <- predRisk(riskmodel1)

predRisk2 <- predRisk(riskmodel2)
```

2. Predicted risks from Cox regression

   The easiest method to generate predicted risks for each individual is using SPSS. Open the data table in SPSS and run Cox regression analysis with all the covariates. Click the save button and check the box "Survival Function." This will save the predicted risk for each individual based on the Cox model. This can now be saved as a text file and imported into R for further analyses.

   Open Table 1 in SPSS, do a Cox regression analysis after performing the standard checks on proportionality assumptions. Save the survival function by clicking the "Save" button and checking the "Survival Function" box. The SPSS table has an additional column which can be renamed to SURV_baseline for the baseline model and redo that survival analysis with GRS included among the covariates and rename the new column as SURV_GRS. Save the SPSS table and this can be opened in R as follows:

```
library(Hmisc)

spss_tbl<-spss.get("spss_table.sav",use.
value.labels=F).
```

3.5 Discrimination Using R (See Note 8)

The following method shows how to generate the C statistic using R:

#Create a survival object using survival time and status using the data frame "t" created earlier

```
library(rms)

S<-with(surv_tbl, Surv(survival, status))
```

#Generate the C Statistic

```
fit<-cph(S ~ Sex + Age + Smoking + BMI + Diabetes
+ Cholesterol + HDL + SystolicBP, x=TRUE, y=TRUE,
surv=TRUE, dxy = TRUE, time.inc=3650, data=d)

set.seed(1)

validate(fit, B=100, dxy=TRUE)
```

This will generate a tabular output, the first line of which is shown below:

	Index.orig	Training	Test	Optimism	Index.corrected	*n*
Dxy	−0.5326	−0.5338	−0.5318	−0.002	−0.5306	100

Dxy is the Somers' Dxy rank correlation and this can be easily converted to C statistic using the formula

$C = (\text{Dxy}/2) + 0.5$ #(the absolute value of Dxy is used)

3.6 Calibration Plot and Hosmer-Lemeshow Goodness-of-Fit Test Statistics

Hosmer-Lemeshow test statistic is a measure of the fit of the model, comparing observed and predicted risks across subgroups of the population. The default number of groups is 10. The function requires the outcome of interest and predicted risks of all individuals.

Example for riskmodel1

specify range of *x*-axis and *y*-axis

```
rangeaxis <- c(0,1)

plotCalibration(data= outc_tbl, cOutcome=
cOutcome, predRisk=predRisk1, groups=groups,
rangeaxis=rangeaxis)
```

This will generate a calibration plot and a *P*-value for the Hosmer-Lemeshow test for goodness-of-fit test.

3.7 Receiver Operating Characteristic Curve (ROC) Plots for Risk Models 1 and 2

specify label of the ROC curve

```
labels <- c("without genetic factors", "with
genetic factors")
```

produce ROC curve

```
plotROC(data= outc_tbl, cOutcome=cOutcome,
predrisk=cbind(predRisk1, predRisk2), labels=
labels)
```

##To produce ROC plots using Cox regression data

```
predRisk1_cox=spss_tbl$SURV_baseline

predRisk2_cox= spss_tbl$SURV_GRS

plotROC(data= spss_tbl, cOutcome=cOutcome,
predrisk=cbind(predRisk1_cox, predRisk2_cox),
labels=labels)
```

3.8 Reclassification NRI and IDI (*See* Notes 9–11)

1. Using PredictABEL
   This generates a reclassification table and computes the net reclassification improvement (NRI) and integrated discrimination improvement (IDI).
   # specify cutoff values for risk categories—in the example below, cutoffs of 10% and 20% are based on clinical decisions

determined by calculated 10-year risks of coronary heart disease <10%, 10–20%, or ≥20%.

#Using predicted risk from logistic regression table

```
cutoff <- c(0,0.1,0.2,1)
reclassification(data= outc_tbl,
cOutcome=cOutcome, predrisk1=predRisk1,
predrisk2=predRisk2, cutoff)
```

#Using predicted risk from Cox regression table.

```
cutoff <- c(0,0.1,0.2,1)
reclassification(data= spss_tbl,
cOutcome=cOutcome, predrisk1=predRisk1_cox,
predrisk2=predRisk2_cox, cutoff)
```

2. Using R

This generates reclassification tables and NRI and IDI using the rms package in R.

#load rms package

```
library(rms)
```

#select the status variable from the survival table

```
Status<-spss_tbl$status

improveProb(predRisk1, predRisk2,t$all.cause.
death)
```

4 Notes

1. R is started by double-clicking on the R icon in Windows. After R is started, there is a console awaiting input.

(a) At the prompt (>), you can enter numbers and perform calculations.

```
1+2 #will return a value 3 after pressing
the enter key.
```

(b) All text after the pound sign "#" within the same line is considered a comment and is ignored by R. In the above command, the text after the # symbol is ignored by R, and after pressing enter, the value 3 will appear as the sum of 1 and 2.

(c) Assign values to variables with the assignment operator "<-" or “=”.

```
x<-2 #assigns value 2 to variable x
```

(d) R functions are invoked by its name, then followed by the parenthesis.

```
x<-c(10,12,15,16,24) # assigns a series of
values (called vector) to x
mean(x) # returns the mean of all the val-
ues in x
```

(e) R provides extensive documentation. For example, entering ?mean or help(mean) at the prompt gives documentation of the function mean in R.

2. R is case sensitive, so take care when typing commands. Install. packages is different from install.packages and the former will throw an error message.
3. For comparing different prediction models, the same individuals need to be included in the different models. It is worthwhile spending some time to ensure the table has no missing covariates. If there are missing covariates, then depending on the model, different numbers of individuals will be included in different models and the results may not be directly comparable.
4. Importing data into R

#if comma-delimited file (csv)

```
surv_tbl<-read.table("datafile.csv",
header=True, sep=",")
```

#or

```
surv_tbl<-csv.get("datafile.csv",
header=True, sep=",")
```

#to read Excel file use the package XLConnect

```
install.packages("XLConnect")
library("XLConnect")
surv_tbl <- ("datafile.xlsx")
```

5. The function na.omit will delete any row that has a missing variable. Imputation strategies will replace missing values with an estimate of the actual value of that case. For example, replacing the missing value by the observed value from another, similar case from the same dataset for which that variable was not missing or replacing the missing value by the mean of the variable in question or using conditional regression mean or expectation maximization (EM) to obtain the best estimates of the true values. Detailed discussion of these methods are beyond the scope of this chapter and requires statistical input.
6. One way to spot collinearity is to put each predictor as a dependent variable, and other predictors as independent variables, determine R^2, and if it's larger than 0.9, we can consider predictor redundant. A more rigorous method is to calculate variance inflation factors.
7. Though a weighted risk score is preferred, it must be emphasized that the effect estimates for associations from GWAS may be biased and of limited utility in risk prediction. Genetic effect estimates from discovery GWAS are likely inflated owing to the "winner's curse," with the actual genetic effect typically smaller than its estimate [20]. Effect estimates from meta-analysis frequently assume "fixed effects" despite important between-study heterogeneity [10]. The case control ascertainment strategy in GWAS can inflate effect estimates as the cases tend to be sampled

from genetic high-risk groups (younger age of onset, positive family history), controls from genetic low-risk groups control subjects have not been sampled by an appropriate sampling strategy [21]. Most GWAS of late onset disease like MI and type 2 diabetes suffer from major potential survival biases, because enrollment into the study is conditioned on survival after onset of disease. For example, 30–70% of MI patients die before admission to the hospital, which means analyses of prevalent MI cases are poorly representative of most incident MIs [22].

8. *See* Harrell et al. [23] review on multivariate prognostic models. For genetic studies, the C statistic is a function of the heritability, the genetic variance explained by the genetic variants, the prevalence of the disease condition, and the minor allele frequency in the population [24]. For CVD, it can be estimated that the upper bounds of the C statistic are ~0.90 for populations with a 10% prevalence of disease and ~0.85 for populations with higher disease prevalence [24, 25]. In genetic risk prediction of CVD, achieving a C statistic of 0.80–0.85 (greater than 0.75 achieved by Framingham Risk Score) will require ~100 uncorrelated genetic variants with relative risks of ~1.5 and minor allele frequencies of 10% that explain ~20% of the heritability of CVD [24]. Current replicated GWAS SNPs have mean relative risks of 1.1–1.2, which means even 100 genetic variants would only explain 1.0–9.1% of the variance of CVD and provide C statistics 0.75 [26], which would be similar to but not much better than current prediction models.

9. A reclassification table indicates the number of individuals who move to another risk category or remain in the same risk category as a result of updating the risk model. The most appropriate setting in which to use reclassification to evaluate risk models is for conditions in which risk strata are clearly defined and closely linked to treatment decisions. For coronary heart disease, risk strata are based on recommendations of the Third Adult Treatment Panel of the National Cholesterol Education Program [27]. Low-, intermediate-, and high-risk categories are based on having predicted 10-year risks of coronary heart disease <10%, 10–20%, or >20%, respectively. It is recommended that individuals in the high-risk category be considered for the same therapies as those with known coronary heart disease.

10. NRI equal to x% means that compared with individuals without outcome, individuals with outcome were almost x% more likely to move up a category than down. A P-value < 0.05 suggests that a significantly greater number are being reclassified appropriately than are being reclassified inappropriately.

11. IDI equal to x% means that the difference in average predicted risks between the individuals with and without the outcome increased by x% in the updated model. This is equivalent to the difference in R^2 between the two models being compared.

References

1. Lloyd-Jones DM (2010) Cardiovascular risk prediction: basic concepts, current status, and future directions. Circulation 121:1768–1777
2. Kannel WB et al (1961) Factors of risk in the development of coronary heart disease—six year follow-up experience. The Framingham Study. Ann Intern Med 55:33–50
3. Pencina MJ et al (2009) Predicting the 30-year risk of cardiovascular disease: the Framingham heart study. Circulation 119:3078–3084
4. Hippisley-Cox J et al (2007) Derivation and validation of QRISK, a new cardiovascular disease risk score for the United Kingdom: prospective open cohort study. BMJ 335:136
5. Aktas MK et al (2004) Global risk scores and exercise testing for predicting all-cause mortality in a preventive medicine program. JAMA 292:1462–1468
6. Khot UN et al (2003) Prevalence of conventional risk factors in patients with coronary heart disease. JAMA 290:898–904
7. Brautbar A et al (2009) Impact of adding a single allele in the 9p21 locus to traditional risk factors on reclassification of coronary heart disease risk and implications for lipid-modifying therapy in the Atherosclerosis Risk in Communities study. Circ Cardiovasc Genet 2:279–285
8. Nambi V et al (2012) The 9p21 genetic variant is additive to carotid intima media thickness and plaque in improving coronary heart disease risk prediction in white participants of the Atherosclerosis Risk in Communities (ARIC) Study. Atherosclerosis 222: 135–137
9. Paynter NP et al (2010) Association between a literature-based genetic risk score and cardiovascular events in women. JAMA 303:631–637
10. Ioannidis JP (2009) Prediction of cardiovascular disease outcomes and established cardiovascular risk factors by genome-wide association markers. Circ Cardiovasc Genet 2:7–15
11. Kathiresan S et al (2008) Polymorphisms associated with cholesterol and risk of cardiovascular events. N Engl J Med 358:1240–1249
12. Ridker PM et al (2007) Development and validation of improved algorithms for the assessment of global cardiovascular risk in women: the Reynolds Risk Score. JAMA 297:611–619
13. Scheuner MT et al (2010) General Cardiovascular Risk Profile identifies advanced coronary artery calcium and is improved by family history: the multiethnic study of atherosclerosis. Circ Cardiovasc Genet 3:97–105
14. Cook NR, Ridker PM (2009) Advances in measuring the effect of individual predictors of cardiovascular risk: the role of reclassification measures. Ann Intern Med 150:795–802
15. Pencina MJ et al (2008) Evaluating the added predictive ability of a new marker: from area under the ROC curve to reclassification and beyond. Stat Med 27:157–172
16. Wang TJ (2011) Assessing the role of circulating, genetic, and imaging biomarkers in cardiovascular risk prediction. Circulation 123:551–565
17. Janssens AC et al (2011) Strengthening the reporting of genetic risk prediction studies: the GRIPS statement. Circ Cardiovasc Genet 4:206–209
18. Wilson PW et al (1998) Prediction of coronary heart disease using risk factor categories. Circulation 97:1837–1847
19. Cook NR (2007) Use and misuse of the receiver operating characteristic curve in risk prediction. Circulation 115:928–935
20. Zollner S, Pritchard JK (2007) Overcoming the winner's curse: estimating penetrance parameters from case-control data. Am J Hum Genet 80:605–615
21. Lubin JH, Gail MH (1984) Biased selection of controls for case-control analyses of cohort studies. Biometrics 40:63–75
22. Thanassoulis G, Vasan RS (2010) Genetic cardiovascular risk prediction: will we get there? Circulation 122:2323–2334
23. Harrell FE Jr, Lee KL, Mark DB (1996) Multivariable prognostic models: issues in developing models, evaluating assumptions and adequacy, and measuring and reducing errors. Stat Med 15:361–387
24. Janssens AC et al (2006) Predictive testing for complex diseases using multiple genes: fact or fiction? Genet Med 8:395–400
25. Wray NR et al (2010) The genetic interpretation of area under the ROC curve in genomic profiling. PLoS Genet 6, e1000864
26. van der Net JB et al (2009) Value of genetic profiling for the prediction of coronary heart disease. Am Heart J 158:105–110
27. (2001) Executive Summary of The Third Report of The National Cholesterol Education Program (NCEP) Expert Panel on Detection, Evaluation, And Treatment of High Blood Cholesterol In Adults (Adult Treatment Panel III). JAMA 285: 2486–2497

Chapter 3

Microarray Analysis of Hypertension

Henry L. Keen and Curt D. Sigmund

Abstract

Hypertension is a complex disorder in which multiple genes, pathways, and organ systems simultaneously interact to contribute to the final level of blood pressure. Fully elucidating these interactions is an important area of hypertension research and one in which high-throughput methods such as microarrays can play a key role. With recent advances in microarray technology, reliable and accurate quantification of all known mRNA transcripts in a sample is now routinely performed. In addition, with improved statistical methods and publicly available tools and resources, robust analysis of the large amount of data generated from microarray experiments is now achievable for all research laboratories as will be outlined in this review.

Key words Hypertension, Blood pressure, Bioinformatics, Microarrays, Computational biology, Gene expression, mRNA

1 Introduction

Hypertension is a multifactorial disease involving different organ systems and a complex interplay between genetics and environment. Determining in a global manner how biological pathways are altered in hypertension is key to both understanding this disease and to developing therapeutic approaches. One approach is to use high-throughput methods such as microarrays in which global gene expression patterns can be identified and analyzed. Studies involving hypertension need not be limited to experimental animal or cell culture models. In fact, gene expression profiling using minimally invasive protocols has been reported for human subjects and there is evidence that blood leukocytes can be used as a biomarker for investigating hypertension [1].

The statistical challenges inherent in analyzing the large amount of data generated in a microarray experiment has led to the creation of new methods to address issues such as sample variation, low sample number and multiple comparison testing. There can be a substantial amount of signal variance from one array to another even when all

Rhian M. Touyz and Ernesto L. Schiffrin (eds.), *Hypertension: Methods and Protocols*, Methods in Molecular Biology, vol. 1527, DOI 10.1007/978-1-4939-6625-7_3, © Springer Science+Business Media LLC 2017

arrays are processed at the same time. Therefore, it is necessary to globally normalize each array (Subheading 3.2) before calculating values for each gene [2]. It is also important that proper procedures are in place to assess the quality of the data generated from the microarray experiment. This can be accomplished by global visualization and clustering of the data (Subheading 3.3) and by experimental replication using an alternative technique such as real-time quantitative RT-PCR (Subheading 3.4), or by genome-wide gene expression profiling by high-throughput RNA sequencing [3].

Visualization of the microarray data is not only useful as part of quality control, but can also provide insight into the overall differences and similarities between experimental models. Traditionally, hypertension has been categorized based on physiological responses (e.g., salt sensitivity, angiotensin II dependence). With the advent of microarray technology, it may be possible to subdivide hypertension into distinct categories based on distinct gene expression profile signatures. A similar methodology has been employed in cancer research to classify and differentiate tumor subtypes that by traditional histological methods are indistinguishable [4]. Common methods of clustering microarray data include principal component analysis (PCA) and hierarchical clustering (HCA). PCA takes microarray data which is of high dimensionality (i.e., expression of thousands of genes) and generates a summary of the global differences between samples as a series of values which can be plotted graphically [5]. HCA involves correlational analysis between and across all samples with the differences among samples represented as a tree graph similar to that used to represent the evolutionary divergence of orthologous proteins [5].

After assessing the global differences between experimental groups, it is important to identify which individual genes (Subheading 3.4) and pathways (Subheadings 3.5 and 3.6) exhibit differential expression. Determination of statistical differences in gene expression in a microarray study is similar to that for any data analysis with two special considerations; the number of genes simultaneously assayed is large and the number of replicate samples is usually relatively small. To overcome these statistical obstacles, a linear modeling approach has been commonly used in the microarray community to assess differential expression in experiments with either simple (e.g., two different groups) or multifactorial designs [6]. In addition to analysis of individual genes, it is important to determine if there are coordinated changes in expression of genes sharing similar functions or part of a common pathway. Gene Set Analysis (Subheading 3.5) can be used to determine if a set of genes, as a whole, is statistically altered in a microarray experiment [7]. One advantage of this approach is that important pathways can be identified when there are clear coordinated alterations in expression of genes in a pathway even though the genes individually exhibit relatively modest changes in expression. An alternative approach (Subheading 3.6) identifies pathways that are statistically enriched in the set of differentially expressed genes.

Once the important genes and pathways in a hypertensive model have been identified, pharmacological agents can be used either as a research tool to dissect underlying mechanisms or as a clinical tool to provide an additional therapeutic approach. This can be accomplished by using specific inhibitors or activators of key pathways. In addition, it should be possible to use pharmacological agents to directly manipulate the gene expression profile to either mimic the hypertensive phenotype or to counteract the molecular changes present in hypertension. A publicly available tool for matching disease and pharmacological profiles has been implemented by the Connectivity Map (CMAP, Subheading 3.7) which combines a compendium of global gene expression profiles from human cell lines treated with a large library of pharmacological compounds with pattern-matching algorithms [8].

In this review, the steps to perform a standard gene expression profiling experiment with microarrays are presented (Fig. 1). We are currently using these methods to investigate the downstream pathways regulated by the transcription factor PPARγ in the vasculature [9]. While the emphasis in this review is on the platform (Affymetrix) used in our laboratory, the general methods outlined are suitable for all array platforms. Moreover, the software tools and resources described do not require knowledge of computer programing or bioinformatics skills, are freely available for use, and in most cases are cross-platform (i.e., Windows, Mac OS, Linux) compatible.

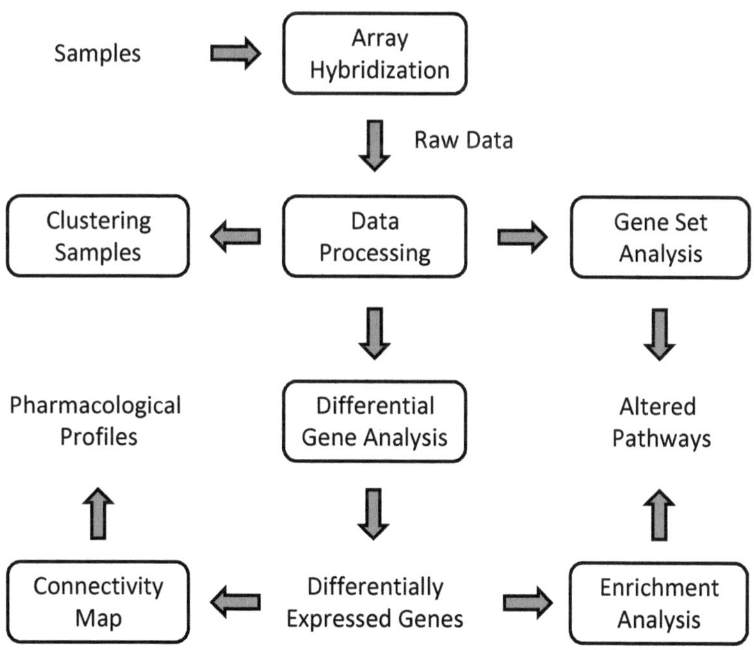

Fig. 1 Schema of the workflow for analysis of microarray data. Each rectangle corresponds to one of the seven sections outlined in Subheading 3

2 Materials

1. A suitable reagent (e.g., Trizol) for RNA isolation.
2. A cleanup kit for generating high quality total RNA free of genomic DNA.
3. A spectrophotometer for quantitation of total RNA.
4. The Agilent Bioanalyzer to assess RNA quality.
5. A real-time quantitative PCR system.
6. A standard personal computer (Windows, Linux, or Mac OS) with a minimum of 4GB RAM and access to the internet.
7. Spreadsheet software such as Microsoft Excel or OpenOffice and a text editor such as Notepad.
8. Java Runtime Environment freely available from Oracle (http://www.oracle.com).

3 Methods

3.1 Samples and Array Hybridization

1. Select samples for RNA isolation (*see* **Note 1**).
2. Isolate total RNA (*see* **Note 2**).
3. Clean up total RNA using a commercially available kit (e.g., RNeasy from Qiagen). It is important to include a DNAse treatment step to eliminate contaminating genomic DNA.
4. Quantitate RNA yield using a spectrophotometer. If the amount of RNA is limiting, a micro-volume spectrophotometer system such as the NanoDrop (Thermo Scientific) can be used. The A260/A280 ratio should be in the range of 1.8–2.0.
5. Assess RNA integrity using the Agilent Bioanalyzer. Both 28S and 18S ribosomal RNA should display prominent bands with no overt evidence of RNA degradation. The minimum RNA Integrity Number (RIN) as calculated by the Bioanalyzer should be in the range of 7–8.
6. Submit 5–10 μg of total RNA per sample to a microarray core facility. If the amount of RNA is limiting, alternative protocols are available (*see* **Note 3**). The submitted total RNA will be used to generate biotin-labeled RNA fragments for hybridization to the array. This step will be followed by washing and scanning of the array. The results generated at this point will be unprocessed data corresponding to the raw signal intensity for each probe set on the array.

3.2 Data Processing

1. Install the R statistics program (freely downloadable from http://www.r-project.org/).
2. For Affymetrix microarrays, install Affymetrix Power Tools (APT; for download go to http://www.affymetrix.com, follow the links to Partners and Programs and then to Developer's Network). Installable binaries and complete source code are freely available.
3. For Affymetrix arrays, put the raw data files (CEL files) and annotation files (available from Developers Network at Affymetrix) in a single directory and make a text file with a header line of "cel_files" followed by the names of all the files to be processed (one name per line).
4. Run the APT command apt-probeset-summarize from the command line to normalize arrays (*see* **Note 4**) and generate signal values for each gene (*see* **Note 5**).
5. The output of **step 4** will consist of text files with processed data, a summary of the data, and a log file. Depending on the number of arrays, this step can take as long as several hours, although the memory demands are not intensive.
6. For Affymetrix exon arrays, the analysis performed in **step 4** can be repeated to perform an exon-specific analysis (*see* **Note 6**).
7. Import the processed data from **step 5** into R using the read. table command. The data will be used in Subheading 3.4 for statistical analysis.
8. Alternative software tools are available for normalizing micro-array data (*see* **Note** 7).

3.3 Clustering Samples

1. Install the programs Cluster 3.0 (http://bonsai.hgc.jp/~mdehoon/software/cluster/index.html) and Maple Tree (http://mapletree.sourceforge.net/). Maple Tree requires installation of the Java Runtime Environment.
2. Use a spreadsheet program to edit the processed microarray data and save as a tab-delimited text file suitable for import into the Cluster 3.0 program.
3. Within the Cluster 3.0 program, import the data and select the clustering analysis (e.g., PCA or HCA) desired. Select the cluster by arrays option (*see* **Note 8**) under the appropriate tab. All the output files should be kept in the same directory.
4. HCA data can be visually inspected using the Maple Tree program by importing the cdt file produced by Cluster 3.0 and the PCA results can plotted in any graphing program (e.g., Microsoft Excel, SigmaPlot).

5. Samples exhibiting an extremely divergent expression pattern (*see* **Note 9**) should be considered outliers and the data processing steps outlined in Subheading 3.2 should be repeated with these samples removed.

3.4 Differential Gene Analysis and Experimental Validation

1. Confirm that the R statistics program is installed (*see* Subheading 3.2).
2. Install the Bioconductor packages limma, Biobase, and qvalue. All Bioconductor packages can be installed from within R (*see* **Note 10**). Under the Package menu, first choose the Bioconductor repository and then select the desired package to install.
3. Use the microarray data previously imported into R (**step 7** of Subheading 3.2) to create an expression set (eSet) object. The eSet object combines expression data with experimental metadata and is created using the ExpressionSet command in the Biobase package.
4. Use the limma package (*see* **Note 11**) to process the eSet object from **step 3**. The limma command lmfit is used to estimate the fold changes and standard errors by fitting a linear model for each gene. Next, information across all genes is used in an empirical Bayes smoothing step (command eBayes) to moderate the standard errors before calculating a *p*-value for each gene.
5. The procedure described in **step 4** can be used in an exon-specific analysis (*see* **Note 12**).
6. Correction for multiple testing can be performed directly within the limma analysis, or can be done using the Bioconductor package qvalue (command qvalue) which takes a list of *p*-values and estimates their respective *q*-values (analogous to a False Discovery Rate).
7. Choose an appropriate statistical cutoff for differential expression. Adjusted *p*-values less than 0.01 or 0.05 are common choices (*see* **Note 13**).
8. Output the table of differentially expressed genes with *p*-values (adjusted and unadjusted) and fold changes to a tab-delimited text file that can be imported into Microsoft Excel (*see* **Note 14**).
9. Selected differentially expressed genes (**step 8**) should be validated using real-time quantitative RT-PCR in the original samples and independently derived samples. The validation set should include both upregulated and downregulated genes over a range of expression changes.
10. In the case of genes with alternative transcripts, the location of the PCR primers should correspond with the locations used for the probes on the microarray (*see* **Note 15**).

11. For the same samples, plot changes in expression (PCR versus microarray). In a successful experiment, these values should be highly correlated and fit a linear curve.

12. Once validation is complete, upload data to a repository such as the Gene Expression Omnibus (GEO; http://www.ncbi.nlm.nih.gov/geo/). To comply with the Minimum Information About a Microarray Experiment (MIAME) guidelines [10], fully describe the experiment, the data files, and analysis steps using template spreadsheets provided by GEO. Next, pack the spreadsheets and data files (raw and normalized) into a single file using software such as WinZip (http://www.winzip.com). Use the Direct Deposit page (login required) to transfer this file to GEO using the GEOarchive option. Data can be kept private until publication.

3.5 Gene Set Analysis to Identify Differentially Expressed Pathways

1. Download the Java based software (*see* **Note 16**) implementing the Gene Set Enrichment algorithm from the Broad Institute (http://www.broadinstitute.org/gsea/index.jsp). The software is platform independent but requires the Java Runtime Environment.

2. Download the Molecular Signatures Database (MSigDB), a collection of annotated gene sets for use with GSEA software, from the GSEA website.

3. Optionally, generate custom-made gene set files (i.e., GMT files) using a standard spreadsheet program or text editor.

4. Generate GCT files containing the microarray data, a class file (CLS) describing the samples, and an annotation file (CHIP) listing each microarray probe and its matching gene symbol or description. This can be done using a standard spreadsheet program or text editor. The GCT and CLS files are mandatory whereas the CHIP file is optional.

5. Run GSEA from the command line (*see* **Note 17**). The run time depends on the number of gene sets analyzed, but generally will require several hours. The minimum number of permutations used for empirical calculation of the *p*-value and false discovery rate is 100, but 1000 is preferred.

6. The output of the GSEA analysis is in the form of navigable HTML files, text files, and Microsoft Excel files. It is recommended that only gene sets having a nominal *p*-value less than 0.05 and a False Discovery Rate less than 25 % be considered for further analysis.

3.6 Enrichment Analysis to Identify Differentially Expressed Pathways

1. For in-depth functional annotation including classification of what types of genes or pathways are altered, use the Database for Annotation, Visualization, and Integrated Discovery (DAVID, http://david.abcc.ncifcrf.gov/) hosted by the National Cancer Institute at the NIH [11].

2. At the DAVID website (**step 5**), import the list of probes found to be differentially expressed (*see* **Note 18**).
3. Choose the background for the enrichment analysis. This is typically from the specific array used in the experiment. If that particular array platform is not listed, the species can be used instead.
4. Choose the Functional Annotation Chart option to perform an enrichment analysis. This analysis determines if there are more expression changes, based on our list of differentially expressed genes, in a particular pathway or functional category than would have been expected by random chance (*see* **Note 19**), thus identifying a set of altered pathways.
5. All reports from DAVID can be downloaded to a format suitable to import into Microsoft Excel.
6. For advanced users, there are additional ways to access the DAVID database (*see* **Note 20**).
7. For additional annotation of the differentially expressed genes go to the Gene Cards website (http://www.genecards.org) and choose the GeneAlaCart option (free registration required).
8. Prepare a text file with a list of all the differentially expressed genes and import into GeneAlaCart. The output will be a text or Excel file with extensive annotation including mapping of genes to descriptions and commonly used aliases (*see* **Note 21**).
9. Basic gene annotation similar to that of **step 3** can be done programmatically (*see* **Note 22**).

3.7 Connectivity Map to Identify Pharmacological Profiles

1. Login to the Connectivity Map (CMAP) website (http://www.broadinstitute.org/cmap/index.jsp). A free registration step is required.
2. Compile the list of differentially expressed genes (i.e., official gene symbols) subdivided based on upregulated or downregulated expression and put into text files.
3. Map the gene symbols to the specific Affymetrix probe sets required by CMAP. This can be done using the NetAffx [12] annotation tool (free registration required) at the Affymetrix website (http://www.affymetrix.com). After login to NetAffx, choose batch query under the 3′ IVT Expression tab and select HG-U133A as array type. Upload the text file from **step 1** and query NetAffx by gene symbol. The output contains a savable list of probe sets for use with CMAP.
4. From the CMAP interface, select the Query tab and using the Quick Query option, upload the probe set lists (**step 2**) and run the analysis (*see* **Note 23**).
5. The results found under permuted results can be sorted, and grouped in a variety of ways before exporting to a Microsoft Excel file.

6. Negative enrichment reflects a match to an expression signature oppositely regulated (i.e., genes that are upregulated have decreased expression in the CMAP data and vice versa, *see* **Note 24**).
7. Detailed information about the pharmacological agents used in the CMAP experiments can be found at PubChem at the NCBI (http://pubchem.ncbi.nlm.nih.gov).

4 Notes

1. It is important that sufficient samples initially be prepared given the likelihood that some samples will not meet the high quality standard required for the microarray experiment.
2. This step typically is done following tissue homogenization in guanidinium isothiocyanate using a variation of the method as described [13]. Total RNA should be prepared instead of poly-A RNA to allow for better assessment of RNA quality.
3. If the amount of RNA is less than that required, samples can be pooled to produce sufficient yield. It is important that each sample within a pool is derived from a separate source and that each pool represents an independent biological replicate. As an alternative to pooling, a preliminary linear amplification step starting with 5–10 ng total RNA be used [14].
4. All arrays must be normalized at the same time. The algorithm frequently used for normalizing microarray data generated from Affymetrix arrays is the Robust Multi-Array Average (RMA) algorithm originally described by Irizarry et al. [2]. For other types of array platforms such as the Illumina Bead chips or dual channel cDNA microarrays, similar algorithms are used and have been implemented in Bioconductor packages available for use in R.
5. By default, all transcripts with sufficient supporting evidence are included in the annotation file used for performing the data analysis. Most genes map to more than one transcript.
6. For Affymetrix exon arrays, the procedures for data normalization are identical for both exon- and gene-level analysis. However, because exon-level analysis is based on a smaller number of probe sets, the level of variance tends to be higher.
7. As an alternative, the algorithms used herein have been implemented in R packages. Using R for this step; however, will generally utilize more memory resources.
8. Optionally, the dataset can be clustered both by genes and by arrays. This is more computationally intensive and should generally be used for clustering a subset of the dataset.

9. There is no consensus on what should be considered an outlier. Generally, if the similarity measure (e.g., correlation coefficient) for the suspected outlier sample is more than 3 standard deviations away from the overall average, then removal of that sample should be considered.
10. Additional information about Bioconductor packages and installable downloads can be found at the Bioconductor website (http://www.bioconductor.org).
11. There are multiple functions available in the limma package to handle high-throughput gene expression profiling data whether the experiment involves microarray (single or dual channel) or alternative methodologies such as RNA sequencing (RNA-Seq). Also, there is graphical version of limma (limmaGUI) available [15].
12. For an exon-specific analysis, the methods of limma can still be used to assess differential expression. However, a preprocessing step is required using a package such as aroma-affymetrix [16], which simultaneously takes into account both gene and exon level changes.
13. There is no consensus on the correct threshold for differential expression. In addition to picking a common *p*-value (adjusted) such as 0.01, some investigators have recommended choosing a *p*-value that is at least tenfold lower than the minimum seen in the set of control probes, which by definition should not be differentially expressed [17]. Alternatively, another approach is to plot log (base 2) fold change in expression versus *p*-value (known as a volcano plot) and determine the *p*-value where the data is best separated (*see* limma vignette for example).
14. By default, fold changes are presented in logarithmic (log2) format. From within Microsoft Excel, these values can be converted into the desired format.
15. The sequences used for designing the array probes are usually available from the manufacturer. These sequences can then be aligned to the genome using tools such as BLAT (http://genome.ucsc.edu) or BLAST (http://www.ncbi.nlm.nih.gov).
16. There is an R version of GSEA implementing the same algorithm. This is generally for more advanced users.
17. There is a graphical user interface available for GSEA.
18. Depending on the specific hypothesis tested, it is often preferable to subdivide the set of differentially expressed genes into upregulated and downregulated lists.
19. A modified Fisher's Exact test is used to determine the *p*-value.
20. For users with a large number of queries, a stand-alone version of the DAVID database called EASE can be downloaded and installed locally. For access from within the Perl or Java programming languages, there is a web service available [18].

21. One example of the importance of identifying gene aliases comes from the gene officially annotated as secreted phosphoprotein 1, commonly known in hypertension research as osteopontin, a key contributor to vascular calcification [19].
22. For programmatic access to annotation databases, use the MySql databases available from the UCSC Genome Browser (http://genome.ucsc.edu).
23. The Quick Query results are only stored temporarily. In order to re-login at a later time and retrieve the results, the Load Signature tool should be selected.
24. Discovery of pharmacological agents that generate an expression signature opposite that seen in hypertension could be a strategy for identifying therapeutics that might actively reverse some of the deleterious effects of hypertensive disease.

Acknowledgment

This work was supported through research grants from the NIH to CDS (HL084207, HL048058, HL061446, HL062984, and NS024621). The authors also gratefully acknowledge the generous research support of the Roy J. Carver Trust.

References

1. Chon H et al (2004) Broadly altered gene expression in blood leukocytes in essential hypertension is absent during treatment. Hypertension 43:947–951, Epub 2004 Mar 08
2. Irizarry RA et al (2003) Exploration, normalization, and summaries of high density oligonucleotide array probe level data. Biostatistics 4:249–264
3. Mortazavi A et al (2008) Mapping and quantifying mammalian transcriptomes by RNA-Seq. Nat Methods 5:621–628
4. Quackenbush J (2006) Microarray analysis and tumor classification. N Engl J Med 354:2463–2472
5. Bergkvist A et al (2010) Gene expression profiling—clusters of possibilities. Methods 50:323–335
6. Smyth GK (2004) Linear models and empirical Bayes methods for assessing differential expression in microarray experiments. Stat Appl Genet Mol Biol 3, 3
7. Subramanian A et al (2005) Gene set enrichment analysis: a knowledge-based approach for interpreting genome-wide expression profiles. Proc Natl Acad Sci U S A 102: 15545–15550
8. Lamb J et al (2006) The Connectivity Map: using gene-expression signatures to connect small molecules, genes, and disease. Science 313:1929–1935
9. Keen HL et al (2009) Bioinformatic analysis of gene sets regulated by ligand-activated and dominant-negative peroxisome proliferator-activated receptor gamma in mouse aorta. Arterioscler Thromb Vasc Biol 30:518–525
10. Brazma A et al (2001) Minimum information about a microarray experiment (MIAME)-toward standards for microarray data. Nat Genet 29:365–371
11. da Huang W, Sherman BT, Lempicki RA (2009) Bioinformatics enrichment tools: paths toward the comprehensive functional analysis of large gene lists. Nucleic Acids Res 37:1–13
12. Liu G et al (2003) NetAffx: Affymetrix probesets and annotations. Nucleic Acids Res 31:82–86
13. Chomczynski P, Sacchi N (1987) Single-step method of RNA isolation by acid guanidinium thiocyanate-phenol-chloroform extraction. Anal Biochem 162:156–159
14. Ginsberg SD (2005) RNA amplification strategies for small sample populations. Methods 37:229–237

15. Wettenhall JM, Smyth GK (2004) limmaGUI: a graphical user interface for linear modeling of microarray data. Bioinformatics 20:3705–3706
16. Purdom E et al (2008) FIRMA: a method for detection of alternative splicing from exon array data. Bioinformatics 24:1707–1714
17. Smyth GK (2005) Limma: linear models for microarray data. In: Gentleman RC et al (eds) Bioinformatics and computational biology solutions using R and bioconductor. Springer, New York, pp 397–420
18. Jiao X et al (2012) DAVID-WS: a stateful web service to facilitate gene/protein list analysis. Bioinformatics 28:1805–1806
19. Scatena M, Liaw L, Giachelli CM (2007) Osteopontin: a multifunctional molecule regulating chronic inflammation and vascular disease. Arterioscler Thromb Vasc Biol 27:2302–2309

Chapter 4

Tissue Proteomics in Vascular Disease

Amaya Albalat, William Mullen, Holger Husi, and Harald Mischak

Abstract

In vascular diseases, as in many other pathophysiological conditions, tissue proteins are subjected to a number of different changes such as protein expression, posttranslational modifications, and proteolytic cleavage. For this reason, the study of the tissue proteome is becoming an increasingly important tool in biological and clinical research. In this chapter, we describe in detail the methodology for the analysis of tryptic digested peptides from aortic tissue extracts from mice with the aim to elucidate differences in the proteome between control and case or vascular diseased tissue samples. The method encompasses the analysis of these complex extracts in a single chromatographic run allowing for increased reproducibility. We also outline the main workflow for the processing of the generated data by statistical and bioinformatic analysis.

Key words Tissue proteomics, FASP method, MS/MS data analysis

1 Introduction

Omics datasets are becoming increasingly relevant in clinical research. Currently, the focus is on three main omics traits: genomics, proteomics, and metabolomics. When placing these into the context, genomics is the by far most advanced technology, in part owed to the relative ease of assessing information. A major advantage in genomics is that the typical target, the DNA, is very stable. In addition, the basic information is encoded by only four nucleic acids, which, further easing assessment, are complementary and can pair via hydrogen bonds.

These properties, and the substantial homogeneity of the nucleic acids on a chemical/molecular level ease assessing the genome, as they allow for duplication and subsequently multiplication, the generation of specific (antisense) probes, and in-depth analysis via enzymatic sequencing.

Unfortunately, the proteome, and the metabolome show much higher chemical diversity, and cannot be analyzed using similar approaches: neither can they be easily duplicated or multiplied in a

Rhian M. Touyz and Ernesto L. Schiffrin (eds.), *Hypertension: Methods and Protocols*, Methods in Molecular Biology, vol. 1527, DOI 10.1007/978-1-4939-6625-7_4, © Springer Science+Business Media LLC 2017

comprehensive way, nor can specific probes, based on a sequence, be rationally generated (it is not possible to easily design antibodies that are really highly specific).

As a result of these issues, genomics is applied much more frequently, and genomics datasets available by far outnumber proteomics or metabolomics datasets.

However, this is in contrast to the biological information contained in these different omics traits. Indeed, due to gene splicing and also due to post-translational modifications one gene does not code for one protein only but for several. Proteins are involved in all cellular functions and cell regulatory mechanisms. This outstanding relevance of proteins is not only due to their key role in physiological processes but also because, as cause or effect they are modified in pathophysiological situations [1]. Therefore, the unbiased study of the tissue proteome is of invaluable importance for the identification of unknown disease mediators. These considerations highlight why comprehensive proteome analysis is becoming an increasingly important tool in biological and clinical research. Previously, tissue proteomics analysis required each extract to be separated into multiple fractions in chromatographic systems and the mass spectral results combined [2]. However, as a result of recent advances in chromatography and mass spectrometry (ultra high pressure nanoflow pumps with 50 cm nanoflow columns linked to high resolution mass spectrometers) a tissue extract can be now adequately analyzed in a single chromatographic run. This allows for greater reproducibility and therefore a lower number of sample replicates are required to identify differential protein expression patterns.

However, this analytical workflow results in a large number of peptides and proteins being identified and the subsequent data analysis requires additional informatics software. A simple bioinformatics solution to the comparison of MS/MS datasets is provided by the software package Scaffold [3]. Using the results generated in Scaffold pathway analysis of the up and down regulated proteins can be attempted in software packages such as Ingenuity Pathway Analysis (IPA), Cytoscape, and Pathway Studio [4].

Vascular diseases including atherosclerosis, intimal hyperplasia, and aneurysms produce, as a consequence or as a cause, changes in the proteome. As outlined in recent viewpoint articles [5, 6], ideally the proteome of the affected entity (tissue) should be assessed as it offers a direct insight into the disease. As also outlined in these articles, such an approach is hindered by the limited availability of tissue, but the technical limitations mentioned are now being addressed. In this chapter we will describe in detail the methodology of the analysis of tryptic digested peptides from aortic tissue extracts from mice with the aim of identifying quantitative differences in the proteome between control and case or diseased tissue samples.

Aortic tissues from mice were prepared according to the *Filter Aided Sample Preparation* (FASP) method [7]. Using this method it is possible to solubilise cellular proteins very efficiently irrespectively of their subcellular location using sodium dodecyl sulfate (SDS) and to obtain protein digests that are suitable for MS-based proteome analysis.

2 Materials

2.1 Sample Preparation Buffers

1. Lysis buffer: 0.1 M Tris–HCl pH 7.6 supplemented with 4% SDS and 0.1 M DTT: Add 1.57 g of Tris–HCl (MW 157.6) into 80 ml of MilliQ water. Adjust pH and bring to volume 100 ml. This buffer is then supplemented with SDS 4% (0.4 g per 10 ml of buffer and 0.1 M of DTT (MW 154.2) (0.154 g of DTT per 10 ml of buffer)).
2. Tris–HCl 0.1 M pH 8.5: Add 3.15 g of Tris–HCl (MW 157.6) into 180 ml of MilliQ water. Adjust pH and bring to volume 200 ml.
3. Urea buffer 8 M in 0.1 M Tris–HCl pH 8.5 (UA): Add 4.8 g urea (MW 60.06) into 6 ml of Tris buffer 0.1 M pH 8.5, mix until urea is dissolved and adjust volume to 10 ml. Prepare 1 ml per 1 sample. This buffer needs to be prepared fresh and used within a day.
4. Iodoacetamide 0.05 M in Urea Buffer (IAA): Add 9.2 mg of iodoacetamide (MW 184.96) into 1 ml of UA buffer. Prepare 0.1 ml per 1 sample. This buffer needs to be prepared fresh and used within a day.
5. ABC Buffer or 50 mM of NH4HCO3 in MilliQ water: Add 0.79 g NH4HCO3 (MW 79.06) into 190 ml of MilliQ water, adjust pH to 8 and volume up to 200 ml.
6. Trypsin Sequencing Grade Modified Trypsin from Promega (Southampton, UK): A bottle of trypsin containing 20 μ g of trypsin is reconstituted with 40 μ l of 25 mM of NH4HCO3 pH 8. This stock solution is therefore at a concentration of 500 ng/μl.
7. Trypsin is reconstituted in 25 mM of NH4HCO3 pH 8 in MilliQ water: Add 0.39 g NH4HCO3 (MW 79.06) into 190 ml of MilliQ water, adjust pH to 8 and volume up to 200 ml.

Note: All reagents unless stated otherwise were from Sigma-Aldrich (Dorset, UK).

2.2 Sample Preparation

1. Tissue homogenizer, Ultra-Turrax T 25 (IKA, Staufen, Germany).

2. Microtube centrifuge, Heraeus, Fresco 17 (Thermo Scientific, UK).
3. Filter units, Microcon YM-30 (Millipore, Watford, UK).

2.3 Nano-LC MS/MS System

1. Dionex Ultimate 3000 RSLS nano flow system (Dionex, Camberly, UK).
2. Nano trap column: Dionex 0.1 × 20 mm 5 μm C18 (Dionex, Camberly, UK).
3. Nano column: Acclaim PepMap C18 nano column 75 μ m × 50 cm, 2 μ m 100 Å (Dionex, Camberly, UK).
4. Proxeon nano spray ESI source (Thermo Fisher, Hemel, UK).
5. Orbitrap Velos FTMS mass spectrometer (Thermo Fisher, Hemel, UK).

2.4 Software

1. Commercial software for the visualization and validation of MS/MS proteomic data: Proteome Discoverer version 1.3 (Thermo Fisher, Hemel, UK), software package Scaffold (http://www.proteomesoftware.com/) (Searle, B. C 2009), Mascot search engine (http://www.matrixscience.com/) and Phenyx (http://www.genebio.com/products/phenyx/). Open source software X! Tandem (http://www.thegpm.org/tandem/index.html), and OMSSA (http://www.ncbi.nlm.nih.gov).
2. Commercial software for bioinformatic pathway analysis: Ingenuity Pathway Analysis (IPA) (http://www.ingenuity.com/) and Pathway Studio (http://www.pathwaystudio.com/). Open source software Cytoscape (http://www.cytoscape.org/).

3 Methods

3.1 Sample Preparation

1. Homogenize mice aorta in lysis buffer (1:10 sample to buffer ratio) using an Ultra-Turrax T 25 (IKA, Staufen, Germany).
2. Incubate lysates at 95 °C for 3 min and clarify them by centrifugation at 16,000 × *g* for 5 min at room temperature. Please note that centrifugation is to be carried out at a temperature above 15 °C in order to avoid precipitation of concentrated SDS.
3. Mix 30 μl of protein extract with 200 μl of UA buffer in the Microcon filter unit and centrifuge at 14,000 × *g* for 15 min.
4. Add 200 μl of UA to the filter unit and centrifuge at 14,000 × *g* for 15 min.
5. Discard the flow-through liquid from the collection tubes.
6. Add 100 μl of IAA solution at mix at 600 rpm for 1 min and incubate without mixing for 20 min.

7. Centrifuge the filter units at 14,000 × *g* for 10 min.
8. Add 100 μl of UA to the filter unit and centrifuge at 14,000 × *g* for 15 min. Repeat this step twice.
9. Add 100 μl of ABC buffer to the filter unit and centrifuge at 14,000 × *g* for 10 min.

   Repeat this step twice.

10. Add 40 μl of ABC buffer containing the trypsin (enzyme to protein ratio 1:100) and mix at 600 rpm for 1 min.
11. Incubate the units in a wet chamber at 37 °C for 4–18 h.
12. Transfer the filter units to new collection tubes.
13. Centrifuge the filter units at 14,000 × *g* for 10 min.
14. Add 40 μl of ABC buffer and centrifuge again at 14,000 × *g* for 10 min.
15. Acidify the filtrates with formic acid.

3.2 Nano-LC M/MS Analysis for Sequencing

1. Tryptic digests were analyzed on a Dionex Ultimate 3000 RSLS nano flow system.

   After loading (5 μ l) onto a Dionex 0.1 × 20 mm 5 μm C18 nano trap column at a flowrate of 5 μ l/min in 98 % 0.1 % formic acid and 2 % acetonitrile, sample was eluted onto an Acclaim PepMap C18 nano column 75 μm × 50 cm, 2 μ m 100 Å at a flow rate of 0.3 μl/min. The trap and nano flow column were maintained at 35 °C. The samples were eluted with a gradient of solvent A: 0.1 % formic acid verses solvent B: 80 % acetonitrile starting at 5 % B rising to 50 % B over 480 min.
2. The eluant was ionized using a Proxeon nano spray ESI source operating in positive ion mode into an Orbitrap Velos FTMS. Ionization voltage was 2.5 kV and the capillary temperature was 200 °C. The mass spectrometer was operated in MS/MS mode scanning from 380–2000 amu. The top 20 multiply charged ions were selected from each scan for MS/MS analysis using CID at 35 % collision energy. The resolution of ions in MS1 was 60,000 and 7500 for CID MS2.
3. MS and MS/MS data files were searched, in this case, against the IPI mouse nonredundant database using SEQUEST (by using Thermo Proteome Discoverer), with trypsin as enzyme specificity. Peptide data were extracted using high peptide confidence and top one peptide rank filters. Alternatively use either the Mascot search engine (Matrix Science) or X! Tandem (The Global Proteome Machine Organization) or Phenyx (GeneBio) or OMSSA (NCBI toolbox) for protein identification. Set Carbamidomethyl (C) as static modification and Oxidation of Methionine and Proline (M, P) as variable modifications and a peptide mass tolerance of ±10 ppm and a fragment mass toler-

ance of±0.5 Da and allow for a maximum of one missed cleavage. Determine the false discovery rates by reverse database searches and empirical analyses of the distributions of mass deviation, whereby Ion Scores can be used to establish score and mass accuracy filters.

3.3 Data Processing by Statistical and Bioinformatic Analysis

Data can be analyzed further by various means. Proteome Discoverer is an ideal solution for preprocessing prior to context, pathway or other downstream analysis. Scaffold software, Ingenuity pathway analysis (IPA) and Pathway studio require some preprocessing of the data, whereas using Cytoscape, and specific plug-ins for this software, necessitates a fair amount of processing prior to the bioinformatics analysis. However, Cytoscape is an ideal solution due to its flexibility and substantial array of analysis tools, which can potentially surpass the other pathway analysis software solutions.

1. Proteome Discoverer: Raw spectra from mass spectrometry measurements can be used directly in this software. It supports multiple dissociation techniques, quantitation technologies, and multiple database search algorithms (Sequest, Mascot, etc.) and combines their outputs to maximize and cross-validate results. It also allows for the determination of the False Discovery Rate (FDR), which can be used to validate protein IDs. Additionally, limited downstream analysis by annotation of identified proteins with GO classifications, PTMs, and literature references from public databases can be used to contextualize a biological significance of the measured samples.
2. Scaffold: This software uses output files generated by various search engines such as Mascot or OMSSA, including Proteome Discoverer. It allows robust statistical validation, label free quantitation and protein homology analysis (Fig. 1). It is also possible to re-query unassigned peptides by expanded database searches, protein quantitation and probability calculations, ROC curves and Venn diagrams, as well as Gene Ontology (GO) annotation analysis and frequency distributions.
3. Ingenuity and Pathway studio: These software solutions cannot handle direct protein ID search results. Either use Proteome Discoverer or manually merge protein identification files from for example Mascot searches to generate a combined sample-by-sample protein ID table. Manual merging is described in the next paragraph below. This list is then used to query underlying databases to find association networks by condition or expression profiling. The underlying databases are prior-knowledge, assembled from existing resources or the literature. The output, in the form of a network or pathway graph, can then be explored further by embedded links to the original source of the information.
4. Cytoscape: Merge all protein identification files containing both the protein ID and cumulative total ion current (TIC) or spectral counts (SC) for the identified protein per sample into

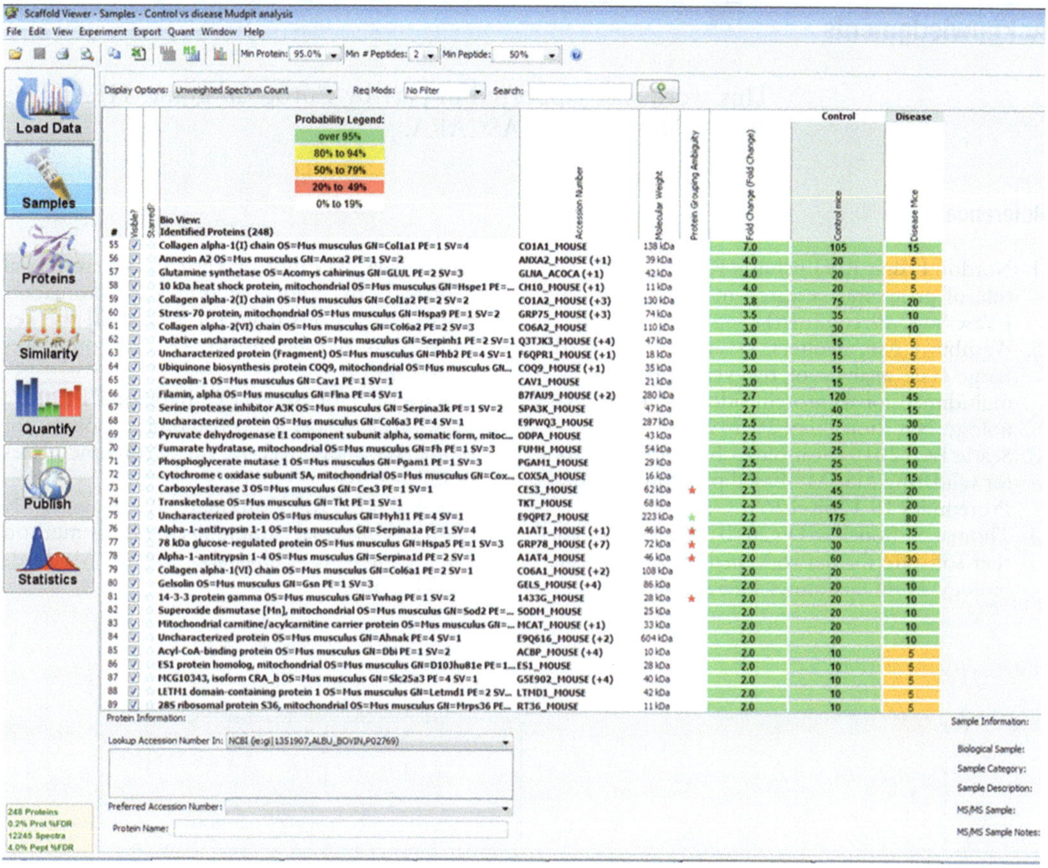

Fig. 1 Print screen output of the data in Scaffold software showing the fold increase changes in proteins between control and case samples

a single spreadsheet based on the protein ID. Missing TIC/SC values for proteins not found in all samples are set to zero. This should result in a table containing a list of identified proteins and columns of TIC/SC values for each sample measured. Optionally, the TIC/SC intensity data per sample can be normalized by summing all TIC/SC values per individual sample and dividing each individual value by this sum. Statistical testing for the relevance of each protein (p-value) is done by Mann–Whitney or *t*-test analysis across all samples. Bonferroni-correction to allow for multiple testing can be applied at this stage. Fold changes are calculated for each individual protein across all samples by averaging the TIC/SC per condition and calculating the fold-change ratio. This output table can then by loaded into Cytoscape and analyzed by keyword distribution (e.g., GO), pathway analysis, contextual databases (disease, literature), etc. as well as distribution diagrams using Cytoscape plug-ins.

Acknowledgments

This work was supported in part by European grant, HEALTH-2011-278249-EU-MASCARA.

References

1. Nordon I, Brar R, Hinchliffe R et al (2009) The role of proteomic research in vascular disease. J Vasc Surg 49:1602–1612
2. Washburn MP, Wolters D, Yates JR (2001) Large-scale analysis of the yeast proteome by multidimensional protein identification technology. Nat Biotechnol 19:242–247
3. Searle BC (2010) Scaffold: a bioinformatic tool for validating MS/MS-based proteomic studies. Proteomics 10:1265–1269
4. Thomas S, Bonchev D (2010) A survey of current software for network analysis in molecular biology. Hum Genomics 4:353–360
5. Good DM, Thongboonkerd V, Novak J et al (2007) Body fluid proteomics for biomarker discovery: lessons from the past hold the key to success in the future. J Proteome Res 6:549–4555
6. Lescuyer P, Hochstrasser D, Rabilloud T (2007) How shall we use the proteomics toolbox for biomarker discovery? J Proteome Res 6:3371–3376
7. Wiśniewski JR, Zougman A, Nagaraj N (2009) Universal sample preparation method for proteome analysis. Nat Methods 6:359–363

Chapter 5

Urine Metabolomics in Hypertension Research

Sofia Tsiropoulou, Martin McBride, and Sandosh Padmanabhan

Abstract

Functional genomics requires an understanding of the complete network of changes within an organism by extensive measurements of moieties from mRNA, proteins, and metabolites. Metabolomics utilizes analytic chemistry tools to profile the complete spectrum of metabolites found in a tissue, cells, or biofluids using a wide range of tools from infrared spectroscopy, fluorescence spectroscopy, NMR spectroscopy, and mass spectrometry. In this protocol, we outline a procedure for performing metabolomic analysis of urine samples using liquid chromatography–mass spectrometry (LC-MS). We outline the advantages of using this approach and summarize some of the early promising studies in cardiovascular diseases using this approach.

Key words Metabolomics, Urine, Hypertension, Mass spectrometry

1 Introduction

Metabolomics is the systematic study of unique chemical fingerprints of small molecules or metabolite profiles that are related to a variety of cellular metabolic processes in a cell, organ, or organism [1, 2]. It is an evolving and promising high-throughput analytic platform in the post-genomic era. The aim of metabolomics is to assay all low molecular weight metabolites, which include sugars, lipids, steroids, vitamins, amino acids, fatty acids, organic acids, and small peptides in biological systems, providing direct and indirect physiologic insights into established and novel metabolic pathways. This enables studies of overall metabolic pathways. The Human Metabolome Project has a central aim to identify, quantify, catalog, and store data on all metabolites that can potentially be found in human tissues and biofluids at concentrations >1 micromolar. Over 8500 metabolites have already been identified and recorded in the Human Metabolome Database, [3] demonstrating the huge challenge faced by researchers in the field of metabolomics. This highlights the biggest challenge in using this platform—chemical entities exist over a wide range of polarities, molecular

Rhian M. Touyz and Ernesto L. Schiffrin (eds.), *Hypertension: Methods and Protocols*, Methods in Molecular Biology, vol. 1527, DOI 10.1007/978-1-4939-6625-7_5, © Springer Science+Business Media LLC 2017

masses, and concentrations that require a range of extraction and chromatographic approaches [2].

1.1 Metabolomics and Urine Analysis

Many biological fluid samples can be used in metabolomic profiling, such as urine, plasma, serum, whole blood, bile, cerebrospinal fluid, saliva, and tissue homogenate. Among these, urine and plasma are most widely used. Plasma analysis has some advantages in that under specific physiological or pathologic conditions, the concentration ratio of macromolecules as well as their small molecule metabolites can be detected. This has a relatively stronger sensitivity in detecting perturbations of health or disease. However, the invasive aspect of obtaining plasma samples is a major disadvantage. Urine analysis has numerous advantages compared with other biological fluid samples. Urine samples can be collected repeatedly in large volumes noninvasively, the processing of urine samples is less complex as it has lower protein content, and the urine metabolites are relatively smaller and thermodynamically stable. Besides, there is also less intermolecular interaction of the metabolites in the urine samples [4]. The disadvantages of urine analysis include the variability in the time intervals for urine sample collection, and procedure to prepare standard solutions for urine samples. Nevertheless, the advantages of urine analysis overweigh its disadvantages [5].

1.2 Approaches of Metabolomics

There are two approaches in metabolomics—untargeted or targeted. The untargeted approach is "open" profiling which is to analyze the data without a specific target, and then generate raw data for further analysis. Untargeted approach of metabolomics is normally used for discovering previously unknown physiological patterns or used as a trial for new methods for the analysis of metabolites. One of many drawbacks about untargeted approach is the issue of reproducibility, because a metabolic profile is not specific to a condition. It varies along with the change in physiological conditions, and is generally affected by a multitude of factors. The identified patterns using an untargeted approach can perhaps help in the hypothesis generation and discover novel pathways or diagnostic tests. On the other hand, targeted approach ("closed" profiling) makes it possible to do a more directed study, focused on a more limited group of metabolites. Thus, a targeted approach is used in the validation of a novel biomarker after its discovery, helping assess reproducibility and enabling better understanding of the mechanism behind the detected pattern of the metabolites.

1.3 Methods for Metabolomics

There are two key techniques used in metabolomics. One is nuclear magnetic resonance (NMR) spectroscopy, and the other one is mass spectrometry (MS). NMR spectroscopy is an analytical technique that uses the magnetic properties of nuclei to identify the chemical entities. NMR has several advantages, for example, the sample preparation needed for NMR spectroscopy is relatively easy, and the structure of the compound presented in NMR spectroscopy is specific and precise. However, NMR spectroscopy is a less sensitive technique. Thus, signals for compounds below a detectable threshold (usually in the nanogram range) may be obscured. MS is an analytical method that is used to detect the mass to charge ratio (m/e or m/z) to identify compounds. MS is generally coupled with separation methods, such as liquid chromatography (LC), gas chromatography (GC), or capillary electrophoresis (CE). This combination is a powerful tool with enhanced sensitivity and high throughput. The choice of different separation methods depends on the character of the analytes, such as their molecular weights and hydrophilicity (or hydrophobicity). For example, LC is mainly used for compounds that are not volatile in solutions; GC is used for nonpolar and volatile compounds; while CE is used for the analysis of chiral compounds. After separation, analytes are required to be ionized before entering MS. Depending on the type of MS detector, different methods for ionization are used, such as electron impact and chemical ionization. MS is considered more sensitive than NMR, due to the former's capability to identify the peaks of numerous compounds even when they are at a relatively much lower concentration range, such as attomole to picomole per liter range.

1.4 Application of Metabolomics in Cardiovascular Research

Large-scale perturbations in metabolism and energetics occur in the heart during the development and progression of heart disease. The majority of studies have looked at plasma metabolites. In patients with stable atherosclerosis, alanine, aspartate, tyrosine, and serine levels were significantly decreased compared to control samples [6]. Two independent studies showed abnormalities in choline metabolism linked to heart disease. A small-scale ischemic heart failure study showed an increase in trimethylamine N-oxide (TMAO) urinary excretion [7]. A larger study of over 1800 subjects showed dose-dependent associations between increased plasma levels of choline, betaine, and TMAO with the presence of cardiovascular disease, and a dose–response relationship between TMAO levels and clinical atherosclerotic plaque burden [8]. However, TMAO production is highly influenced by diet, with TMAO higher in meat eaters than vegetarians and higher in fish eaters than meat eaters; thus its specificity for atherosclerosis is questionable [9]. Three metabolites of the dietary lipid phosphatidylcholine–choline, trimethylamine N-oxide (TMAO), and betaine–were identified and then shown to predict risk for CVD in an independent large clinical cohort [8]. The urinary profiles of 4630 individuals from the UK, the USA, China, and Japan were examined by 1H-NMR spectroscopy and a number of common metabolites (including formate, hippurate, and alanine), many associated with diet, were found to be highly correlated with blood pressure [10]. In the Framingham heart study, 2422 normoglycemic individuals followed for 12 years had amino acids, amines, and other polar metabolites profiled in baseline specimens by liquid chromatography–tandem mass spectrometry (LC-MS). Five branched-chain and aromatic amino acids showed highly significant associations with future diabetes: isoleucine, leucine, valine, tyrosine, and phenylalanine [11]. In a linked genome wide association study and plasma metabolomic study of around 3000 individuals, significant associations were observed between single nucleotide polymorphisms in the glucokinase regulator gene, plasma mannose/glucose ratio, and cardiometabolic syndrome, between fatty acid desaturase 1, plasma ratio of long chain fatty acids and resting heart rate, and between UDP-glucuronosyl transferase, plasma oleoylcarnitine/bilirubin ratio, and coronary artery disease [12].

Metabolomics is a relatively new field and the high-throughput with relatively short experimental times needed for analysis makes it a front-runner in translational studies. In this protocol, we describe a generic procedure for urinary metabolomic studies.

2 Methods

1. Collection of urine samples: Urine is collected over a 24 h period, kept at 4 °C and then aliquoted and stored at −80 °C until use (*see* **Note 1**).
2. Reagents
   (a) Reagents for liquid chromatography - mass spectrometry (LC-MS) procedure.
      - High purity deionized water
      - Acetonitrile

   (b) Reagents for sample extraction
      High purity deionized water
      Chloroform
      Methanol

(*see* **Note 2**).

3. Urine extraction: Metabolites are extracted using a slightly modified version of the Folch method [13]. Chloroform is used as the nonpolar and methanol as the polar extracting solvents along with water, allowing the extraction of both nonpolar and polar, water-soluble, and organic-soluble metabolites. Samples are maintained on ice at all intervals.

(a) Thaw each sample and take out an aliquot of 30 μl

(b) Add 90 μl of methanol and 30 μl of chloroform to a final ratio of 1:3:1 (urine:methanol:chloroform).

(c) Mix vigorously at 4 °C for 1 h.

(d) Centrifuge for 3 min at 13,000 ×*g*, at 4 °C.

(e) Store supernatant at −80 °C until analysis by LC-MS

(*see* **Note 3**).

4. LC-MS procedure

(a) LC. Metabolites are separated by polarity and hydrophilicity using a ZIC-HILIC 4.6 mm × 15 cm column (Merck SeQuant, Sweden) running at 300 μl/min, on a UltiMate 3000 Rapid Separation LC system (Thermo Fisher, UK). Separation is based on weak electrostatic interactions occurring between hydrophilic metabolites and the zwitterionic stationary phase. Mobile phase gradient runs from 20% H_2O-80% ACN to 80% H_2O-20% ACN in 30 min, followed by a wash at 5% ACN-95% H_2O for 6 min and equilibration at 20% H_2O-80% ACN for 8 min.

(b) MS. Eluted metabolites are directed via heated electrospray ionization (ESI) to an Orbitrap Exactive mass analyser (Thermo Fisher), which exhibits ultrahigh mass accuracy and resolution and is operated in both positive and negative ion modes (30 s switch).

5. Data analysis: Raw MS data from Orbitrap Exactive is processed using mzMatch/IDEOM Excel interface tools [14, 15], a standard pipeline suitable for getting meaningful metabolomic information from LC-MS raw data.

(a) Extract raw MS files using Xcalibur software.

(b) Manually sort raw files (.raw) into folders according to study group.

(c) Using IDEOM:

- Use msconvert to convert MS raw data (.raw) into a functional format (.mzXML) and split polarity.
- Run XCMS library [16] (R-package) to pick peaks and convert files into .peakML format.
- Run mzMatch [15] to combine data, apply several filters, and relate annotated peaks.
- Import mzMatch data into IDEOM and enter grouping information (e.g., treatment, control, blank, etc.)
- Update IDEOM Database sheet with retention times of authentic standards. We use a list of more than 200 standards that are re-analyzed/run in every experiment.

- Run identification of metabolites by mass and retention time, based on the authentic standards list and online metabolite databases (e.g., KEGG, BioCyc, HMDB). At this stage, metabolite quantification and additional filtering for contaminants, isotopes/adducts also takes place.
- Combine positive and negative polarity datasheets. If a metabolite gives peaks in both polarities, the one with the highest intensity will be automatically chosen.
- Compare all sets to apply univariate statistical analysis and visualize the data. All groups are compared against the "control" group. Pair-wise comparisons between only two groups can be performed by excluding the other groups.

(d) Use PeakML Viewer program [15] for rapid inspection of data quality (peak shape, intensity, confidence levels) and dataset comparisons (*see* **Note 4**).

(e) Normalize the intensity levels of each metabolite to the total intensity of metabolites in the sample and/or to the creatinine levels.

(f) Filter for significance employing the Rank Products non-parametric statistical test [17], which is based on ranks of fold changes (FC) and multiple testing. Significance cutoff is set to 0.05 (False discovery rate, FDR < 0.05).

(g) Upload datasets containing KEGG identifiers, corresponding expression values, and FDR onto Ingenuity Pathway Analysis software (Ingenuity® Systems, www.ingenuity.com). Each identifier is mapped to the corresponding metabolite in the Ingenuity® Knowledge Database. A cut-off (FDR < 0.05) is set to identify significantly changing molecules, called Network Eligible molecules. When overlaid to a global molecular network generated by Ingenuity® Knowledge Database, Networks of Network Eligible molecules are algorithmically generated based on their connectivity. Individual metabolites and networks are associated with metabolic processes/pathways and biomarker search.

(h) Metabolites exhibiting the most significant changes are validated to authentic individual standards by MS/MS fragmentation, using the same LC-MS analysis.

3 Notes

It is critical that all the samples/replicates are collected and treated following the exact same protocol, as metabolome is highly unstable, thus changes rapidly throughout the entire collection/extraction/analysis process.

1. Replicates are essential for data analysis. A minimum of $N=5$ biological replicates is recommended. Avoid thaw/freeze circles. It is preferable to use a new aliquot each time.
2. All the reagents used must be of high purity for mass spectrometry.
3. Before starting the extraction procedure, set centrifuge and thermomixer to 4 °C. If precipitate is observed in the tubes immediately after the addition of the extraction solvent, repeat using fresh reagents. If thermomixer is not available, just tape a tube-rack onto a vortex in the cold room. If shipping of extracts is required, use dry ice for transport. Always prepare a control sample using the extraction solvent (follow **steps b–e**) to allow removal of solvent contaminants at the data-analysis stage. In this case mix solvent with water instead of urine.
4. Full mzMatch/IDEOM/PeakML Viewer documentation can be found at http://mzmatch.sourceforge.net. Before start using IDEOM download and install R packages and Msconvert (links available on the IDEOM excel spreadsheet). Also, ensure these programs are in folders that do not contain spaces in their name (e.g., avoid "Program Files"). Detailed help for the IDEOM template/Macro can be found on the excel spreadsheet. To start working on IDEOM first enable Macros in excel (click the bar at the top of the screen). To process data, follow numbered processing steps by clicking the macro buttons. Further analysis can be done on the "Identification," "Comparison," and "allBasePeaks" sheets.

References

1. Heather LC et al (2012) A practical guide to metabolomic profiling as a discovery tool for human heart disease. J Mol Cell Cardiol. doi:10.1016/j.yjmcc.2012.12.001
2. Griffin JL et al (2011) Metabolomics as a tool for cardiac research. Nat Rev Cardiol 8:630–643
3. Wishart DS et al (2009) HMDB: a knowledgebase for the human metabolome. Nucleic Acids Res 37:D603–D610
4. Kemperman RF et al (2007) Comparative urine analysis by liquid chromatography-mass spectrometry and multivariate statistics: method development, evaluation, and application to proteinuria. J Proteome Res 6:194–206
5. Ryan D et al (2011) Recent and potential developments in the analysis of urine: a review. Anal Chim Acta 684:8–20
6. Teul J et al (2009) Improving metabolite knowledge in stable atherosclerosis patients by association and correlation of GC-MS and 1H NMR fingerprints. J Proteome Res 8:5580–5589
7. Kang SM et al (2011) (1)H nuclear magnetic resonance based metabolic urinary profiling of patients with ischemic heart failure. Clin Biochem 44:293–299
8. Wang Z et al (2011) Gut flora metabolism of phosphatidylcholine promotes cardiovascular disease. Nature 472:57–63
9. Zhang AQ, Mitchell SC, Smith RL (1999) Dietary precursors of trimethylamine in man: a pilot study. Food Chem Toxicol 37:515–520
10. Holmes E et al (2008) Human metabolic phenotype diversity and its association with diet and blood pressure. Nature 453:396–400
11. Wang TJ et al (2011) Metabolite profiles and the risk of developing diabetes. Nat Med 17:448–453
12. Suhre K et al (2011) Human metabolic individuality in biomedical and pharmaceutical research. Nature 477:54–60
13. Folch J, Lees M, Sloane Stanley GH (1957) A simple method for the isolation and purifica-

tion of total lipides from animal tissues. J Biol Chem 226:497–509

14. Creek DJ et al (2012) IDEOM: an Excel interface for analysis of LC-MS-based metabolomics data. Bioinformatics 28:1048–1049
15. Scheltema RA et al (2011) PeakML/mzMatch: a file format, Java library, R library, and toolchain for mass spectrometry data analysis. Anal Chem 83:2786–2793
16. Smith CA et al (2006) XCMS: processing mass spectrometry data for metabolite profiling using nonlinear peak alignment, matching, and identification. Anal Chem 78:779–787
17. Breitling R et al (2004) Rank products: a simple, yet powerful, new method to detect differentially regulated genes in replicated microarray experiments. FEBS Lett 573:83–92

Chapter 6

Systems Biology Approach in Hypertension Research

Christian Delles and Holger Husi

Abstract

Systems biology is an approach to study all genes, gene transcripts, proteins, metabolites, and their interactions in specific cells, tissues, organs, or the whole organism. It is based on data derived from high-throughput analytical technologies and bioinformatics tools to analyze these data, and aims to understand the whole system rather than individual aspects of it. Systems biology can be applied to virtually all conditions and diseases and therefore also to hypertension and its underlying vascular disorders. Unlike other methods in this book there is no clear-cut protocol to explain a systems biology approach. We will instead outline some of the most important and common steps in the generation and analysis of systems biology data.

Key words Systems biology, Genomics, Transcriptomics, Proteomics, Metabolomics, Bioinformatics, Pathway analysis, Data integration

1 Introduction

Systems biology is an approach to study biological processes in their full complexity. It aims to study all genes, gene transcripts, proteins and metabolites, and most crucially, the interaction between these molecules. Associated disciplines therefore include genomics, transcriptomics, proteomics, and metabolomics (Fig. 1), but a number of other "omics" disciplines have been defined more recently (http://omics.org). There is no unifying definition of systems biology, but an approach to a definition was made by Kirschner in 2005 (Textbox) [1]. Systems biology can have a number of facets, including the qualitative analysis of large networks of genes, proteins, and metabolites; the detailed quantitative analysis of smaller systems such as cells; and the less detailed modeling of larger systems such as tissues, organs, or the whole organism. Systems biology can be applied to virtually all conditions and diseases and therefore also to hypertension [2, 3] and its underlying vascular disorders [4].

The workflow of systems biology data analysis is illustrated in Fig. 2. It is obvious that this work relies on high-quality data, in the first instance from the wet lab experiments, and in the second

Rhian M. Touyz and Ernesto L. Schiffrin (eds.), *Hypertension: Methods and Protocols*, Methods in Molecular Biology, vol. 1527, DOI 10.1007/978-1-4939-6625-7_6, © Springer Science+Business Media LLC 2017

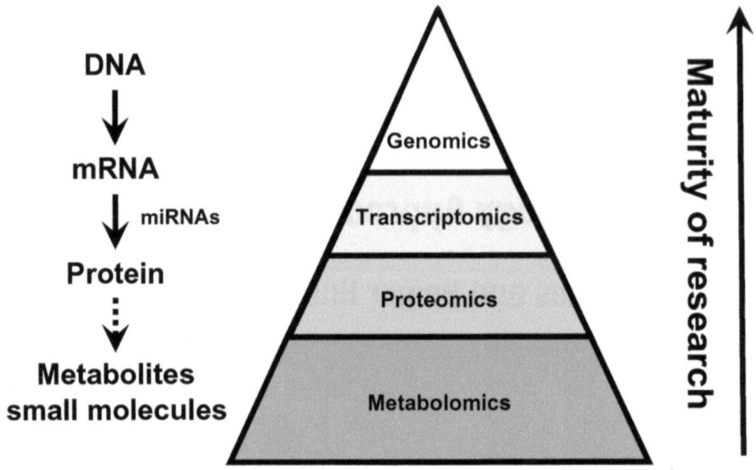

Fig. 1 Disciplines associated with systems biology. The main disciplines genomics, transcriptomics, proteomics, and metabolomics are based on the classic paradigm of molecular biology: transcription of DNA to messenger RNA (mRNA), translation to proteins, and regulation of the metabolism by these proteins. The complexity of the disciplines grows from the top to the bottom of the pyramid while the maturity of research methods is going in the opposite direction [4]. The more recent discovery of the crucial role that non-coding RNAs such as microRNAs (miRNAs) play in the regulation of gene transcription is just one example of the complexity of the system

instance from analysis using databases and software tools to generate a database format for higher level analysis. Important steps in a "systems" analysis involve group/keyword analysis, pathway analysis, gene network analysis, interactome analysis, and disease analysis followed by integration of all results.

Group/keyword analysis is based on gene ontology (GO) to identify relevant biological processes, molecular function, and cellular compartments. Kyoto Encyclopedia of Genes and Genomes (KEGG), REACTOME, and BioCarta keywords allow definition of relevant pathways for further exploration. *Pathway analysis* maps genes and proteins onto existing pathway maps, e.g., metabolic or signalling maps. Tools that are used for pathway analysis include KEGG and PathVisio. *Gene network analysis* can use the NCBI Medical Subject Headings (MESH) to study diseases and pathways. *Interactome analysis* is based on the assumption that similar cellular involvement tends to cluster together through physical interactions. Based on shared biological function signalling cascades can be assembled and interactions that are not related to prior functional tagging can be developed. In *disease analysis* the relevant features will be mapped to human disease descriptors and compared to physiological data (Fig. 3).

For *data integration*, all data analyses will be assembled and merged based on overlapping results. Systems biology analysis tends to focus on networks rather than single proteins/genes; therefore,

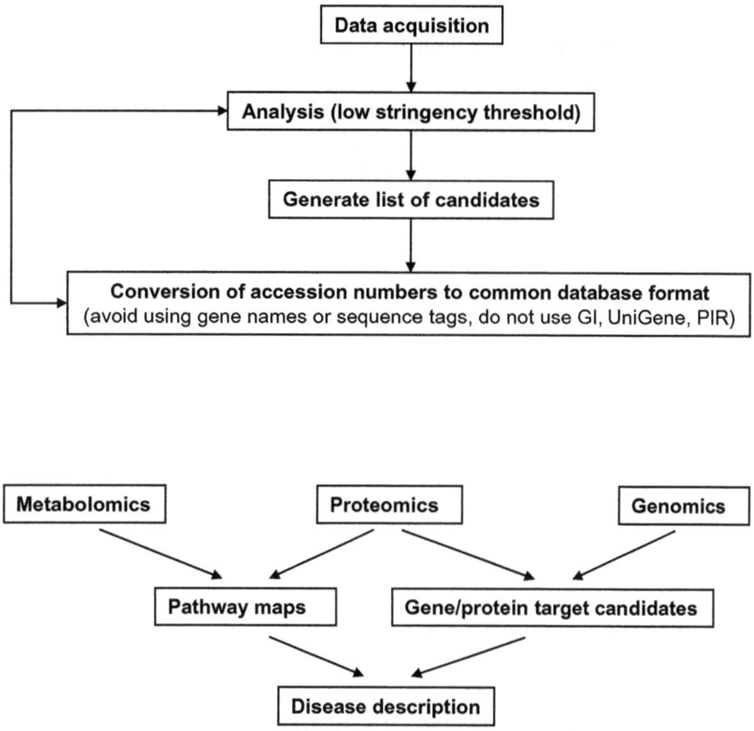

Fig. 2 Systems biology workflow. The top panel shows the key steps of data acquisition, data analysis, generation of candidate lists, and the conversion of accession numbers of individual modalities into a common database format (see Notes). Names and sequence tags as well as GI (GenInfo Identifier) numbers, UniGene references, and PIR (Protein Information Source) are not suitable as they are not used uniformly across the collaborating databases. The bottom panel shows how data from different disciplines can be integrated using pathway maps and target candidates to describe diseases or other physiological or patho-physiological conditions

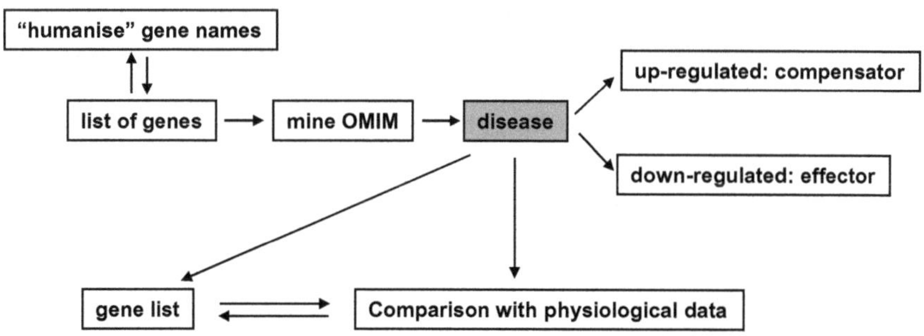

Fig. 3 Disease analysis. Concepts of disease analysis include a generation of gene names as a result of the systems biology analysis and matching with specific diseases. A comparison with (patho)physiological data and clinical and subclinical phenotypes in disease models is mandatory to validate the findings

every set of molecules from the analysis needs to be integrated and cross-correlated. However, independent findings can be used to validate the analysis (or a certain aspect of the analysis).

Table 1
Requirements for systems biology data analysis

Process	Target database	Use	Time
Data shifting (accession numbers)	To SwissProt	Blast and manual	500–1000 entries/day (manual) batch 10 min
Data sifting (combine repeats)		AWASH software	Minutes
Data extraction	ENSEMBL, KEGG, etc.	UniProt db Rapier software	Minutes for db interconversion ½ day
Functional group cluster analysis	PADB tags SwissProt tags	Manual Tag extraction	1000/day ½ day
Group/keyword analysis	Ensembl	ClueGO	10 min
Pathway analysis	UniProt KEGG	PathVisio KEGG	1 h 1 day
Gene network analysis	Gene names (human)	GPEC	1 h
Interactome analysis	UniProt	MiMI	Minutes
Disease analysis	Gene names (human)	iRefScape	Minutes
Integration of all results	UniProt/KEGG/other	?	???

The table gives an indication of the time required for key steps in systems biology data analysis

Due to the complexity of systems biology and the multitude of associated disciplines there is no unifying approach to perform systems biology studies. Unlike other chapters in this book we will not be able to provide readers with clear-cut protocols. Instead, we will describe some of the most important issues related to data handling and will provide an example of one of our recent studies using a proteomics-based approach in diabetes-related vascular disease that could also be applied to models of hypertension. Table 1 gives an overview of the key steps and estimated times for these procedures. For details on the wet lab methods we would like to refer to other chapters describing, for example, genomic and proteomic studies.

2 Materials

We provide a list of databases and software tools that we routinely use to process and analyze systems biology data (for general issues relating to these tools see Notes).

2.1 *AWASH*

A batch processing software to cross-index accession numbers from one database to another, as well as merging datasets based on common handles such as accession numbers. Available through the PADB database (holgerhusi@padb.org) or through the authors of this chapter.

2.2 BioCarta

It depicts molecular relationships from areas of active research in an open source approach: http://www.biocarta.com.

2.3 BLAST (Basic Local Alignment Search Tool)

It enables sequence similarity search. Servers are at UniProt (http://www.uniprot.org), NCBI (http://blast.ncbi.nlm.nih.gov), or ExPASy (http://web.expasy.org/blast).

2.4 ClueGO

A Cytoscape plug-in that visualizes the nonredundant biological terms for large clusters of genes in a functionally grouped network [5]: http://www.ici.upmc.fr/cluego.

2.5 COPaKB (Cardiac Orgamellar Protein Atlas Knowledgebase)

A specialized protein knowledge base of cardiovascular proteome biology and medicine: http://www.heartproteome.org.

2.6 Cytoscape

An open source software platform for visualizing complex networks and integrating these with any type of attribute data [6]: http://www.cytoscape.org.

2.7 Ensembl

A software system that produces and maintains automatic annotation on selected eukaryotic genomes [7]: http://www.ensembl.org.

2.8 Genenames

A curated online repository of HGNC-approved gene nomenclature and associated resources including links to genomic, proteomic and phenotypic information, as well as dedicated gene family pages [8]: http://www.genenames.org.

2.9 GO (Gene Ontology)

A bioinformatics initiative with the aim of standardizing the representation of gene and gene product attributes across species and databases [9]: http://www.geneontology.org.

2.10 iRefScape

A plugin for Cytoscape that exposes iRefIndex data as a navigable graphical network [10]: http://irefindex.uio.no/wiki/iRefIndex.

2.11 KEGG (Kyoto Encyclopedia of Genes and Genomes)

A database resource for understanding high-level functions and utilities of the biological system, from molecular-level information, especially large-scale molecular datasets generated by genome sequencing and other high-throughput experimental technologies [11]: http://www.genome.jp/kegg.

2.12 Mascot

A powerful search engine that uses mass spectrometry data to identify proteins from primary sequence databases [12]: http://www.matrixscience.com.

2.13 MiMI (Michigan Molecular Interactions)

It provides access to the knowledge and data merged and integrated from numerous protein interactions databases and augments this information from many other biological sources. MiMI merges data from these sources with "deep integration" into its single database [13]: http://mimi.ncibi.org/MimiWeb.

2.14 MSblender

A statistical tool for merging database search results from multiple database search engines for peptide identification based on a multivariate modeling approach [14]: http://polaris.icmb.utexas.edu/index.php/MSblender.

2.15 OMIM (Online Mendelian Inheritance in Man)

A comprehensive, authoritative, and timely compendium of human genes and genetic phenotypes: http://www.ncbi.nlm.nih.gov/omim.

2.16 OMSSA (Open Mass Spectrometry Search Algorithm)

An efficient search engine for identifying MS/MS peptide spectra by searching libraries of known protein sequences [15]: http://pubchem.ncbi.nlm.nih.gov/omssa.

2.17 PADB (Proteomics Analysis DataBase)

A gateway for the analysis of large-scale biochemical and mass spectrometry screens of biological materials by bioinformatics and systems biology: http://www.padb.org.

2.18 PathVisio

A tool for displaying and editing biological pathways [16]: http://www.pathvisio.org.

2.19 Proteome Discoverer

A flexible, expandable platform for the analysis of qualitative and quantitative proteomics data: http://portal.thermo-brims.com.

2.20 Rapier

A purpose written software to dissect SwissProt/UniProt ".dat" files and to transform these files into a tabulated format. Available through the PADB database (holgerhusi@padb.org) or through the authors of this chapter.

2.21 Reactome

An open-source, open access, manually curated, and peer-reviewed pathway database [17]: http://www.reactome.org.

2.22 RefSeq (Reference Sequence Collection)

A comprehensive, integrated, nonredundant, well-annotated set of sequences, including genomic DNA, transcripts, and proteins: http://www.ncbi.nlm.nih.gov/RefSeq.

2.23 UniProt (Universal Protein Resource)

A central database of protein sequence and function created by joining the information contained in Swiss-Prot, TrEMBL (Translated EMBL [European Molecular Biology Laboratory]), and PIR (Protein Information Resource). UniProt is a high-quality, manually annotated, nonredundant protein sequence database [18]: http://www.uniprot.org.

3 Methods

Here, we provide an example of analysis of proteomic data from aortic tissue from mice with streptozotocin-induced diabetes and control animals. Samples were prepared and conditioned according to our standard protocols, followed by proteolytic digestion and LC-MS/MS analysis (see the chapter on proteomics). Peptide/

protein IDs were assigned using Proteome Discoverer (alternatives: MASCOT, OMSSA, MSblender).

These data have been published recently [19] and illustrate the analysis levels and the types of outputs that results from individual analysis steps. The starting point is an expression analysis matrix with accession numbers and measured intensities.

1. Fetch sequence and unify accession numbers from redundant to nonredundant.

   This might require extensive BLAST searching. An example for accession numbers for "Isoform 1 of Ras-related protein Rab-6A" in different databases is: COPaKP: IPI00116697 → UniProt: P35279 → SwissProt reviewed: RAB6A_MOUSE. If necessary, use alternative reviewed species to obtain a unique handle or define/declare unique parent molecule). An alternative is to use a pre-clustered/unified database; a human dataset (PADB) but currently no pre-clustered mouse datasets are available.

2. Assemble alternative accession numbers required for analysis (e.g., Ensembl, RefSeq, genenames, etc.).

   This can be done using the batch procedure implemented in the UniProt database.

3. Merge original dataset based on nonredundant key (sum or average intensities of entries from the same sample).

4. Calculate *P*-values, fold changes, false discovery rates, etc.

5. Apply and decide on analysis criteria ($P < 0.05$, minimum peptide count, relevant fold change, etc.)

   P-values can be calculated in various ways; however, we use both Mann-Whitney-Wilcoxon and *t*-test values and analyze datasets with both 0.05 and 0.1 values as cutoffs to avoid biased stringencies. Additionally, Bonferroni/Bonhoeffer correction is applied to all values to allow for multiple testing.

6. Functional group cluster analysis (PADB).

   Group clusters: in our data we found, for example, over-representation of transport molecules in the up-regulated dataset, whereas the enzyme class is over-represented in the down-regulated dataset. Other major shifts were observed in the inhibitor and scaffolder classes in the down-regulated dataset.

   Subtractive clusters: in our data we found, for example, up-regulation of muscle-proteins (in transport and cytoskeletal classes), and a general down-regulation of enzymes, scaffolders, and inhibitors.

7. Group analysis (ClueGO).

   - GO cellular component: in our data we found, for example, an up-regulation of myofibrillar molecules (e.g., muscle cells) in the disease model.

- GO biological process: this is associated with up-regulation of proteins involved in muscle function, down-regulation of scaffolders (protein targeting), inhibitors (response to stimulus), and mainly enzymatic processes involved in pentose-phosphate shunt (metabolic, fatty acid pathway).
- GO molecular function: our data correspond to down-regulation of transferases (pentose-phosphate pathway) and oxidoreductases (fatty acid and pentose phosphate pathway).
- KEGG pathways: in associated pathways we found up-regulation of tight-junction molecules (myosins), and down-regulation of fatty acid, pentose phosphate and PPAR signalling pathway molecules and proteins involved in cell cycle regulation.

8. Pathway analysis (PathVisio).

   In our data pathway analysis demonstrates a general down-regulation of molecules involved in fatty acid metabolism, and, together with an indication of adipocytokine signalling reduction.

9. Interactome analysis (MiMI)

   We performed interactome cluster analysis and found:

   - down-regulated: pronounced clusters involve glycolysis and fatty acid metabolism as well as oxidative phosphorylation and MAPK signalling pathways based on the composition of the interactome-clusters. Additionally, a down-regulation of translation and developmental clusters was found.
   - up-regulated: the interactome analysis shows two separate clusters, one that is almost uniquely involved in cellular development, and one that encompasses mainly cytoskeletal and adhesion processes with transcriptional control elements, protein transport and respiration/apoptotic modules.
   - Using protein-protein interaction analysis we found:
   - down-regulated: abundance and orchestrated down-regulation of proteins involved in fatty acid/carbohydrate (glycolysis) metabolism.
   - up-regulated: a marked up-regulation of proteins mainly found in muscle tissue as well as transcriptional elements.

10. Disease analysis (iRefScape).

    In our data this analysis shows that the major non-compensated mechanisms are in the "neurological" and "fat" categories, as well as the "metabolic" category. Please *see* Fig. 3 for illustration of the process.

11. Physiology

    Systems biology data will then be interpreted against a (patho)physiological background with phenotypes such as aortic thickening, weight loss, or glycemia.

12. Further steps.

    Depending on the experimental model and data structure further work will be required, including integration of all data (accession number independent); extraction and comparison of/with external data (PubMed, other datasets); and further testing (immunohistochemistry, western blots, etc.).

4 Notes

As there is no standard pathway to perform systems biology analysis, there can be a multitude of challenges depending on the experimental model, disease or condition, data structure, data analysis, and data integration. We will highlight a few of the more common challenges with databases and suggest relevant solutions. We will also provide some indication of the time required for systems biology-based data analysis.

Potential Problems with Databases and Accession Numbers

1. *Constant data drift.* New literature data, for example new sequence data of genes or proteins, lead to changes in databases and new versions of databases. As a consequence, accession numbers within databases will change.
2. *Accession numbers, gene, and protein numbers are not stable.* Names are subject to changes with new versions of specific databases and may be different between different types of databases.
3. *Analysis tools may require old versions of accession numbers.* Analysis tools are often based on specific versions of databases, and updated accession numbers can sometimes not be interpreted.
4. *Different analysis tools may require different versions of databases.* This is particularly challenging when integrative analysis across different modalities (e.g., genomic and proteomic data) using different analysis tools is performed.

Possible Solutions

1. Define common database so that all entries use this database (either PADB or UniProt/SwissProt).
2. Map source data to this database (batch mapping at UniProt, or extensive BLAST searching (manual).
3. Acquire additional data (batch mapping of accession numbers, gene and protein name extraction from FASTA files, additional data from batch download of UniProt files, and taking this file apart using own software (e.g., Rapier).

4. Cross-mapping and merging using own specific software (e.g., AWASH) or own scripts.
5. Statistical analysis using own software (Mann-Whitney-Wilcoxon statistical testing) or Excel in-built functions.

Definition of Systems Biology

Systems biology is the study of the behavior of complex biological organization and processes in terms of the molecular constituents. It is built on molecular biology in its special concern for information transfer, on physiology for its special concern with adaptive states of the cell and organism, on developmental biology for the importance of defining a succession of physiological states in that process, and on evolutionary biology and ecology for the appreciation that all aspects of the organism are products of selection, a selection we rarely understand on a molecular level. Systems biology attempts all of this through quantitative measurement, modeling, reconstruction, and theory.

Marc W Kirschner [1].

Acknowledgments

Work in our laboratory is supported by grants from the European Union ("EU-MASCARA," grant agreement 278249; and "PRIORITY," grant agreement 279277) and by the Scottish Government (Strategic Research Development Grant "Biomarkers for Battling Chronic Disease").

References

1. Kirschner MW (2005) The meaning of systems biology. Cell 121:503–504
2. Fung MM, Zhang K, Zhang L et al (2011) Contemporary approaches to genetic influences on hypertension. Curr Opin Nephrol Hypertens 20:23–30
3. Thongboonkerd V (2005) Genomics, proteomics and integrative "omics" in hypertension research. Curr Opin Nephrol Hypertens 14:133–139
4. Gerszten RE, Wang TJ (2008) The search for new cardiovascular biomarkers. Nature 451: 949–952
5. Bindea G, Mlecnik B, Hackl H et al (2009) ClueGO: a cytoscape plug-in to decipher functionally grouped gene ontology and pathway annotation networks. Bioinformatics 25:1091–1093
6. Smoot ME, Ono K, Ruscheinski J et al (2011) Cytoscape 2.8: new features for data integration and network visualization. Bioinformatics 27:431–432
7. Flicek P, Ahmed I, Amode MR et al (2012) Ensembl 2013. Nucleic Acids Res 41:D48–D55
8. Seal RL, Gordon SM, Lush MJ et al (2011) genenames.org: the HGNC resources in 2011. Nucleic Acids Res 39:D514–D519

9. Ashburner M, Ball CA, Blake JA et al (2000) Gene ontology: tool for the unification of biology. The Gene Ontology Consortium. Nat Genet 25:25–29
10. Razick S, Magklaras G, Donaldson IM (2008) iRefIndex: a consolidated protein interaction database with provenance. BMC Bioinformatics 9:405
11. Kanehisa M, Goto S, Sato Y et al (2012) KEGG for integration and interpretation of large-scale molecular data sets. Nucleic Acids Res 40:D109–D114
12. Perkins DN, Pappin DJ, Creasy DM et al (1999) Probability-based protein identification by searching sequence databases using mass spectrometry data. Electrophoresis 20:3551–3567
13. Tarcea VG, Weymouth T, Ade A et al (2009) Michigan molecular interactions r2: from interacting proteins to pathways. Nucleic Acids Res 37:D642–D646
14. Kwon T, Choi H, Vogel C et al (2011) MSblender: a probabilistic approach for integrating peptide identifications from multiple database search engines. J Proteome Res 10:2949–2958
15. Geer LY, Markey SP, Kowalak JA et al (2004) Open mass spectrometry search algorithm. J Proteome Res 3:958–964
16. van Iersel MP, Kelder T, Pico AR et al (2008) Presenting and exploring biological pathways with PathVisio. BMC Bioinformatics 9:399
17. Croft D, O'Kelly G, Wu G et al (2011) Reactome: a database of reactions, pathways and biological processes. Nucleic Acids Res 39:D691–D697
18. UniProt Consortium (2012) Reorganizing the protein space at the Universal Protein Resource (UniProt). Nucleic Acids Res 40:D71–D75
19. Husi H, Van Agtmael T, Mullen W, Bahlmann FH, Schanstra JP, Vlahou A, Delles C, Perco P, Mischak H (2014) Proteome-based systems biology analysis of the diabetic mouse aorta reveals major changes in fatty acid biosynthesis as potential hallmark in diabetes mellitus-associated vascular disease. Circ Cardiovasc Genet. 7(2):161–70.doi:10.1161/CIRCGENETICS.113.000196.

Chapter 7

Measurement of Angiotensin Peptides: HPLC-RIA

K. Bridget Brosnihan and Mark C. Chappell

Abstract

The renin-angiotensin system (RAS) is a complex circulating and tissue-based system. There are multiple pathways for the formation and degradation of peptides. In order to understand the functions of the system, characterization of angiotensin peptides (products and substrates) is important. Radioimmunoassays with the requisite specificity and sensitivity have been developed to allow for the characterization and quantification of circulating and tissue angiotensins. Here, we describe the appropriate methods for collecting the tissue and blood, the extractions steps required to partially purify and remove larger molecular weight-interfering proteins from tissue and plasma, and the radioimmunoassay of three of the peptides of this system (Ang I, Ang II, and Ang-(1-7)), as well as the verification of immunoreactive identity for Ang II and Ang-(1-7) by combined high-performance liquid chromatography—RIA analysis.

Key words Radioimmunoassay, Angiotensin I, Angiotensin II, Angiotensin-(1-7), HPLC, Extraction, Homogenization

1 Introduction

Since 1987 our group has been involved in the determination of angiotensin peptides in plasma and tissue [1]. This characterization included a detailed assessment of the necessity of using a cocktail of protease inhibitors to prevent the endogenous generation and degradation of peptides during sample collection and sample handling [2]. The original inhibitor cocktail was modified when it was reported by Campbell et al. [3] that the aspartyl protease inhibitor pepstatin was not sufficient to prevent the exogenous generation of angiotensin I (Ang I) from renin, requiring the inclusion of a specific renin inhibitor in addition to pepstatin to block this pathway.

The ongoing characterization of the bioactive peptides of the RAS, angiotensin II (Ang II), and Ang-(1-7), has revealed contrasting actions on blood pressure [4], cell growth [5], angiogenesis [6], and inflammation [7]. Thus, to determine their physiological role, it is important to quantify these peptides in tissue and plasma as a first step toward understanding the agonist/antagonistic balance of the

Rhian M. Touyz and Ernesto L. Schiffrin (eds.), *Hypertension: Methods and Protocols*, Methods in Molecular Biology, vol. 1527, DOI 10.1007/978-1-4939-6625-7_7, © Springer Science+Business Media LLC 2017

RAS. Indeed, we recently published an evaluation of angiotensin quantification methods and the expected peptide values in plasma, urine, and various tissues [8]. The predominant method used to characterize the peptides involves direct radioimmunoassays (RIA) characterized by the selective immunoreactivity against the three C terminal products, Ang I [Ang-(1-10)], Ang II [Ang-(1-8)]), and Ang-(1-7) that differ by 1-3 amino acids (Fig. 1). With the specificity of these C-terminally directed antibodies, which do not cross react with each other, the use of direct RIAs is capable of demonstrating the overall pattern of metabolism among the major peptides of the system in various tissues. Moreover, the cross reactivity of each antibody with its amino-terminal fragments allowed for the complete characterization of the angiotensin profile by combining high-performance liquid chromatography (HPLC) separation with RIAs. The validity, however, of using the direct RIAs became apparent when it was discovered that the predominant peptide of each peptide is the parent peptide with the amino-terminal fragments comprising a minority of the overall immunoreactivity [9, 10] (Fig. 4).

2 Materials

1,10-Phenanthroline monohydrate (o-PT, Sigma-Aldrich, St. Louis, MO, # P-1294), pepstatin (Peninsula Labs, San Carlos, CA, # 4039, Na p-hydroxymercuribenzoate (NaHMB, Sigma-Aldrich,

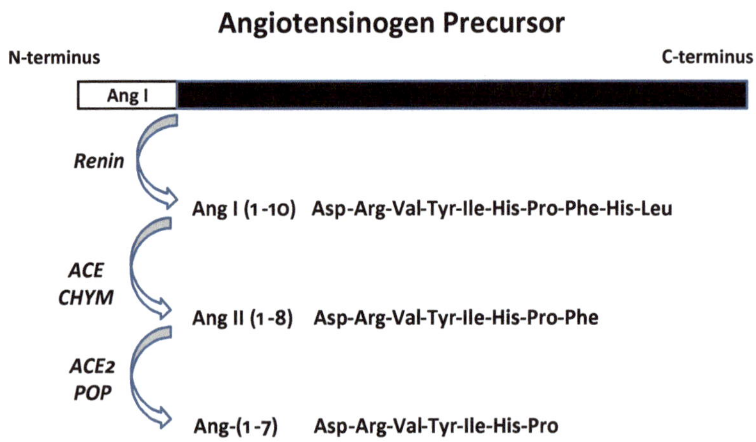

Fig. 1 Scheme for the processing of the precursor protein angiotensinogen to the bioactive peptides angiotensin II (Ang II) and Ang-(1-7). The enzyme renin cleaves angiotensinogen at the N-terminus to form the decapeptide Ang I. Processing of Ang I to the octapeptide Ang II involves angiotensin converting enzyme (ACE) and chymase (CHYM). Subsequent processing to the heptapeptide Ang-(1-7) from Ang II occurs through ACE2 and prolyl oligopeptidase (POP). Note the shared N-terminal sequence among all three peptides but the unique C-terminal sequence that dictates the specificity of C-terminus directed antibodies utilized for radioimmunoassays

Milville NY, #H0642), rat renin inhibitor (AnaSpec Inc. Fremont CA, #WFML-1), sodium (tetra) ethylenediamine tetraacetate acid (EDTA, Fisher, Pittsburgh, PA, # S657-500), Tris base (Sigma-Aldrich, #T1503), Na Azide (Sigma-Aldrich, #S-2002); NaCl (Sigma-Aldrich, #S-3014), glacial acetic acid (Fisher #A35-500), Sep-Pak C18 3 cc Vac cartridges (Waters, Milford, MA, # WAT020805); *n*-heptafluorobutyric acid (Fisher #25003), bovine serum albumin (BSA, Sigma # A7888), Ang I radioimmunoassay kit (Peninsula Laboratories, Inc. San Carols, CA 94070 # 2067), Ang II radioimmunoassay kit (ALPCO, Windham, NH # RK-A22), Iodine-125 10 mCi per 0.1 ml (Perkin Elmer, Waltham, MA, NEZ033A010MC), trifluoroacetic acid (TFA, HPLC grade, Pierce, Dallas TX, CAS 76-05-01), chloramine T (Sigma #C9887), sodium metabisulfite (Sigma-Aldrich, #S-9000), Methanol HPLC grade (Fisher #A412), phosphoric acid (Sigma-Aldrich #215104), acetonitrile HPLC grade (Fisher, #A998), Ang-(1-7), Ang-(2-7), Ang-(3-7), Ang II, Ang-(2-8), Ang-(3-8), Ang-(4-8) (Bachem, King of Prussia, PA).

3 Methods

3.1 Blood

3.1.1 Materials for Blood Sample Collection

1. Preparation of inhibitor cocktail for collection of blood and tissue samples. In one beaker, dissolve 0.36 g 1,10-phenanthroline monohydrate (o-PT, Sigma-Aldrich # P-1294) in 115 ml ultrapure water (New England Reagent Laboratory # 0015). In another beaker, dissolve 0.302 g pepstatin (Peninsula Labs # 4039, mol weight 686 g/l) in 60 ml pure ethyl alcohol. Mix both solutions on magnetic stirrer for 4–5 h at room temperature. Add contents of beakers and continue mixing. Add 1.32 g Na p-hydroxymercuribenzoate (NaHMB, Sigma-Aldrich, #H0642) and allow to dissolve for 10–15 min. Mixture will become less cloudy. Aliquot 10 ml into large glass tubes, cap and store in a refrigerator.
2. Vortex inhibitor cocktail and then add to EDTA tubes prior to collection: 50 μl per ml of blood to be collected.
3. *For rat and mice blood, RAT RENIN INHIBITOR is added to the blood.* Dissolve 0.001 g rat renin inhibitor (AnaSpec Inc. #WFML-1) in 1 ml ultrapure water (1 mM) (New England Reagent Laboratory # 0015). Aliquot into 125 μl portions and store at −20 °C. Dilute × 10 with ultrapure water (0.1 mM). Unused diluted inhibitor can be aliquoted and stored at −20 °C.
4. Add 100 μl of 0.1 mM rat renin inhibitor to EDTA tube prior to 3 ml blood collection.
5. For human blood, no rat renin inhibitor is added to blood.
6. *15% EDTA:* Dissolve 15 g EDTA (Fisher # S657-500) in 100 ml distilled water and store in a refrigerator. The EDTA is used to rinse funnels when collecting blood by decapitation.

3.1.2 Method for Collection of Blood

1. Add the appropriate amount of well-mixed inhibitor cocktail and rat renin inhibitor to a lavender (EDTA) top sample tube according to the following proportions: 3 ml of blood, 0.150 ml of inhibitor cocktail, and 0.100 ml of 0.1 mM rat renin inhibitor.
2. Prechill the sample tube in an ice water slush bath prior to collection.
3. Collect the sample and gently invert the tube to mix a number of times. Immediately return tube to the ice bath.
4. Centrifuge sample at 2000 × *g* for 10 min in refrigerated centrifuge.
5. Transfer plasma into a prechilled conical centrifuge tube and centrifuge at 2000 × *g* again for 10 min under refrigeration.
6. Harvest plasma into polypropylene tubes, label and store frozen at −80 °C.

Note: If collecting samples with syringe or by decapitation, rinse syringe or funnel with 15 % EDTA solution prior to use.

3.1.3 SepPak Separation of Plasma Peptides

Materials for SepPak for Plasma Samples

1. *Elution solvent.* Add 7 ml Ultra Pure Water to 43 ml ethanol, pour into bottle and mix well. Mix 48 ml of this solution with 2 ml glacial acetic acid. The final mixture is used for elution. Keep at room temperature.
2. *4% Glacial Acetic Acid.* Add 2 ml glacial acetic acid to 48 ml ultra pure water and mix. Keep at room temperature while seppaking, store remaining solution in refrigerator (can be stored for up to 2 weeks).
3. *125 I Ang II for spiking samples*—Add radioactivity to Pro Buffer in amounts needed to achieve a count rate of approximately 500 cpm/50 μl. Ensure adequate amount of radioactivity for TC (total count) tubes to use to count the recovery of your seppak samples.
4. *NOP Buffer (no protein buffer).* Weigh and dissolve the following in approximately 900 ml room temperature distilled water: 12.1102 g of Tris base (Sigma-Aldrich, #T1503), 0.5000 g Na Azide (Sigma-Aldrich, #S-2002); 5.0000 g NaCl (Sigma-Aldrich, #S-3014), 4.3800 g EDTA (Fisher #BP 120-500). Adjust the pH to 7.4 using glacial acetic acid (Fisher #A35-500) (approximately 4.4 ml are needed). Bring the final volume to 1000 ml with distilled water, mix and store in the refrigerator.
5. *Pro Buffer (Protein buffer). Add 0.1 g BSA to* 100 ml NOP buffer. (Freeze remainder in small aliquots).
6. SepPak columns: Sep-Pak C18 3 cc Vac cartridges. From Waters cat# WAT020805.

Methods for SepPak for Plasma (1 ml Total Volume Applied to Column)

1. Thaw samples in ice water and centrifuge at 4 °C for 30 min, then aliquot 1 ml samples into glass prechilled 16 × 100 tubes. 1 ml is sufficient to use for the single determination of Ang I, Ang II, and Ang-(1-7). If sample volume is less than 1 ml, use as much sample as possible and record actual volume.
2. Add Ang II radioactivity to sample.
3. Place Sep-Pak columns on manifold equipped with stopcocks. Unless noted otherwise, the reagents are applied to the columns in a manner that allows the reagents to drip through the column without drying the column. Allow each solution to go through all of the columns on the manifold before applying the next solution.
4. Apply 5 ml elution solvent to each column.
5. Apply 5 ml methanol solvent to each column.
6. Empty waste in reservoir into used solvent container.
7. Apply 5 ml water to each column. (Procedure may be stopped at this point if needed, leave some water on column).

The next steps should continue without stopping.

8. Apply 5 ml 4 % acetic acid to each column.
9. Add sample to column.
10. Add 4 ml ultra pure water to the cold sample tubes, rinse tubes, and add water to column.
11. Remove sample tubes from ice and add another 4 ml ultra pure water, rinse and add to column.
12. Push water through column and apply 2 ml acetone to each column. When acetone has gone through, turn the vacuum on slightly and remove the remaining acetone from each column. (Turn on vacuum to columns one at a time to approx. 5-mmHg for 5 s.) DO NOT ALLOW THE COLUMN TO DRY.
13. *Collect Eluates in appropriate glass tubes after applying elution solvent in the following manner*:
14. Apply 1 ml elution solvent and let absorb on the column.
15. Apply 1 ml elution solvent and let absorb on the column.
16. Apply additional 1.3 ml elution solvent to each column to each column.
17. After the final application has been absorbed onto the column, increase vacuum slightly to allow the release of the elution solvent from the columns.
18. Weigh the elution fraction collected and record weight.
19. Mix content of tubes thoroughly and quantitatively pipette 0.5 ml of the elution fraction into appropriately labeled small (12 × 75) glass tubes for Ang II, 0.5 ml for Ang I, and 2 ml for Ang-(1-7).

20. Dry tubes in Savant without heat.
21. *After samples are dry, reconstitute as follows*:

    For Ang II—0.6 ml Alpco Kit RIA Buffer (assay volume = 0.5 ml).

    For Ang I—0.125 ml fresh Pro Buffer (assay volume = 0.100 ml).

    For Ang-(I-7)—0.225 ml fresh Pro Buffer (assay volume = 0.200 ml). These volumes allow for a single RIA determination for each peptide.
22. After allowing time for samples to dissolve, count tubes in the gamma counter along with total count tubes.

    Freeze samples and calculate extraction efficiencies.
23. FOR TOTAL COUNT TUBES: Add the appropriate amount of radioactivity (i.e., 50 μl) into three tubes and bring volume to 1.333 ml.

3.2 Tissue

3.2.1 Materials for Tissue Homogenization

1. 0.1 N HCl: Add 0.17 ml HCl to volume of 20 ml ultra pure water.
2. Acid Ethanol: 80 ml ethanol + 20 ml ultra pure water + 0.83 ml 0.1 N hydrochloric acid.
3. 15% EDTA: add 150.0 g sodium (tetra) ethylenediamine tetraacetate technical powder to volume of 1000 ml distilled H_2O.
4. Inhibitor: 150 μl cocktail inhibitor (see above) + 100 μl rat renin inhibitor (1 mM) in each tube.
5. Radioactivity: ^{125} I-Ang II for spiking samples—Add radioactivity to Pro Buffer in amounts needed to achieve a count rate of approximately 500 cpm/100 μl (450–550 μl).
6. *1% HFBA*: Add 1 ml *n*-heptafluorobutyric acid (HFBA Fisher Cat #25003) to 99 ml ultra pure water.
7. *NOP Buffer* (no protein buffer): Weigh and dissolve the following in approximately 900 ml room temperature distilled water (do not use water that has been sitting overnight or longer at room temperature): Tris base (Sigma-Aldrich, #T1503) 12.1102 g; Na Azide (Sigma-Aldrich, #S-2002) 0.5000 g; NaCl (Sigma-Aldrich, #S-3014) 5.0000 g; EDTA (Fisher #BP 120-500) 4.38 g.

    Adjust the pH to 7.4 using glacial acetic acid (Fisher #A35—500). (Approximately 4.4 ml is needed). Bring the final volume to 1000 ml with distilled water, mix and store in the refrigerator.
8. *Pro Buffer*: Dissolve 0.1 g BSA (Sigma Cat # A7888) per 100 ml NOP Buffer. Make fresh each use.

3.2.2 Methods for Tissue Homogenization

Day 1

1. Prepare dry ice container and an ice water slush bath.
2. Place 50 ml plastic conical tubes in ice bath labeled for each sample and add the following: 10 ml Acid Ethanol, 100 μl 15 % EDTA, 100 μl Inhibitor Cocktail; 50 μl rat renin inhibitor 1 mM; 100 μl Ang II radioactivity—Store remainder to use for counting recovery.
3. Label weight boats and place them in dry ice (Tare the weight of the boat).
4. Place tissue in boats: cut tissue if large (~300 mg for duplicates, ~100 mg for single determination).
5. Weigh frozen tissue and record weight. Place back on dry ice to keep frozen until sample is homogenized.
6. Place clean homogenizer blade in a homogenizer and rinse with 50/50 mixture of ethanol/water mixture.
7. Add tissue to an appropriately labeled 50 ml tube and immediately homogenize; Homogenize at 20,000 × *g* for 30 immersions.
8. Between each sample homogenizer blade must be rinsed with methanol to remove any remaining tissue.
9. Remove 500 μl of the sample and transfer to a 12 × 75 mm tube and store at −20 °C for protein determinations.
10. Transfer remaining sample to a centrifuge tube (16 ml Nalgene) and spin at 12,000 × *g* for 20 min at 4 °C (Sorvall Super-speed RC-2B automatic refrigerated centrifuge).
11. After spin put samples at −20 °C overnight (do not discard supernatant).

Day 2

1. All steps are done on ice.
   Recentrifuge samples at 12,000 × *g* for 20 min at 4 °C.
2. Transfer supernatant to a 15 ml conical tube and add 5 ml of 1 % HFBA.
3. Discard pellet.
4. Place samples at −20 °C for 24 h.

Day 3

1. Spin samples at 3000 × *g* for 15 min at 4 °C.
2. Pour off about 4 ml of the supernatant into a 12 × 75 glass tube and dry in Savant down to 1 ml.
3. Repeat this step until 1 ml of solution is left. Transfer supernatant to a 15 ml conical tube. (Do not transfer any pellet).
4. Add 9 ml of 0.1 % HFBA to the remaining sample.

5. Vortex.
6. Sep-Pak as soon as possible.

3.2.3 Sep-Pak Protocol for Tissue

Materials Solutions for Tissue SepPak

1. Acid MeOH: add 80 ml of MeOH, 20 ml of H_2O, and 100 μl of HFBA.
2. 0.1 % HFBA: Add 100 μl and 99.9 ml of H_2O.
3. SepPak columns: Sep-Pak C18 3 cc Vac cartridges. From Waters cat# WAT020805.

SepPak Methods for Tissues

1. Label columns and tubes (Waters sep-pak vac 3 cc [200 mg] part # wat 854945).
2. Prepare column by applying the following solutions: (allow to gravity feed) 5 ml of acid MeOH-Close column after application: 10 ml of 0.1 % HFBA (do not let the column dry out); close column after application; 10 ml of 0.1 % HFBA (do not let the column dry out). Close column after application.
3. Apply the sample (allow to gravity feed). Close column after application.
4. Wash column with 10 ml of 0.1 % HFB. Add 5 ml to tube sample in ice bath and rinse then apply cold to column. Remove from ice bath.
5. Close column after application. Add remaining 5 ml to the same tube and apply to column. Close column after application.
6. Wash column with 5 ml of H_2O. Close column after application. Gently push air through the column to remove any remaining water. (I use a 5 cc syringe and push air 2×).
7. Discard waste.
8. Place glass tubes (16 × 100) in sep-pak manifold labeled appropriately. Sequentially add 1 ml of acid MeOH (apply very slight vacuum only to get eluate started to flow then allow to gravity to elute solvent). Close column, add 1 ml of acid MeOH Close column; Add 1.3 ml of acid MeOH. Close column. Allow to gravity feed.
9. After all the solution has been absorbed onto the column, push air through to completely empty to column.
10. Weigh samples.
11. Vortex and separate as follows:
    (a) For duplicate determination: Label 6 12 × 75 PS conical tubes for each sample. Pipetter 0.5 ml into each tube.
    (b) For single determination: Label 3 12 × 75 PS conical tubes for each sample. Pipette 1 ml into each tube.
12. Dry in savant without heat.

13. When dry, count recovery.
14. Store at 4 °C until assayed.

3.3 Radio immunoassays

The tissue and plasma extracts are separated and measured by three radioimmunoassays.

3.3.1 Ang I Radioimmunoassay

1. Commercially available kit. Peninsula Laboratories, Inc. San Carols, CA 94070 Catalog # 2067. 125 tubes.
2. Standard Curve: 0.25 pg/tube–640 pg/tube.
   Assay volume: 100 μl.
   Sensitivity: 0.250 pg/tube.
3. C-terminal directed antibody, thus, cross reacts with Ang I, Ang-(2-10), Ang-(3-10). Little or no cross reactivity with Ang II or Ang-(1-7).
4. To convert to fmol/ml, multiply pg/ml by 0.772. (MW Ang I = 1296).

3.3.2 Ang II Radioimmunoassay

1. Commercially available kit. ALPCO, Windham, NH 03087. Catalog # RK-A22. 100 tubes.
2. Standard Curve: 2–500 pg/ml.
   Assay volume: 500 μl.
   Sensitivity: 0.8 pg/ml.
3. 2 day assay.
4. C-terminal directed antibody, thus, cross reacts with Ang II, Ang-(2-8), Ang-(3-8). Little or no cross reactivity with Ang I or Ang-(1-7).
5. To convert to fmol/ml, multiply pg/ml by 0.953 (MW Ang II = 1049).

3.3.3 Ang-(1-7) Radioimmunoassay

1. Hypertension Core Laboratory developed assay.
2. Standard Curve: Ang-(1-7) (Bachem, King of Prussia PA).
   Range of Standard Curve: 2.5–2000 pg/tube.
   Assay volume: 100 μl.
   Sensitivity: 1.25 pg/tube.
3. 2 day assay.
4. C-terminal directed antibody, thus, cross reacts with Ang-(1-7), Ang-(2-7), and Ang-(3-7). Little or no cross reactivity with Ang I or Ang-(1-7).
5. To convert to fmol/ml, multiply the corrected pg/ml by 1.115 (MW for Ang-(1-7) = 897 g/l).
6. Values obtained from the RIAs are corrected for recovery, assay volume, concentration and dilution of extraction and homogenization procedures.

(a) For plasma, values are expressed for plasma as pg/ml (fmol/ml).

(b) For tissue, values are pg/mg protein (fmol/mg protein) or pg/g tissue weight (fmol/g tissue weight).

3.4 Iodination of Peptides

The radioimmunoassay requires preparation of ^{125}I-labeled peptides.

3.4.1 Materials for Ang-(1-7) Iodination

1. Iodine-125 10 mCi per 0.1 ml (Perkin Elmer NEZ033A010MC).
2. MilliQ Plus ultra pure water system with distilled water input (Millipore Q Pak cartridges #CPMO004D2).
3. Chloramine T (Sigma #C9887) 1 mg/ml in MilliQ ultra-pure water, *prepare fresh.*
4. Sodium metabisulfite (Sigma #S-9000) 3 mg/ml in MillQ water, *prepare fresh.*
5. Phosphate buffered saline (PBS).
6. Ang-(1-7) (Bachem) 1 mM in MillQ water.
7. SepPak columns: Sep-Pak C18 3 cc Vac cartridges (Waters # WAT020805).
8. Trifluoroacetic acid (TFA, HPLC grade, Pierce CAS 76-05-01) 0.1 % solution. 0.1 ml TFA in 100 ml MillQ water.
9. Methanol (HPLC grade, Fisher #A412), 80 % solution in 0.1 % TFA. Add 0.1 ml TFA to 80 ml methanol and bring to a final volume of 100 ml with MilliQ water.
10. 15 ml conical tubes (Starstedt #62.554.002).

3.4.2 Method of Iodination

Peptide iodination and purification on SepPak C18 column is performed in a certified chemical hood. Use multiple pairs of gloves and a lead apron during the iodination procedure. Store iodine behind lead bricks or lead shielding.

1. Activate SepPak column.
   (a) Flush 5 ml of 80 % methanol/0.1 % TFA through column using a 10 ml syringe that fits into column at approximately one drop per second.
   (b) Flush 10 ml 0.1 % TFA through column at one drop per second. Cap the column outflow and leave approximately 200 μl 0.1 % TFA in column bed.
2. To a 0.5 ml microcentrifuge tube at room temperature, add in the following order:
   (a) 10 μl Ang-(1-7).
   (b) 20 μl PBS.

(c) 10 μl Iodine-125. Pierce septum of container with a Hamilton 50 μl syringe (#81460) to transfer iodine-125. Avoid opening container to air.

(d) 10 μl Chloramine T to initiate iodine-125 incorporation. Incubate for 30 s.

(e) 50 μl sodium metabisulfite to terminate reaction.

(f) 200 μl 0.1 % TFA to transfer reaction contents.

3. SepPak Purification

(a) Uncap column and place activated SepPak within the 1st 15 ml tube.

(b) Transfer iodinated material to column. Rinse reaction vial twice with 200 μl 0.1 % TFA and transfer to column. Add 3.0 ml 0.1 % TFA to column and allow content to flow through column into tube.

(c) Transfer column to 2nd 15 ml tube. Wash column with 10.0 ml 0.1 % TFA using a syringe.

(d) Transfer column to 3rd 15 ml tube and wash with 10.0 ml MillQ water using a syringe. Completely push all the water through the column prior to the elution step.

(e) Elute ^{125}I-peptide with 80 % methanol/0.1 % TFA into 1.5 ml centrifuge tubes. Collect 1.0 ml per tube.

4. Determine iodination efficiency

(a) Remove 5 μl from each collection tube and count in a gamma counter. Calculate the total counts per ml based on the volume of each collection tube.

(b) Unreacted iodine-125 is not retained by the column and is collected in the 1st 15 ml tube. The 2nd and 3rd 15 ml collection tubes should contain little radioactivity.

(c) The ^{125}I-peptide is completely eluted by methanol in the 1st and 2nd 1.5 ml microcentrifuge tubes. The highest counts per ml should be in the 1st 1.5 ml collection tube.

(d) Evaporate the methanol solution in a vacuum centrifuge (Savant SpeedVac #100H with Welch Dry Fast pump #2044 and activated carbon filter to trap evaporated iodine-125) prior to final purification by HPLC.

3.5 HPLC Purification of ^{125}I-Peptides

HPLC purification is necessary to separate the unlabeled and the mono- and di-^{125}I forms of the peptide. These forms are not separated by the SepPak C18 extraction column. The SepPak column efficiently removes the unreacted iodine-125 and iodination reagents.

3.5.1 HPLC Equipment and Buffers (See Fig. 2)

1. Shimadzu LC20AD system with binary pumps, CTO-20A column oven, and DGU-20A3 degassing system.

2. Shimadzu #SPD-10A UV-VIS Absorbance Detector, 220 nm for peptides.
3. Rheodyne ceramic manual injectors #9125 with 500 μl PEEK injector loop.
4. Rheodyne switching valves #7025 to direct solvent flow to multiple injectors and columns.
5. Bioscan Dual Channel Flow Counter #FC-2000 with PMT detector #B-FC-3100 for detection of ^{125}I-peptides.
6. NovaPak C18 narrow bore columns, 2.1 × 150 mm (Waters #WAT023655) with Synergy guard columns 2.1 × 10 mm (Waters #WATO23655).
7. Gilson FC204 fraction collectors.
8. Mobile phase A: Phosphoric acid (Sigma Aldrich #215104), 0.1 % solution. Add 1 ml phosphoric acid to 1000 ml degassed MillQ water and filter (GE #R02SP04700, 0.2 μm, 47 mm Nylon membrane).
9. Mobile phase B: Acetonitrile (Fisher, HPLC Grade #A998), 80 % solution. Add 1 ml phosphoric acid to 800 ml acetonitrile and bring to a final volume of 1000 ml with degassed MillQ water and filter (GE #R02SP04700).
10. Tris–HCl, 1 M, pH 8.0 at 4 °C (Sigma, #T1503); titrate pH with HCl.
11. Bovine serum albumin (BSA, Sigma #A6003), 0.1 % in 1 M Tris–HCl, pH 8.0.

3.5.2 HPLC Purification (See Figs. 2 and 3)

1. Equilibrate HPLC system at a flow rate of 0.35 ml/min 8.0 % mobile phase B at 25 °C. Direct solvent flow through injector and column 1 via switching valve (*see* Fig. 2).
2. The programmed gradient for ^{125}I-Ang-(1-7) purification is:

   Step 1: 8–28 % B linear gradient for 25 min.

   Step 2: 28 % B isocratic conditions for 10 min.

   Step 3: 28 to 8 % B linear gradient for 15 min.

   Step 4: 8 % B isocratic for 10 min.
3. Reconstitute ^{125}I-peptide with 0.5 ml 8.0 % mobile phase B and inject solution onto the HPLC. Initiate gradient and fraction collector for 1 min (0.35 ml) fractions.
4. Pool the two fractions that contain the major peak of radioactivity corresponding to mono- ^{125}I-Ang-(1-7). Typical elution time for the mono ^{125}I-form is 15 min. The second smaller peak corresponds to di-^{125}I-Ang-(1-7) and is discarded.
5. Dilute the pooled fractions 1:1 with 1 M Tris–HCl/0.1 % BSA and store at 4 °C in a lead container.

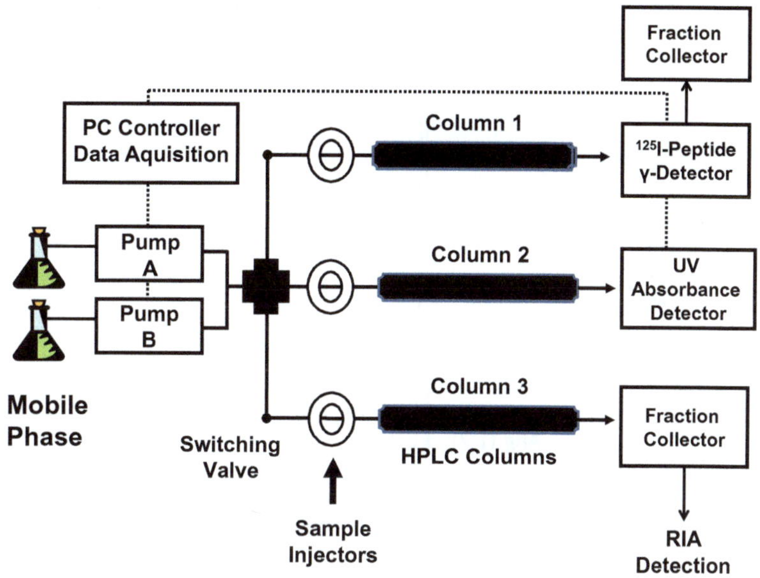

Fig. 2 High-performance liquid chromatography (HPLC) system for separation and detection of angiotensin peptides. The system consists of a PC-based controller for operation of the solvent gradient and data acquisition/analysis from the radioactive and UV detectors (▪▪▪▪); a switching valve to input solvent flow to the sample injectors and their respective HPLC columns #1-3 that output into an inline ^{125}I-peptide gamma detector, a UV absorbance detector or directly into a fraction collector. Column 1 is utilized for purification of ^{125}I-labeled peptides or analysis of ^{125}I-peptide metabolism products and identification of peptidase activities [11, 12]; column 2 is exclusively for standardization and analysis of unlabeled angiotensin peptides; column 3 is exclusively utilized for separation of endogenous angiotensins and subsequent detection by RIA

6. Flush the injector with 80% mobile phase B and run a gradient to 80% B to remove residual radioactivity from the column. Store the column between purifications in 100% acetonitrile.

3.6 HPLC Verification of Endogenous Angiotensins

The HPLC separation of angiotensins can be combined with RIA detection of endogenous peptides in collected fractions to verify the identity of immunoreactive peptides.

3.6.1 HPLC Equipment and Buffers (See Fig. 2)

1. Shimadzu HPLC system as described in Subheading 3.5.
2. Mobile phase A: HFBA (Pierce Sequanal Grade, #25003), 0.1% solution. Add 1 ml HFBA to 1000 ml degassed MillQ water and filter (GE #R02SP04700, 0.2 μm, 47 mm Nylon membrane).
3. Mobile phase B: Acetonitrile (Fisher, HPLC Grade #A998), 80% solution. Add 1 ml HFBA to 800 ml acetonitrile and bring to a final volume of 1000 ml with degassed MillQ water and filter (GE #R02SP04700).

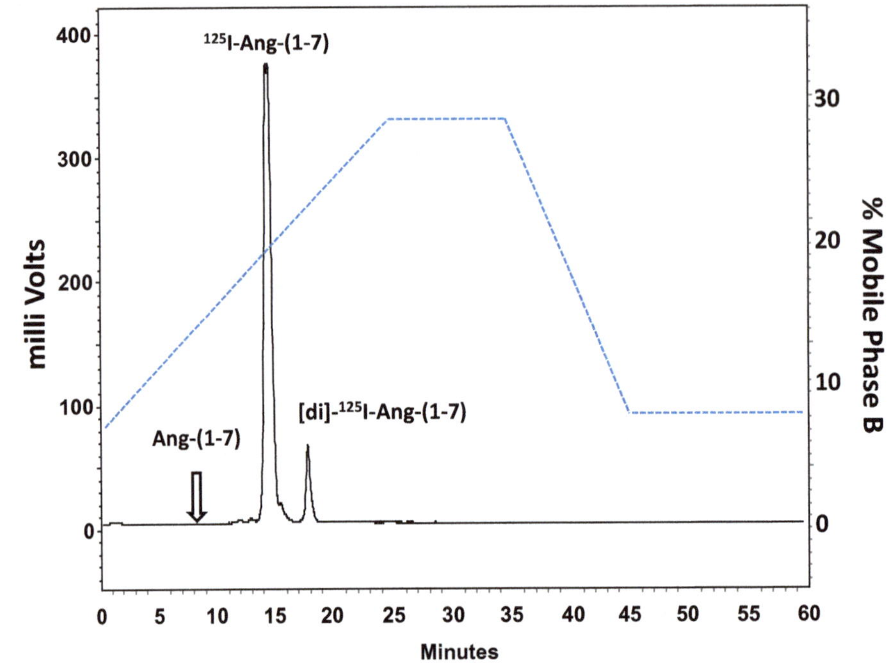

Fig. 3 Chromatograph of ^{125}I-Ang-(1-7) purification by high-performance liquid chromatography (HPLC) following peptide iodination and SepPak C18 extraction. The major peak of radioactivity corresponds to mono-^{125}I-Ang-(1-7) that elutes at a retention time of 15 min. The second radioactive peak corresponds to di-^{125}I-Ang-(1-7) that elutes later in the gradient. Although not detected by the flow-through gamma detector, the unlabeled peak of Ang-(1-7), designated by the open arrow, elutes earlier than the iodinated forms of the peptide. The right axis illustrates the gradient change (....) for mobile phase B (80 % acetonitrile/0.1 % phosphoric acid) versus time in the HPLC purification. Gradient conditions are 8–28 % B linear over 25 min, 28 % B isocratic for 10 min, 28 to 8 % B linear for 10 min, 8 % isocratic for 15 min at a flow rate of 0.35 ml/min at 25 °C

4. Chromtech 0.45 μm PTFE filter vial system (#FV-2045).
5. Starstedt conical 4.5 ml collection and RIA tubes (#57.477).
6. Angiotensin standards, Bachem 1 mM in MillQ water.
   (a) Ang-(1-7).
   (b) Ang-(2-7).
   (c) Ang-(3-7).
   (d) Ang II.
   (e) Ang-(2-8).
   (f) Ang-(3-8).
   (g) Ang-(4-8).

3.6.2 HPLC Standardization

1. Equilibrate HPLC system at a flow rate of 0.35 ml/min 15.0 % mobile phase B at 25 °C. Direct solvent flow through injector, column 2 and UV absorbance detector via switching valve (*see* Fig. 1).

2. The programmed gradient for Ang-(1-7) and Ang II separation is:
   Step 1: 15–40% B linear gradient for 20 min.
   Step 2: 40% B isocratic conditions for 20 min.
   Step 3: 40–15% B linear gradient for 10 min.
   Step 4: 15% B isocratic for 20 min.
3. Inject angiotensin standards (10 nmol each) and initiate the gradient. Ensure that the column and gradient achieve baseline separation of angiotensin peptides as indicated by the UV absorbance profile. Note the elution times of the standard angiotensin peptides.
4. Switch the valve to injector and column 3 connected directly to the fraction collector. Inject 500 μl of 15% B and initiate the gradient. Collect 1 min fractions (0.35 ml) for 40 min (@ 40 fractions) for subsequent RIA analysis.
5. Once the HPLC returns to baseline conditions, inject Ang-(1-7) and Ang II standards (250 fmol each) in 500 μl of 15% B and initiate the gradient. Collect 1 min fractions for 40 min (@ 40 fractions) for subsequent RIA analysis.
6. Completely evaporate the HPLC fractions from the previous runs in a vacuum centrifuge (Savant SpeedVac). Assay tubes 1 to 20 from each run with the Ang-(1-7) RIA. Assay tubes 21–40 with the Ang II RIA. The RIA is performed directly in the HPLC collection tubes.
7. Ensure that the collected fractions from the blank solvent injection do not exhibit immunoreactive peaks by the Ang-(1-7) or Ang II RIAs. Establish that injection of the angiotensin standards reveals baseline separation of the peptides. Plot the immunoreactive values for the Ang-(1-7) and Ang II RIAs versus time to construct a standard chromatograph. Note the order of elution for the peptides is Ang-(3-7), Ang-(1-7), Ang-(2-7), Ang-(4-8), Ang-(3-8), Ang II, Ang-(2-8).
8. Rinse the injector with 80% mobile phase B. Once HPLC equilibrates, inject 500 μl 80% B and run gradient to remove residual peptide standards.

3.6.3 HPLC Procedure: Sample (Fig. 4)

1. The immunoreactive content of the sample should be determined prior to the HPLC step to ensure detection of the peptide. We recommend that the sample for HPLC contain a minimum of 250 fmol of immunoreactive Ang-(1-7) or Ang II. Either an individual sample or a pooled sample can be fractioned by HPLC.
2. Equilibrate HPLC system at a flow rate of 0.35 ml/min 15% mobile phase B at ambient temperature. Inject 500 μl of 15% B, initiate gradient, and collect 40 × 1 min fractions. These fractions

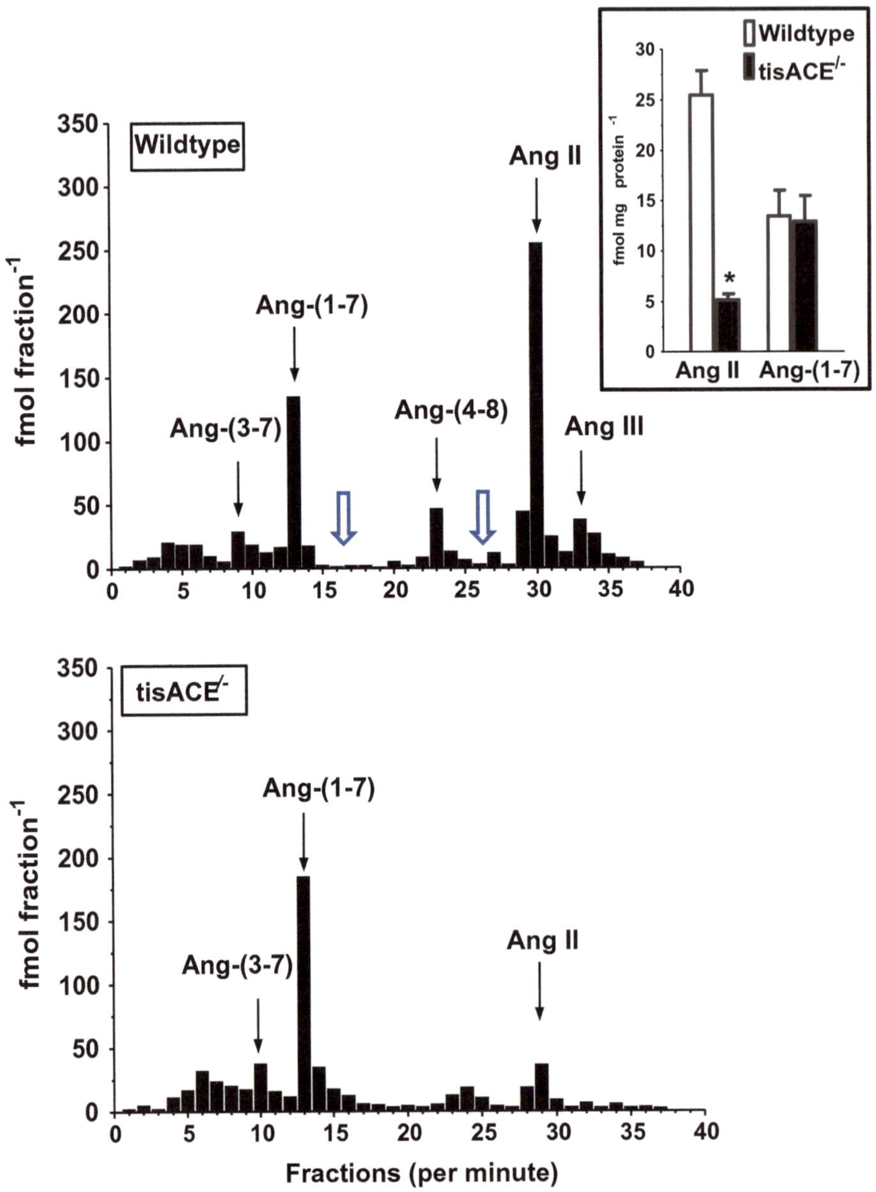

Fig 4 Combined high-performance liquid chromatography (HPLC) separation and RIA analysis of pooled kidney extracts from wildtype and tissue ACE knockout (tisACE$^{-/-}$) mice. The collected HPLC fractions were completely evaporated and assayed by the Ang-(1-7) RIA (fractions 1-20) and the Ang II RIA (fractions 21–40). The HPLC solvent system is 0.1 % HFBA (mobile phase A) and 80 % acetonitrile/0.1 % HFBA (mobile phase B). Gradient conditions for Ang-(1-7) and Ang II separation were: 15–40 % B linear over 20 min; 40 % B isocratic for 20 min; 40–15 % B linear for 10 min, 15 % isocratic for 20 min at a flow rate of 0.35 ml/min at 25 °C. The *arrows* indicate the elution peaks for Ang-(3-7), Ang-(1-7), Ang-(4-8), Ang II, and Ang-(2-8) (Ang III). The *open arrows* indicate expected elution times for Ang-(2-7) and Ang-(3-8), respectively. *Inset*: intrarenal concentration of Ang II and Ang-(1-7) (fmol/mg protein) in wildtype ($n=8$) and *tis*ACE$^{-/-}$ mice ($n=8$); *$P<0.001$ versus wildtype. Figure adapted with permission from Modrall et al. [9]

from the blank solvent are assayed to ensure there is no background material prior to the HPLC analysis of the sample.

3. Reconstitute the sample in 15 % B to completely dissolve material. To facilitate this process, sample vials can be placed in a sonicating water bath (Branson Ultrasonic Bath, B200R-1). Centrifuge samples at 30,000 × *g* for 10 min to pellet insoluble material and filter on a Chromtech 0.45 μm PTFE filter vial (#FV-2045).
4. Inject 500 μl of sample onto the HPLC, begin gradient, and collect 40 × 1 min fractions.
5. Following equilibration of the HPLC, inject 500 μl of 80 % B and run gradient to remove residual sample contaminants.
6. Either additional samples can be injected on the HPLC (with blank solvent injections between each run) or the mixture of angiotensin peptides for RIA detection is run to calibrate the current separation.
7. The HPLC fractions are evaporated in the vacuum centrifuge and subjected to the Ang-(1-7) and Ang II RIAs.
8. Plot the immunoreactive content of the HPLC fractions versus time for each sample to display the profile of angiotensin peptides (*see* Fig. 4).
9. Store the HPLC and column in 100 % acetonitrile when not in use.

4 Notes

1. The iodination procedure is applicable for angiotensin peptides, their peptide receptor antagonists, and other peptides provided they contain a tyrosine residue.
2. The short reaction time (30 s) with Chloramine T and the high peptide to iodine ratio ensures predominant mono-iodination of the peptide. Longer reaction times will result in greater formation of di-^{125}I-Ang-(1-7).
3. The efficiency of iodination is typically 60–80 %. Reduced efficiency or absence of peptide iodination usually indicates the need to replace the Chloramine T reagent.
4. Note that the Tris–HCl buffer is temperature sensitive and the final pH of the buffer should be adjusted at the appropriate temperature.
5. We find that the immediate use of the iodine-125 results in optimal iodination of angiotensin peptides. We recommend obtaining the iodine-125 from the supplier as soon as the product is synthesized.

6. The ^{125}I-Ang-(1-7) can be repurified by HPLC after 1 to 2 months storage. The ^{125}I-peptide must be initially extracted on the SepPak column to remove the Tris–HCl/BSA buffer that interferes with the HPLC purification.
7. The use of other HPLC C18 columns configured in narrow or conventional bore (2–4 mm; internal diameter) may be applicable in the purification of ^{125}I-Ang-(1-7) or other peptides; however, the gradient conditions should be optimized for each column with the appropriate peptide standards to ensure resolution and recovery of the ^{125}I-peptide.
8. Alternative HPLC buffers such as TFA or HFBA (0.1 %) can be utilized for the purification of ^{125}I-Ang-(1-7) and other angiotensin peptides. These buffers may necessitate modification of the gradient conditions.
9. It is imperative that the HPLC fractions are completely evaporated and dry prior to assay by RIA. Although both HFBA and acetonitrile are volatile, any residual amount of the acid or solvent will significantly interfere with the RIA and may yield false-positive values.
10. The use of two injectors and identical columns ensures that the UV absorbance calibration with the angiotensin standards on one column does not contribute to immunoreactive carryover on the endogenous peptide column. The column calibration by UV absorbance requires markedly higher peptide concentrations than RIA detection (nmol vs. fmol range—a 10^6-fold difference in sensitivity). For example, 0.001 % carryover of 10 nmol Ang II standard would be detected as a significant immunoreactive peak of 100 fmol the by Ang II RIA.
11. Given the high sensitivity of the angiotensin RIAs, all reagents should be of the highest quality and used solely for the HPLC-RIA application to ensure no interference with the assay.
12. Other HPLC C18 columns configured in narrow or conventional bore (2–4 mm internal diameter, respectively) may be applicable for the characterization of endogenous angiotensins. The gradient separation conditions must be optimized for each column with the appropriate peptide standards.
13. Peptide analysis by HPLC should be performed on samples that have undergone extensive extraction to remove potential contaminating material that may interfere with the RIAs employed and/or compromise the HPLC separation.
14. For a large number of samples, we typically perform direct RIAs to obtain the mean values and subsequently analyze a sample pool to characterize their immunoreactive identity. As shown in Fig. 4 (inset), direct RIAs of Ang II and Ang-(1-7) revealed a lower Ang II content in kidneys of ACE knockout

mice, but no change in Ang-(1-7). The HPLC-RIA analysis of pooled kidney samples demonstrates lower immunoreactive peaks corresponding to Ang II and Ang-(4-8) in the ACE knockout mice; however, the peak of Ang-(1-7) is not reduced. The HPLC analysis confirms the direct RIA results for kidney content of Ang II and Ang-(1-7), as well as demonstrates that Ang II and Ang-(1-7) are the predominant immunoreactive forms in the kidney as detected by their respective RIAs.

Acknowledgment

Support was provided in part by the National Institutes of Health, NHLBI-P01 HL51952, HL56932, HD084227, Unifi, Inc. Greensboro, NC and Farley-Hudson Foundation, Jacksonville, NC.

References

1. Chappell MC, Brosnihan KB, Diz DI, Ferrario CM (1989) Identification of angiotensin-(1-7) in rat brain. Evidence for differential processing of angiotensin peptides. J Biol Chem 264:16518–16523
2. Kohara K, Tabuchi Y, Senanayake P, Brosnihan KB, Ferrario CM (1991) Reassessment of plasma angiotensins measurement: effects of protease inhibitors and sample handling. Peptides 12:1135–1141
3. Campbell DJ, Kladis A, Valentijn AJ (1995) Effects of losartan on angiotensin and bradykinin peptides and angiotensin-converting enzyme. J Cardio Pharm 26:233–240
4. Sampaio WO, Nascimento AAS, Santos RA (2003) Regulation of cardiovascular signaling by kinins and products of similar converting enzyme systems. Systemic and regional hemodynamic effects of angiotensin-(1-7) in rats. Am J Physiol Heart Circ Physiol 284:H1985–H1994
5. Tallant EA, Clark MA (2003) Molecular mechanisms of inhibition of vascular growth by angiotensin-(1-7). Hypertension 42:574–579
6. Machado RD, Santos RA, Andrade SP (2000) Opposing actions of angiotensins on angiogenesis. Life Sci 66:67–76
7. Capettini LS, Montecucco R, Mach R, Stergiopulos N, Santos RA, da Silva RF (2012) Role of renin-angiotensin system in inflammation, immunity and aging. Curr Pharm Des 18:963–970
8. Chappell MC (2016) Biochemical evaluation of renin-angiotensin system: the good, bad and absolute? Am J Physiol Heart Circ Physiol 310:H137–H152
9. Modrall JG, Sadjadi J, Brosnihan KB, Gallagher PE, Yu CH, Bernstein KE, Chappell MC (2004) Depletion of tissue angiotensin-converting enzyme differentially influences the intrarenal and urinary expression of angiotensins. Hypertension 43:849–853
10. Kohara K, Brosnihan KB, Ferrario CM (1993) Angiotensin-(1-7) in the spontaneously hypertensive rat. Peptides 14:883–891
11. Westwood BM, Chappell MC (2012) Differential metabolism of angiotensin-(1-12) in the circulation and kidney of the mRen2. Lewis congenic rat. Peptides 35:190–195
12. Yamaleyeva L, Gilliam-Davis S, Almeida I, Brosnihan KB, Lindsey SH, Chappell MC (2012) Differential regulation of circulating and renal ACE2 and ACE in hypertensive mRen2.Lewis with early onset diabetes. Am J Physiol Renal Physiol 302:F1374–F1384

Chapter 8

Measurement of Angiotensin Converting Enzyme 2 Activity in Biological Fluid (ACE2)

Fengxia Xiao and Kevin D. Burns

Abstract

Angiotensin-converting enzyme 2 (ACE2) is a recently described member of the renin-angiotensin system that hydrolyzes angiotensin (Ang) II to Ang-(1-7), and may thereby protect against cardiovascular and renal diseases. ACE2 is a type 1 integral membrane protein and contains a catalytically active ectodomain that can be shed from the cell surface into the extracellular space, via cleavage by a disintegrin and metalloproteinase-17 (ADAM-17). ACE2 enzymatic activity and protein can be detected in biological fluids, including urine, plasma, and conditioned cell culture media. We present a detailed method for measurement of ACE2 activity in biological fluids, using hydrolysis of an intramolecularly quenched fluorogenic ACE2 substrate, in the absence or presence of the ACE2 inhibitors MLN-4760 or DX600. Recombinant human or mouse ACE2 is used to generate standard curves for this assay, with ACE2 detection ranging from 1.56 to 50 ng/ml. While MLN-4760 potently inhibits the activity of both human and mouse ACE2, DX600 (linear form) only effectively blocks human ACE2 activity in this assay. In biological samples of human and mouse urine, cell culture medium from mouse proximal tubular cells, and mouse plasma, the mean intra- and inter-assay coefficients of variation (CVs) of the assay range from 1.43 to 4.39%, and from 7.01 to 13.17%, respectively. We present data on the time and substrate concentration dependence of the assay, and show that exogenous d-glucose, creatinine, urea, and albumin do not interfere with its performance. In biological fluids, this assay is a simple and reliable method to study the role of ACE2 and its shed fragments in cardiovascular and renal diseases.

Key words Angiotensin-converting enzyme 2, Substrate, Fluorescence, Plasma, Urine, Proximal tubule

1 Introduction

Angiotensin-converting enzyme 2 (ACE2), a zinc-metallopeptidase, is a recently identified member of the renin-angiotensin system that degrades angiotensin (Ang) II to Ang-(1-7) [1, 2]. ACE2 is also a receptor for the coronavirus that causes severe acute respiratory syndrome (SARS) [3]. Although ACE2 is found in many tissues, it is highly expressed in the kidney, particularly within cells of the proximal tubule [4, 5]. Because it decreases levels of the vasoconstrictor Ang II and generates the vasodilator Ang-(1-7), ACE2

Rhian M. Touyz and Ernesto L. Schiffrin (eds.), *Hypertension: Methods and Protocols*, Methods in Molecular Biology, vol. 1527, DOI 10.1007/978-1-4939-6625-7_8, © Springer Science+Business Media LLC 2017

may protect against hypertension [6] and renal disease [7, 8]. ACE2 has also been shown to prevent acute lung injury [9].

ACE2 is shed at its carboxy-terminus from the plasma membrane in cells via "a disintegrin and metalloproteinase-17" (ADAM-17) pathway [10, 11]. Recently, soluble ACE2 has been detected in certain biological fluids, including urine, plasma, and cell culture medium, by enzyme-linked immunosorbent assay (ELISA), enzyme activity assay, or western analysis [10, 12, 13]. In this chapter, we describe a detailed method for measurement of ACE2 enzyme activity in biological fluids using a commercially available synthetic fluorogenic substrate for ACE2. We provide a practical, cost-effective, and high-throughput method to study the potential role of ACE2 shedding in renal and cardiovascular disease.

2 Materials

The following reagents must be prepared and brought to room temperature before starting the assay.

1. *Assay buffer:* 50 mM 2-(*N*-Morpholino)ethanesulfonic acid (MES), 300 mM NaCl, 10 μM $ZnCl_2$, adjust pH to 6.8. Store at 4 °C when not in use.
2. *Fluorogenic ACE2 substrate:* Mca-Ala-Pro-Lys(Dnp)-OH (AnaSpec, San Jose, CA, USA, Catalog Number: 60757), reconstitute in 1 % NH_4OH to 15 mM. Aliquoted samples can be stored at −20 °C for at least 3 months or −80 °C for at least 6 months.
3. *Protease inhibitors: N*-ethylmaleimide (NEM, 100 mM stock in double-distilled H_2O [ddH_2O]) and phenylmethylsulfonyl fluoride (PMSF, 100 mM stock in ethanol). Aliquot and store at −20 °C.
4. *ACE2 inhibitor:* MLN-4760 (10^{-5} M stock in ddH_2O, also called GL1001, provided by Ore Pharmaceuticals, Cambridge, MA, USA, and commercially available from Calbiochem, San Diego, CA, USA, Catalog Number: 530616) or DX600 (linear form, 10^{-5} M stock in ddH_2O, AnaSpec, Catalog Number: 62337).
5. *ACE inhibitor:* Captopril (10^{-4} M stock in ddH_2O, Sigma-Aldrich, St. Louis, MO, USA).
6. *ACE2 Standard:* Recombinant human ACE2 (human rACE2, R&D Systems Inc., Minneapolis, MN, USA, Catalog Number: 933-ZN) and recombinant mouse ACE2 (mouse rACE2, R&D Systems Inc., Catalog Number: 3437-ZN). Reconstitute with phosphate-buffered saline (PBS) to 10 μg/ml. Aliquots are stable for at least 3 months at −20 °C and at least 6 months at −80 °C.

7. *96-well Microplate (black).*
8. *Fluorescence Microplate Reader:* We use the FLUOstar Galaxy fluorometer (BMG Labtechnologies, Durham, NC, USA), detecting emission at 405 nm with excitation at 320 nm.

3 Methods

In the following section, we describe the ACE2 activity assay. First, we present the generation of the standard curve (Subheading 3.1), followed by measurement of ACE2 activity in biological fluids (Subheading 3.2).

3.1 Generation of Standard Curves Using Human or Mouse rACE2

3.1.1 Preparation of ACE2 Substrate/Assay Buffer Solution

Calculate the amount of working reagents to use. Add fluorogenic ACE2 substrate and protease inhibitors to the assay buffer (*see* Subheading 2, **item 1**) immediately before each experiment, to generate the ACE2 substrate/Assay buffer solution, to achieve concentrations as follows: 15 μM ACE2 substrate, 1 mM NEM, and 1 mM PMSF (Table 1). Seventy-five micro liter of the ACE2 substrate/assay buffer solution will be used in each reaction (*see* below Subheading 3.1.3). The protease inhibitors are added to prevent substrate hydrolysis in biological solutions [14]. For the standard curve generation, we also routinely add protease inhibitors to the assay buffer.

3.1.2 Preparation of ACE2 Standard Dilutions

Dilute 10 μg/ml stock of human or mouse rACE2 1:30 in assay buffer to a concentration of 333.33 ng/ml for standard #1 (Table 2). Perform 1:2 serial dilutions of the preceding ACE2 standard in assay buffer for standards #2-6, with the lowest concentration at 10.42 ng/ml. Standard #7 is a blank that should contain no rACE2 (instead add 15 μl assay buffer alone). Add 15 μl/well of the serially diluted ACE2 standards into a total volume of 100 μl of ACE2 enzymatic reaction solution (see Table 2) to

Table 1
ACE2 substrate/assay buffer solution[a]

Components (stock solutions)	Volume (μl)	Conc. in substrate/assay buffer mix
ACE2 substrate (15 mM in 1% NH_4OH)	1	15 μM
NEM (100 mM in ddH_2O)	10	1 mM
PMSF (100 mM in ethanol)	10	1 mM
Assay buffer (*see* Subheading 2, **item 1**)	979	–
Total volume (μl)	1000	

NEM *N*-ethylmaleimide, *PMSF* phenylmethylsulfonyl fluoride, *Conc* concentration
[a]1000 μl provides sufficient buffer for 3 measurements performed in duplicate (75 μl per well)

Table 2
Components of ACE2 activity standard curve solution (per well)[a]

rACE2 standard	Diluted rACE2 conc. (ng/ml)	rACE2 volume/well (μl)	ACE2 inhibitor[b] or ddH_2O volume/well (μl)[c]	ACE2 substrate/ assay buffer (μl)	Total volume/ well (μl)	Final rACE2 conc. (ng/ml)
1	333.33	15	10	75	100	50
2	166.66	15	10	75	100	25
3	83.33	15	10	75	100	12.5
4	41.67	15	10	75	100	6.25
5	20.83	15	10	75	100	3.13
6	10.42	15	10	75	100	1.56
7	0	15[d]	10	75	100	0

rACE2 recombinant ACE2, *ddH2O* double-distilled H_2O, *Conc* concentration

[a]The volume of each component listed is for each well, to give a total volume of 100 μl of ACE2 enzymatic reaction solution, on a 96-well microplate. Each reaction is performed in duplicate

[b]ACE2 inhibitor: MLN-4760 or DX600

[c]For each dilution, one duplicate reaction is performed in ddH_2O (10 μl), and another duplicate is performed with the addition of ACE2 inhibitor MLN-4760 or DX600 (10 μl, from stock of 10^{-5} M)

[d]Standard #7 is a blank, with the addition of assay buffer alone, instead of rACE2

achieve final ACE2 concentrations of 50, 25, 12.5, 6.25, 3.13, and 1.56 ng/ml.

3.1.3 Measurement of ACE2 Activity in Standard Dilutions

Set up the plate configuration on a 96-well black microplate: the standards are run in duplicates, along with a blank control that contains no rACE2. For each concentration of ACE2 standard, two wells are used for total ACE2 activity, and two wells are used for measurement of activity in the presence of the ACE2 inhibitor MLN-4760 or DX600. The volumes of each individual component per well are shown in Table 2. The final volume of the ACE2 enzymatic reaction is 100 μl/well, and the sequence of addition of components to the plate is as follows:

1. Add 10 μl of ddH_2O into each of the total enzymatic activity reaction wells of a 96-well microplate. For the inhibitor wells, instead add 10 μl of ACE2 inhibitor solution (10^{-5} M MLN-4760 or 10^{-5} M DX600 stock).
2. Add 75 μl of the ACE2 substrate/assay buffer (*see* Subheading 3.1.1) to all wells.
3. Add 15 μl of diluted ACE2 standards to each well, thereby achieving a total reaction volume of 100 μl for each well.
4. Cover the plate with microplate sealing film, followed by aluminum foil to prevent access to light, and incubate the plate at room temperature for 16 h on a plate shaker.

5. Read the 96-well plate on a fluorescence reader with excitation wavelength of 320 nM and emission wavelength of 405 nM.
6. For determination of the percentage of inhibition of ACE2 activity by MLN-4760 or DX600, subtract the Relative Fluorescence Unit (RFU) reading of the substrate blank from the readings for each well. The ACE2-specific activity for each standard is determined by subtracting the RFU obtained in the presence of MLN-4760 or DX600 from the reading in the absence of inhibitor.

3.1.4 Generation of Standard Curves

Construct a standard curve by plotting the known concentrations (*X* axis) of rACE2 standards versus the RFUs (*Y* axis) of rACE2 standards (Fig. 1). A highly linear relationship is observed between the RFU and rACE2 concentration for both human rACE2 ($R^2=0.9998$, $p<0.001$ for MLN-4760, $R^2=0.9999$, $p<0.001$ for DX600, Fig. 1a) and mouse rACE2 ($R^2=0.9976$, $p<0.001$ for MLN-4760, Fig. 1b), with a range of ACE2 detection from 1.56 to 50 ng/ml. The linear equations generated for human and mouse rACE2 are used to convert the RFU to ACE2 concentrations in human or mouse biological fluids, respectively. In our hands, the RFU signal reaches saturation when the rACE2 concentration is greater than 50 ng/ml. The RFU signal becomes very weak or undetectable when the rACE2 concentration is less than 1.56 ng/ml. This range approximates the detection limits for human ACE2 using a commercial ELISA, which we previously reported to range from 0.39 to 25 ng/ml [13].

3.2 Measurement of ACE2 Activity in Biological Fluids

3.2.1 Initial Preparation of Biological Samples

Using this assay, we have measured ACE2 activity in human urine samples collected from renal transplant recipients [13]. We have also measured ACE2 activity in urine samples from male FVB/N mice, with and without streptozotocin (STZ)-induced diabetes, and in conditioned culture medium collected from primary cultures of mouse proximal tubular (PT) cells, after up to 72 h incubation in medium. Mouse proximal tubule (PT) cells derived from C57BL6 mice were grown in a defined medium of DMEM-F12 (1:1), supplemented with insulin (5 μg/ml), transferrin (5 μg/ml), selenium (5 ng/ml), hydrocortisone (50 nM), and 3,3′,5-triiodo-*L*-thyronine (2.5 nM), without fetal bovine serum (FBS). Serum has previously been demonstrated to contain ACE2 enzymatic activity, and should be avoided in this assay [15]. All biological samples are collected and placed on ice, aliquoted and then centrifuged at 12,000 × *g* for 5 min at 4 °C. Supernatants are collected, and stored at −80 °C until the assay is performed.

We also have measured ACE2 activity in plasma, from mice with or without STZ-induced diabetes [8]. Blood is collected in chilled eppendorf tubes, and plasma is separated by centrifugation at 3000 × *g* for 10 min at 4 °C, and stored at −80 °C until time of the assay.

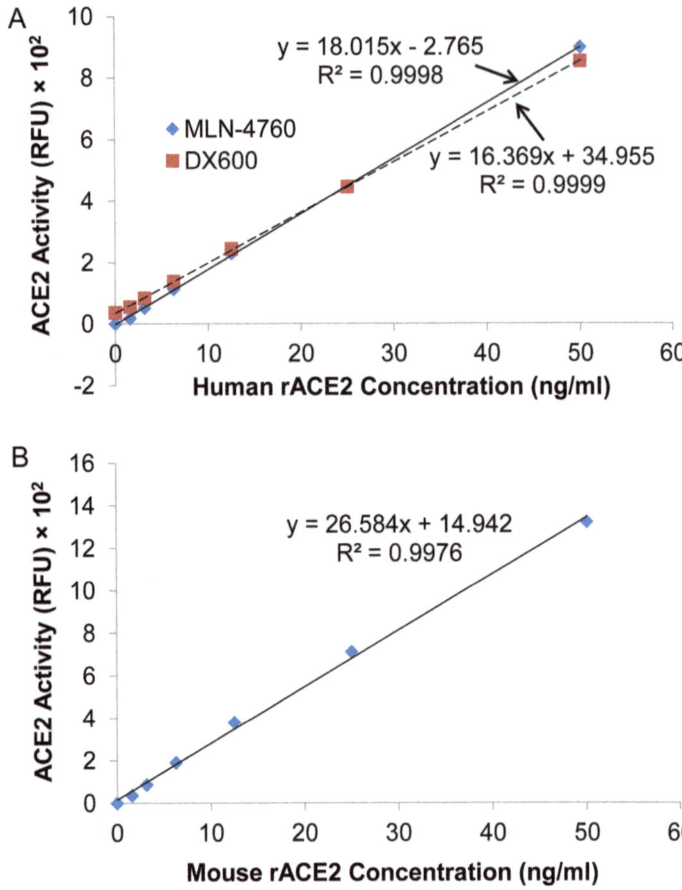

Fig. 1 Standard curves for ACE2 activity assay. The assay was performed for 16 h incubation. Graph shows the concentrations of recombinant ACE2 (rACE2) versus the ACE2 activity (RFU). (**a**) Standard curves generated for human rACE2. The ACE2 inhibitors MLN-4760 (10^{-6} M) or DX600 (10^{-6} M) were used. The relationship is highly linear for rACE2 concentrations between 0 and 50 ng/ml ($R^2 = 0.9998$, $p < 0.001$ for MLN-4760, $R^2 = 0.9999$, $p < 0.001$ for DX600). (**b**) Standard curve generated for mouse rACE2. The ACE2 inhibitor MLN-4760 (10^{-6} M) was used. A highly linear relationship exists for rACE2 concentrations between 0 and 50 ng/ml ($R^2 = 0.9976$, $p < 0.001$)

3.2.2 Assay Conditions

1. We dilute urine samples at least 1:2 and plasma samples 1:7.5 with assay buffer. For conditioned cell culture medium, undiluted samples are used. For each well on the 96-well plate, use 15 μl of diluted urine (e.g., 7.5 μl urine plus 7.5 μl assay buffer), 15 μl of diluted plasma (2 μl plasma plus 13 μl assay buffer), and 15 μl undiluted culture medium in a final volume of 100 μl of enzymatic reaction. If ACE2 activity falls outside the detection limits of the assay, a lower or higher dilution may be required.

2. Measure the ACE2 activity (RFU) in biological fluids by following the same experimental procedure described for ACE2 standards (*see* Subheading 3.1.3).
3. Calculate the ACE2 concentrations from the RFU in biological fluids using the linear equations generated for human or mouse rACE2, as appropriate (Fig. 1). The ACE2 concentrations must be corrected for the dilution factor to obtain the actual concentrations in the undiluted samples. ACE2 concentration in biological fluids is typically expressed as ng/ml.
4. The amount of urinary ACE2 can be corrected for the creatinine concentration in the urine samples, as a control for urinary dilution, and reported as ng/μg creatinine. ACE2 activity in culture medium can be corrected for the cell protein amounts on the culture dishes, and reported as ng/μg protein.

3.2.3 Intra- and Inter-Assay Coefficients of Variability (CV) in Biological Fluids

We have determined the intra- and inter-assay CVs of the ACE2 activity assay for biological samples, and the results support the reliability of this assay. Three samples each of human and mouse urine, mouse PT cell culture medium, and mouse plasma were assayed on six separate occasions in duplicate. The mean intra-assay CV for the assay is 4.39 ± 0.74 % in human urine, 3.04 ± 0.61 % in mouse urine, 1.43 ± 0.20 % in cell culture medium, and 3.84 ± 0.63 % in mouse plasma. The mean inter-assay CV value is 13.17 ± 0.77 % in human urine, 7.01 ± 1.04 % in mouse urine, 9.47 ± 0.22 % in cell culture medium, and 10.92 ± 1.88 % in mouse plasma (Table 3).

4 Notes

We have determined the extent of inhibition of ACE2 activity by MLN-4760 (10^{-6} M) or DX600 (10^{-6} M, linear form, AnaSpec), using human and mouse rACE2. Specificity can also be assessed, and in this regard we have used the ACE inhibitor captopril. At concentrations of human and mouse rACE2 ranging from 0 to 400 ng/ml, ACE2 enzymatic activity (measured after 16 h) is not blocked by captopril (10^{-5} M) (Fig. 2). Indeed, as an internal control, one may add captopril (10^{-5} M) or another ACE inhibitor to each reaction well (as a component of the assay buffer) in the ACE2 assay.

Both MLN-4760 and DX600 strongly inhibit the activity of human rACE2 over a wide range of concentrations of the recombinant enzyme (1.56–400 ng/ml), with the degree of inhibition ranging from 74.5 to 99.0 % for MLN-4760, and from 62.2 to 100 % for DX600 (Fig. 2a). At high concentrations of human rACE2 (100–400 ng/ml), MLN-4760 has a more potent inhibitory effect (98.7–99.0 %) compared to DX600 (62.2–90.0 %).

Table 3
Intra- and inter-assay coefficients of variability (CV)

Samples		Volume/well (μl)	Mean ACE2 activity (ng/ml)	Intra-assay CV (%)[a]	Inter-assay CV (%)[b]
Human urine	1	7.5	57.65	5.87	11.70
	2	7.5	167.28	3.64	14.29
	3	7.5	151.49	3.67	13.51
	Mean ± SE			4.39 ± 0.74	13.17 ± 0.77
Mouse urine	1	7.5	402.82	1.86	5.52
	2	7.5	159.50	3.36	6.49
	3	7.5	175.34	3.90	9.01
	Mean ± SE			3.04 ± 0.61	7.01 ± 1.04
Culture medium	1	15	74.76	1.76	9.38
	2	15	69.35	1.06	9.88
	3	15	100.72	1.49	9.14
	Mean ± SE			1.43 ± 0.20	9.47 ± 0.22
Mouse plasma	1	2	420.47	4.99	8.88
	2	2	400.10	3.69	9.20
	3	2	162.49	2.83	14.67
	Mean ± SE			3.84 ± 0.63	10.92 ± 1.88

CV coefficient of variability, *SE* standard error of the mean
[a]The intra-assay CV is an average value of the individual CVs for the duplicates in six measurements
[b]The inter-assay CV is calculated for each sample by dividing the standard deviation of six measurements by the mean ACE2 activity of six measurements

It is important to note that only MLN-4760 (and not DX600) significantly blocks the activity of mouse rACE2, with the degree of inhibition ranging from 87.6 to 98.2% (Fig. 2b). DX600 exerts no inhibitory effect on mouse rACE2 activity in this assay. Indeed, DX600 (10^{-6} M) actually enhanced RFU at lower levels of mouse rACE2 (3.13–50 ng/ml). In this regard, Pedersen et al. [16] measured the dissociation constant (*K*i) between DX600 and human or mouse ACE2 in activity assays with the same ACE2 substrate, and reported the *K*i for human ACE2 to be significantly lower (0.040 ± 0.005 μM) than the *K*i for mouse ACE2 (0.36 ± 0.03 μM), suggesting that DX600 has higher affinity for human ACE2. The inhibitory effect of another commercially available conformational variant of DX600 (cyclic form) on ACE2 has not yet been tested in our assay. However, Ye et al. have reported that the disulfide bridged cyclic variant of DX600 (Bachem) had no inhibitory effect

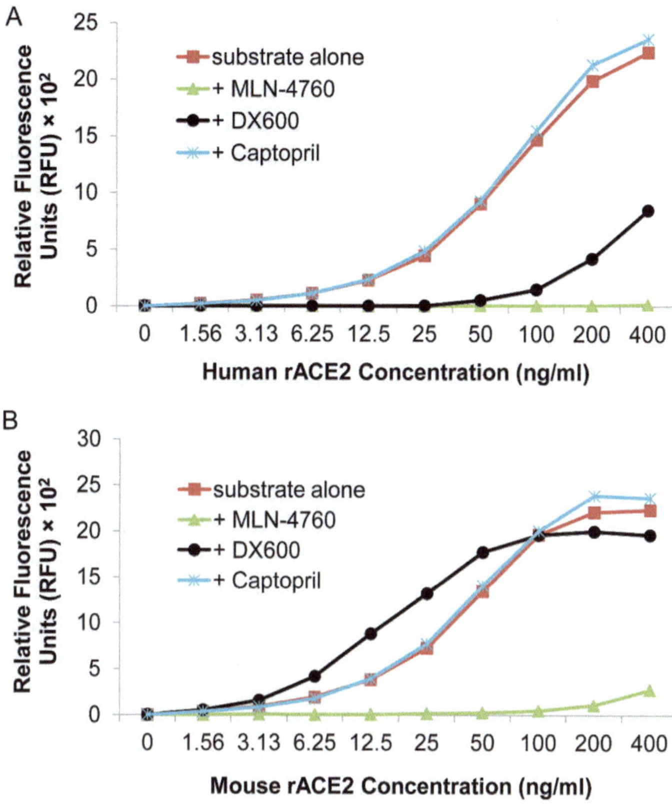

Fig. 2 Effect of ACE2 inhibitors MLN-4760 (10^{-6} M), DX600 (10^{-6} M), and ACE inhibitor captopril (10^{-5} M) on ACE2 enzyme activity. The assay was performed for 16 h incubation. Graph depicts the concentrations of recombinant ACE2 versus the Relative Fluorescence Units (RFU). A background RFU value (67.5 RFU for **a**, 62.0 RFU for **b**) of the substrate blank control was subtracted from the readings for each well. (**a**) Effect of MLN-4760, DX600, and captopril on human rACE2 activity. (**b**) Effect of MLN-4760, DX600, and captopril on mouse rACE2 activity

on mouse or rat ACE2, even at high concentrations, but effectively inhibited human rACE2 [17].

We have also examined the dose-dependent effects of MLN-4760 and DX600 (linear form) on ACE2 activity (measured at 16 h), using mouse rACE2 at concentrations from 0 to 50 ng/ml. An increase in MLN-4760 concentration from 10^{-6} to 10^{-5} M does not significantly enhance the assay characteristics (97.1–100% inhibition for 10^{-5} M, 95.0–99.3% for 10^{-6} M). Indeed, a highly linear relationship between the ACE2 activity (RFU) and mouse rACE2 concentration is observed for both concentrations of MLN-4760 (R^2=0.9950, p<0.001 for 10^{-5} M; R^2=0.9954, p<0.001 for 10^{-6} M). In contrast, DX600 has no significant inhibitory effect on mouse rACE2 activity even at concentrations as high as 10^{-5} M. Similarly, two groups have reported that 10^{-6} M DX600 (purchased from Phoenix Pharmaceuticals, Belmont, CA, USA) only partly (and ineffectively) blocks mouse recombinant or mouse kidney ACE2 activity [16, 17]. However, significant inhibition of mouse ACE2 has been observed with DX600 at 10^{-5} M using an assay buffer maintained at pH 6.5 (16). In rat PT segments, we have used the linear form of DX600 (10^{-6} M) (obtained from Phoenix Pharmaceuticals) to demonstrate inhibition of Ang-(1-7) formation from Ang-(1–10), suggesting inhibition of rat ACE2 [5]. In rat kidney cortex, Ye et al. showed that DX600 (10^{-6} M) only partly inhibited ACE2 activity, measured at pH 6.5 [17]. Accordingly, because of the relatively poor inhibition of rodent ACE2 by DX600, for mouse biological samples we use 10^{-6} M of MLN-4760 for all experiments. For the ACE2 activity assay in human biological fluids, either MLN-4760 or DX600 can be used.

To determine if concentrations of ACE2 fluorogenic substrate lower than 11.25 μM can be used for the assay, we have studied the effect of various substrate concentrations (ranging from 1.41 to 11.25 μM) on mouse rACE2 enzyme activity (Fig. 3). At low substrate concentrations (1.41 μM and 2.81 μM), mouse rACE2 activities are reduced to only 0–25 % of values obtained at 11.25 μM substrate concentration (Fig. 3a). On the other hand, a highly linear relationship between the activity (RFU) and rACE2 concentration is observed for substrate concentration of 5.63 μM or 11.25 μM ($R^2=0.9994$, $p<0.001$ for 11.25 μM; $R^2=0.9903$, $p<0.001$ for 5.63 μM), with the same detection limits (1.56–50 ng/ml) (Fig. 3b). Accordingly, in our assays with biological samples, we routinely use at least 11.25 μM of the ACE2 substrate, although use of 5.63 μM substrate concentration would be acceptable. However, we would not recommend use of ACE2 substrate concentrations lower than this.

Is it necessary to incubate samples for 16 h prior to measurement of fluorescence? We have addressed this question by measuring ACE2 activity at different time points (2, 6, 16, and 24 h incubation), with mouse rACE2 concentrations ranging from 0 to 200 ng/ml (Fig. 4a). A time-dependent increase in ACE2 activity is observed for all mouse rACE2 concentrations. By 16 h of incubation, the RFU signal has reached saturation for mouse rACE2 concentrations between 100 and 200 ng/ml. The linear detection range for ACE2 with 16 h incubation is between 1.56 and 50 ng/ml (Fig. 4b). In contrast, for a 2 h incubation time, a linear relationship still exists between ACE2 activity and ACE2 concentration for mouse rACE2 between 100 and 200 ng/ml (Fig. 4a). Thus, the detection limit of the assay for 2 h incubation is extended between 1.56 and 200 ng/ml ($R^2=0.9981$, $p<0.001$), although RFU values are significantly lower at all ACE2 concentrations (*see* Fig. 4). In our lab, we routinely select 16 h as an incubation time for the assay, since ACE2 activity in most biologic samples we have studied is within the 16 h detection limit (i.e., up

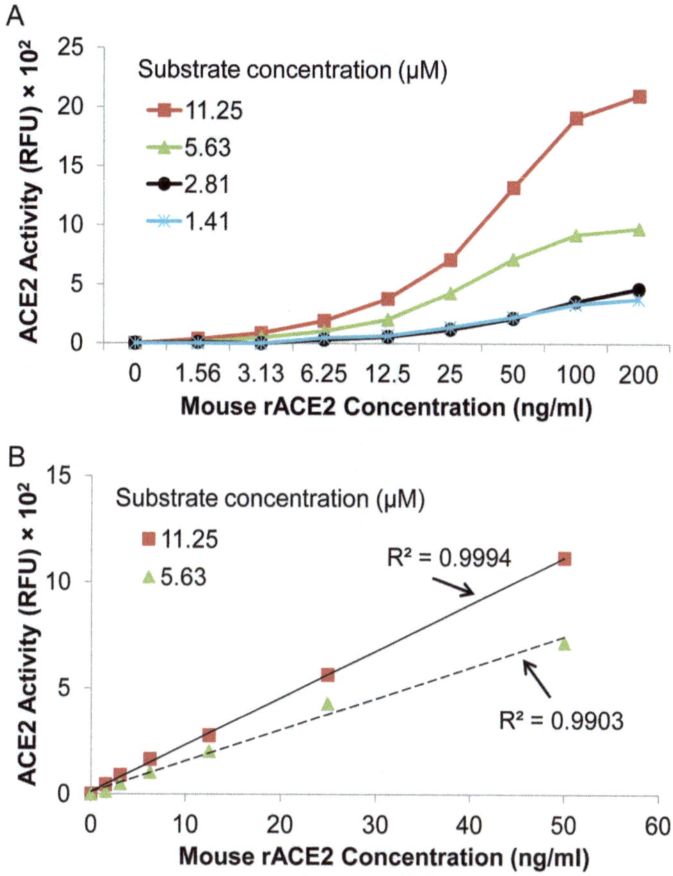

Fig. 3 Effect of substrate concentrations on ACE2 activity. (**a**) The assay was performed with different ACE2 substrate concentrations (11.25, 5.63, 2.81, and 1.41 μM) for 16 h incubation using mouse rACE2 concentrations between 0 and 200 ng/ml. Graph depicts the concentrations of mouse rACE2 versus the activity (RFU) at different substrate concentrations. (**b**) Standard curves generated for mouse rACE2 with 11.25 or 5.63 μM ACE2 substrate concentrations. A highly linear relationship between mouse rACE2 and the RFU exists for both substrate concentrations ($R^2 = 0.9994$, $p < 0.001$ for 11.25 μM; $R^2 = 0.9903$, $p < 0.001$ for 5.63 μM)

to 50 ng/ml). If there is a relatively high ACE2 protein level in the biological fluid of interest, the incubation time can be reduced to as short as 2 h.

As noted, using this assay we perform endpoint RFU measurements, calculate the ACE2 protein concentrations from standard curves, and typically record this value in ng/ml for biological fluids, and not as ACE2 activity per se. ACE2 activity can also be reported as RFUs per volume of sample per unit time (RFU/ml/min or RFU/ml/h). To present data as ACE2 enzymatic activity, the 96-well plate should be read on a fluorescence reader in kinetic

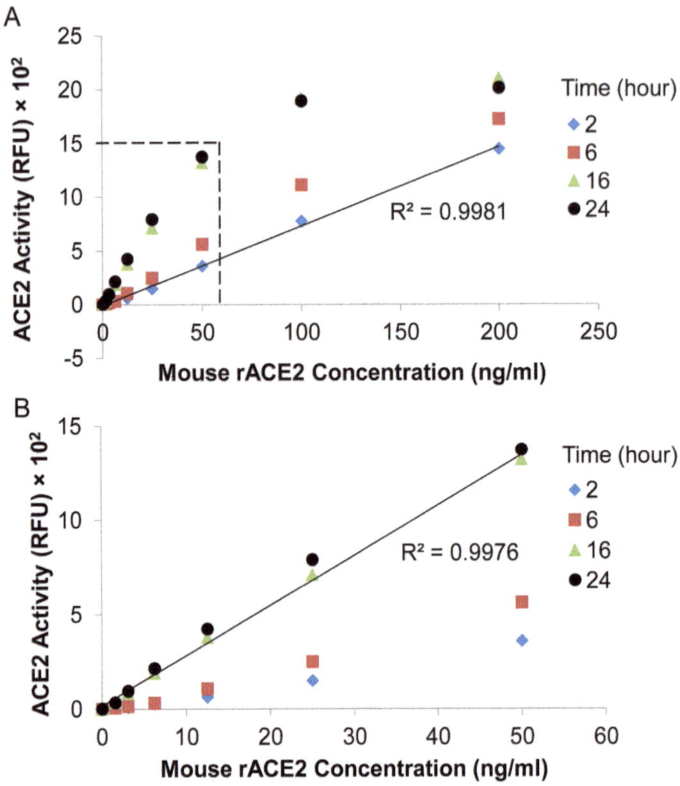

Fig. 4 Time course of ACE2 activity assay. ACE2 activity was measured for 2, 6, 16, and 24 h incubation, with mouse rACE2 concentrations ranging from 0 to 200 ng/ml. Graph depicts the concentrations of mouse rACE2 versus the ACE2 activity (RFU) at different time points. (**a**) Standard curve generated for mouse rACE2 for 2 h incubation. A highly linear relationship exists for rACE2 concentrations from 0 to 200 ng/ml ($R^2 = 0.9981$, $p < 0.001$). The area marked with dashed lines is shown in **b**. (**b**) Standard curve generated for mouse rACE2 for 16 h incubation. The relationship is highly linear for rACE2 concentrations between 0 and 50 ng/ml

mode. The maximum velocity (V_{max}, RFU/min) in each sample can be determined, and adjusted for the inhibitor-containing wells. Specific ACE2 activity (pmole/min) is then calculated from the adjusted V_{max} using a conversion factor (pmol/RFU), determined from a calibration standard curve constructed using a fluorescent peptide fragment (MCA-Pro-Leu-OH, Bachem, Bubendorf, Switzerland, Catalog number M-1975). Final ACE2 enzymatic activity in biological fluids can be corrected for the sample dilution factor, and expressed as pmole/ml/min.

Pedersen et al. [16] have reported that activity assays of human, rat, and mouse ACE2 are highly pH-dependent, with maximal hydrolysis rate of ACE2 substrate at assay buffer pH 6.5, and minimal activity at pH 8.0 [16]. We use an assay buffer at pH 6.8 for our ACE2 activity assay, and we recommend measuring the pH of biological samples prior to conduct of the assay. To limit any effect of pH of biological samples on the assay, we advise diluting samples with the assay buffer as much as possible.

For measurement of plasma ACE2 activity, avoidance of chelators such as EDTA in the blood collection tubes is recommended, since chelation could inhibit the activity of the metallopeptidase ACE2.

Urine samples may have significant background fluorescence at 405 nm. For example, in undiluted urine samples from mice with gene deletion of ACE2, we typically obtain background fluorescence readings greater than 2000 RFU for 7.5 μl urine in the assay. Because such autofluorescence may interfere with the fluorescence signal and reduce the ability to detect ACE2, we suggest dilution of urine samples (e.g., in wild-type mice we typically dilute the urine sample 1:15 with assay buffer to 15 μl/well).

Does freeze/thaw of biological fluids affect ACE2 activity? We have measured ACE2 activity in samples of human and mouse urine, and mouse PT cell culture medium after as many as three freeze/thaw cycles. Interestingly, we found no significant difference in ACE2 activity between any freeze/thaw cycle for all three sample categories (data not shown, $p > 0.05$). Nonetheless, for biological samples it is likely prudent to restrict use of repetitive freeze/thaw for this assay. Furthermore, we do not recommend repetitively freezing and thawing recombinant ACE2 protein, as we found that ACE2 activity can be significantly lost after a second freeze-thaw cycle.

In previous studies, we reported that urinary ACE2 activity is enhanced in renal transplant patients with diabetes, using this enzyme activity assay [13]. In preliminary data, we also found that incubation of mouse PT cells with high glucose concentrations enhances ACE2 activity in the culture medium, suggesting increased shedding of ACE2 from the cell membrane (data not shown). Accordingly, we have determined if high glucose concentrations alone can affect the assay. As shown in Fig. 5a, ACE2 activity in mouse PT cell culture medium with a high d-glucose concentration (25 mM) is not significantly different from that in the same medium with a normal d-glucose concentration (7.8 mM) ($p > 0.05$, $n = 3$).

We have also studied the effect of increasing concentrations of creatinine (Sigma-Aldrich) and urea (Sigma-Aldrich) on the assay, since these substances are relatively abundant in urine. Using mouse rACE2, we found that neither creatinine (0.01–3.75 mM) nor urea (1.5–300 mM) had any significant effect on ACE2 activity when added to assay buffer (Fig. 5b, c).

Finally, since we reported a correlation between urinary protein and urinary ACE2 levels [13], we have examined the effect of

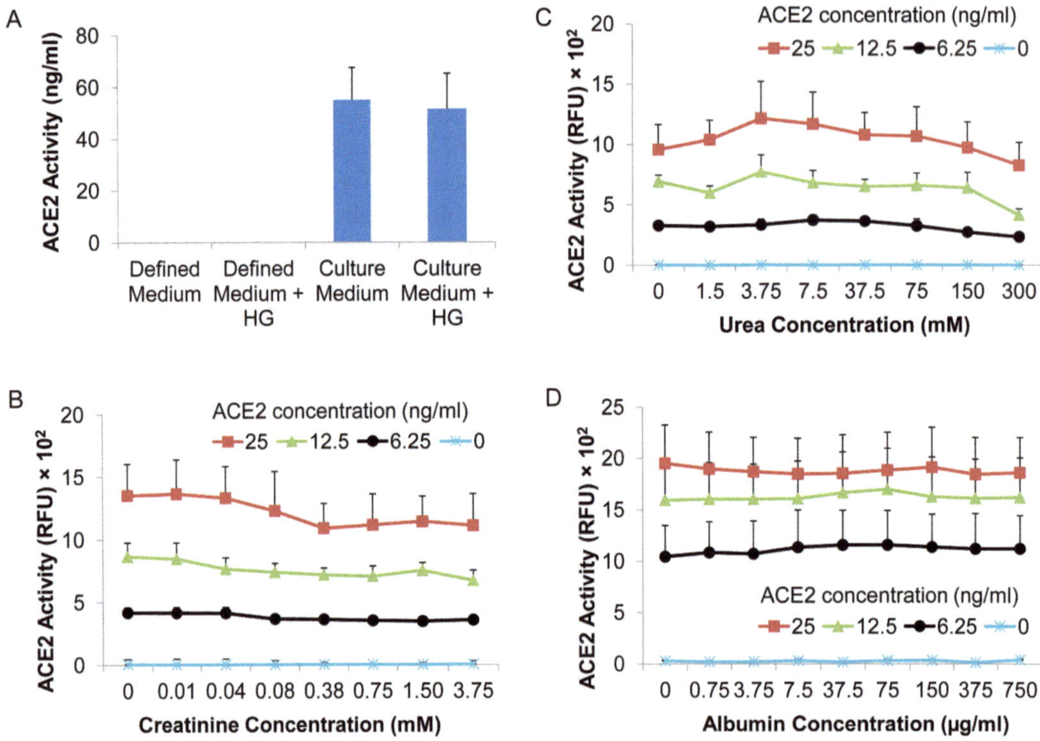

Fig. 5 Effect of potential modulators on ACE2 activity assay. The assay was performed for 16 h incubation. (**a**) Graph shows ACE2 activity in defined medium (not incubated with mouse PT cells), and culture medium collected from primary cultures of mouse PT cells after 72 h incubation, in the presence of normal (7.8 mM) or high concentrations of d-glucose (HG, 25 mM). No ACE2 activity is detected in the defined medium. Results are means ± SEM; $p > 0.05$, culture medium vs culture medium + HG; $n = 3$. (**b**) Graph depicts the effect of addition of various concentrations of creatinine on ACE2 activity (RFU) at different mouse rACE2 concentrations. Results are means ± SEM; $p > 0.05$ for all graphs; $n = 3$. (**c**) Graph depicts the effect of addition of various concentrations of urea on ACE2 activity (RFU) at different mouse rACE2 concentrations. Results are means ± SEM; $p > 0.05$ for all graphs; $n = 3$. (**d**) Graph depicts the effect of addition of exogenous albumin on ACE2 activity (RFU) at different mouse rACE2 concentrations. Albumin at the indicated concentrations was added to urine samples (1 μl) from mice with gene deletion of ACE2. Results are means ± SEM; $p > 0.05$ for all graphs; $n = 3$

exogenous albumin on the ACE2 activity assay. For these experiments, increasing concentrations of albumin (Cohn Fraction V, Sigma-Aldrich, Catalog number A8806) were added to urine samples (1 μl/well) from C57BL6 mice with ACE2 gene deletion, and ACE2 activity was measured following incubation with increasing concentrations of mouse rACE2 (0–25 ng/ml). For these experiments, the average albumin concentration in the urine samples from mice with ACE2 gene deletion was 0.15 μg/ml. As shown in Fig. 5d, addition of exogenous albumin (0.75–750 μg/ml) had no effect on rACE2 activity.

Acknowledgments

We thank Dr. Susan B. Gurley (Duke University Medical Center, Durham, NC, USA) for providing the ACE2 gene knockout mice. We also thank Ore Pharmaceuticals (Cambridge, MA, USA) for providing the ACE2 inhibitor MLN-4760.

References

1. Donoghue M, Hsieh F, Baronas E et al (2000) A novel angiotensin-converting enzyme-related carboxypeptidase (ACE2) converts angiotensin I to angiotensin 1-9. Circ Res 87:E1–E9
2. Tipnis SR, Hooper NM, Hyde R et al (2000) A human homolog of angiotensin-converting enzyme. Cloning and functional expression as a captopril-insensitive carboxypeptidase. J Biol Chem 275:33238–33243
3. Li W, Moore MJ, Vasilieva N et al (2003) Angiotensin-converting enzyme 2 is a functional receptor for the SARS coronavirus. Nature 426:450–454
4. Ye M, Wysocki J, Naaz P et al (2004) Increased ACE 2 and decreased ACE protein in renal tubules from diabetic mice: a renoprotective combination? Hypertension 43:1120–1125
5. Li N, Zimpelmann J, Cheng K et al (2005) The role of angiotensin converting enzyme 2 in the generation of angiotensin 1-7 by rat proximal tubules. Am J Physiol Renal Physiol 288:F353–F362
6. Wysocki J, Ye M, Rodriguez E et al (2010) Targeting the degradation of angiotensin II with recombinant angiotensin-converting enzyme 2: prevention of angiotensin II-dependent hypertension. Hypertension 55:90–98
7. Oudit GY, Liu GC, Zhong J et al (2010) Human recombinant ACE2 reduces the progression of diabetic nephropathy. Diabetes 59:529–538
8. Nadarajah R, Milagres R, Dilauro M et al (2012) Podocyte-specific overexpression of human angiotensin-converting enzyme 2 attenuates diabetic nephropathy in mice. Kidney Int 82:292–303
9. Imai Y, Kuba K, Rao S et al (2005) Angiotensin-converting enzyme 2 protects from severe acute lung failure. Nature 436:112–116
10. Iwata M, Silva Enciso JE, Greenberg BH (2009) Selective and specific regulation of ectodomain shedding of angiotensin-converting enzyme 2 by tumor necrosis factor alpha-converting enzyme. Am J Physiol Cell Physiol 297:C1318–C1329
11. Jia HP, Look DC, Tan P et al (2009) Ectodomain shedding of angiotensin converting enzyme 2 in human airway epithelia. Am J Physiol Lung Cell Mol Physiol 297:L84–L96
12. Mizuiri S, Aoki T, Hemmi H et al (2011) Urinary angiotensin-converting enzyme 2 in patients with CKD. Nephrology (Carlton) 16:567–572
13. Xiao F, Hiremath S, Knoll G et al (2012) Increased urinary angiotensin-converting enzyme 2 in renal transplant patients with diabetes. PLoS One 7, e37649
14. Tikellis C, Bialkowski K, Pete J et al (2008) ACE2 deficiency modifies renoprotection afforded by ACE inhibition in experimental diabetes. Diabetes 57:1018–1025
15. Lubel JS, Herath CB, Velkoska E et al (2008) Angiotensin converting enzyme 2 (ACE2) activity in fetal calf serum: implications for cell culture research. Cytotechnology 58:119–126
16. Pedersen KB, Sriramula S, Chhabra KH et al (2011) Species-specific inhibitor sensitivity of angiotensin-converting enzyme 2 (ACE2) and its implication for ACE2 activity assays. Am J Physiol Regul Integr Comp Physiol 301:R1293–R1299
17. Ye M, Wysocki J, Gonzalez-Pacheco FR et al (2012) Murine recombinant angiotensin-converting enzyme 2: effect on angiotensin II-dependent hypertension and distinctive angiotensin-converting enzyme 2 inhibitor characteristics on rodent and human angiotensin-converting enzyme 2. Hypertension 60:730–740

Chapter 9

Determining the Enzymatic Activity of Angiotensin-Converting Enzyme 2 (ACE2) in Brain Tissue and Cerebrospinal Fluid Using a Quenched Fluorescent Substrate

Srinivas Sriramula, Kim Brint Pedersen, Huijing Xia, and Eric Lazartigues

Abstract

Angiotensin-converting enzyme 2 (ACE2) is a component of the renin-angiotensin system (RAS) which plays an important role in the regulation of blood pressure and volume homeostasis. Accumulating evidence shows alterations in ACE2 expression and activity in several hypertensive animal models, as well as in patients with hypertension. In order to assess the role of brain ACE2 in hypertension, a specific ACE2 assay is required. Based on a quenched fluorescent substrate, we describe an easy-to-use method for determining ACE2 activity in brain tissue and cerebrospinal fluid. The method can further be adapted for other tissues, plasma, cell extracts, and cell culture supernatants.

Key words ACE2, Quenched fluorescent substrate, Mca-APK(Dnp), DX600, Hypertension, Brain ACE2, CSF

1 Introduction

1.1 Background

Angiotensin-converting enzyme 2 (ACE2) is a component of the renin-angiotensin system (RAS) which plays an important role in the regulation of blood pressure and volume homeostasis [1, 2]. ACE2 is a metallo-carboxypeptidase that hydrolyzes the octapeptide angiotensin-II (Ang-II) to the heptapeptide angiotensin-(1-7) (Ang-(1-7)). ACE2 can also hydrolyze several other peptides unrelated to the RAS, such as apelin 13, apelin 36, neurotensin, kinetensin, dynorphin, [des-Arg^9]-bradykinin, and [Lys-des-Arg^9]-bradykinin [3]. The expression and distribution of ACE2 was predominantly identified in the testis, heart, and kidney [4]. However, tissue distribution of ACE2 is now considered widespread in the body including in the liver, intestine, lung, pancreas, adipose tissue, uterus, ovary, placenta, and brain [2, 5]. ACE2 is a type 1 transmembrane protein with the N-terminus located extracellularly and an intracellular C-terminus [6]. The extracellular domain including its catalytic site can be cleaved from the cell

Rhian M. Touyz and Ernesto L. Schiffrin (eds.), *Hypertension: Methods and Protocols*, Methods in Molecular Biology, vol. 1527, DOI 10.1007/978-1-4939-6625-7_9, © Springer Science+Business Media LLC 2017

membrane by peptidases such as ADAM17 [7]. Thus, ACE2 can be found not only in tissues but also in plasma [8] and cerebrospinal fluid (CSF) [9]. It is now well established that ACE2 is an important component of the brain RAS. In animal models, ACE2 mRNA expression, protein expression, and activity are decreased in the brain during several cardiovascular diseases including hypertension [2, 10, 11]. Circulating ACE2 activity is elevated in patients with heart failure and correlates with disease severity [8]. It has been shown that ACE2 expression can be altered at the posttranscriptional level where ACE2 protein and enzymatic activity are altered without any change at the mRNA level [12].

ACE2 activity can be measured by assessing the Ang-(1-7) formation from radioactively labeled Ang-II [13]. However, this method requires sophisticated equipment such as high-performance liquid chromatography or mass spectrometry [14]. ACE2 activity can conveniently be measured using quenched fluorescent substrates such as (7-methoxycoumarin-4-yl)acetyl-Tyr-Val-Ala-Asp--Ala-Pro-Lys(2,4-dinitrophenyl)-OH [Mca-YVADAPK(Dnp)] and (7-methoxycoumarin-4-yl)acetyl-Ala-Pro-Lys(2,4-dinitrophenyl)-OH [Mca-APK(Dnp)] [3]. ACE2 hydrolyzes the peptide bond between the proline and lysine residues of Mca-APK(Dnp). This removes the quenching effect of the dinitrophenyl group on the fluorescence of the methoxycoumarin moiety (Fig. 1a). These quenched fluorescent substrates are not specific for ACE2 as they can also be hydrolyzed by other enzymes such as ACE, caspase 1, and prolyl endopeptidase [12, 15, 16]. Non-specific hydrolysis of the quenched fluorescent substrates is determined as the hydrolysis rate in the presence of an ACE2-specific inhibitor, such as DX600 [17]. However, the sensitivity of ACE2 inhibition by DX600 depends on the species [10]. Therefore, an optimized assay is essential in order to measure the ACE2 activity accurately. Here we describe an easy-to-use method for ACE2 measurement in brain tissue and CSF that can further be adapted for other tissues, plasma, cell extracts, and cell culture supernatants. It is based on the hydrolysis of Mca-APK(Dnp) in the absence and presence of DX600.

1.2 Example 1: ACE2 Activity in Hypothalamus

Expression of a human ACE2 transgene under the control of the synapsin promoter (Syn-hACE2 mice) results in robust overexpression of ACE2 mRNA and protein in the brain as determined by real-time qRT-PCR and Western blot analysis, respectively [18]. Here we demonstrate that Syn-hACE2 mice have markedly higher ACE2 activity in the hypothalamus than wild-type non-transgenic C57BL/6 J mice. The hypothalamus was isolated from wild-type and Syn-hACE2 mice, and ACE2 extracts were prepared. Extracts containing 10 μg protein were used for hydrolysis of Mca-APK(Dnp) in the presence and absence of DX600. Figure 1b shows the time courses of fluorescence development. The hydrolysis rates are calculated as the slopes of the regression lines between

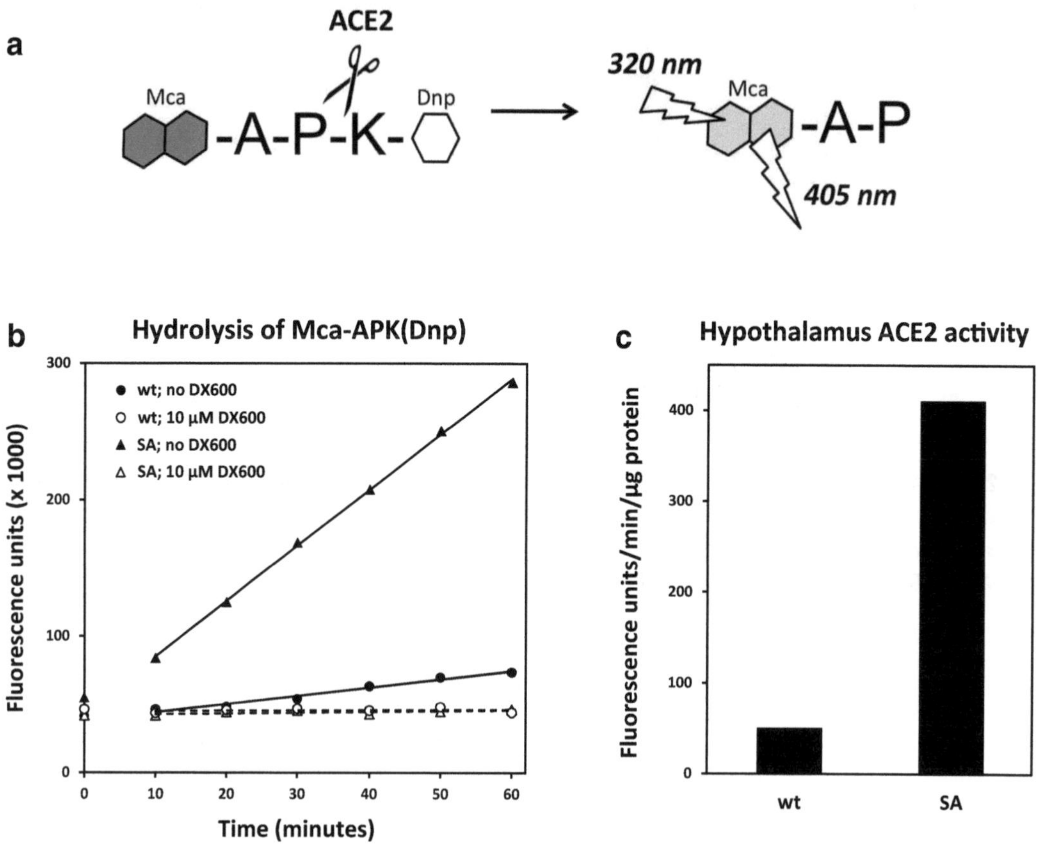

Fig. 1 ACE2 activity assay for hypothalamus of non-transgenic wild-type (wt) and Syn-hACE2 (SA) mice. (**a**) Cleavage of Mca-APK(Dnp) by ACE2 is determined by fluorescence at 405 nm after excitation at 320 nm. (**b**) Hydrolysis rates of 10 μM Mca-APK(Dnp) by hypothalamus extracts in the absence and presence of 10 μM DX600 are calculated as the slopes of the regression lines. (**c**) The difference of hydrolysis rates in the absence and presence of DX600 gives the true ACE2 activity which is expressed as fluorescence units/min/μg of protein

the 10 and 60 min time points. In the absence of DX600, the hydrolysis rates are 606 and 4078 fluorescence units (FU)/min for wild-type and Syn-hACE2 mice, respectively. In the presence of DX600, the rates are 23 and 60 FU/min. The hydrolysis rates due to ACE2 are then 606-23 = 583 and 4078-60 = 4018 FU/min. Dividing the hydrolysis rates by the amount of protein yields the final ACE2 activity measurement which is depicted in Fig. 1c. The human ACE2 transgene thus leads to an approximately sevenfold increase in ACE2 activity in the hypothalamus.

1.3 Example 2: ACE2 Activity in Cerebrospinal Fluid

Very limited amount of CSF (<10 μL) can be obtained from mice using puncture techniques. We therefore used a perfusion/microdialysis method that provides a larger volume (typically 300 μL/day). However, the components of the CSF will be diluted in the

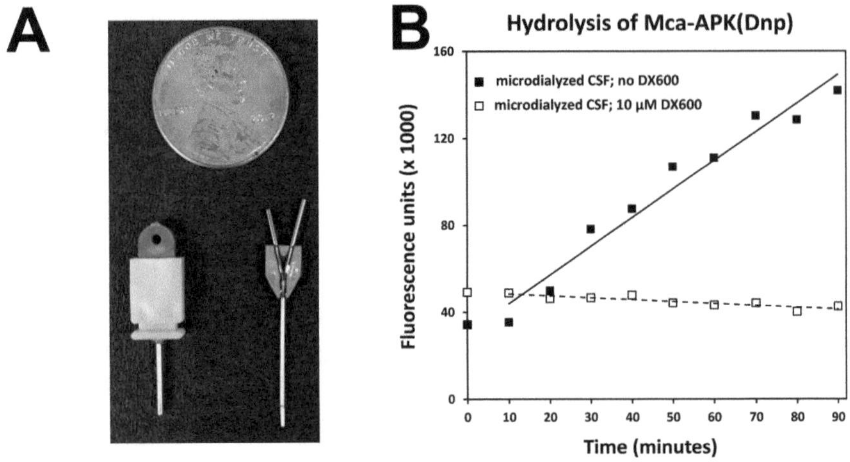

Fig. 2 ACE2 activity in mouse CSF. (**a**) The cannula guide at the left was implanted intracerebroventricularly. Following recovery of the mouse, the top part of the cannula guide was removed, and the microdialysis probe at the right was inserted. A US penny is shown for size. (**b**) Hydrolysis of Mca-APK(Dnp) by dialyzed CSF that was concentrated by freeze-drying was determined in the absence and presence of 10 μM DX600

perfusate. We dialyzed CSF with a microdialysis probe which is shown in Fig. 2a. No ACE2 activity could be detected using crude microdialyzed CSF isolated from C57BL/6J mice. We concentrated the dialyzed CSF five times by freeze-drying and resuspension in a smaller volume. The concentrated dialyzed CSF has clear Mca-APK(Dnp)-hydrolyzing activity that can be inhibited by DX600 (Fig. 2b) demonstrating that ACE2 has become shed into the CSF.

2 Materials

2.1 Solutions

Solutions are prepared at room temperature using deionized water.

1. 500 mM Tris base: Dissolve 60.57 g Tris base in H_2O to a total volume of 1000 mL.
2. 500 mM Tris–HCl: Dissolve 78.78 g Tris–HCl in H_2O to a total volume of 1000 mL.
3. Mix 500 mM Tris base and 500 mM Tris–HCl in a ratio of 2.75:100 (v/v). With a pH-meter, check that pH in an aliquot is 6.5 ± 0.1 (*see* **Note 1**).
4. 2 M NaCl: Dissolve 116.886 g NaCl in H_2O to a total volume of 1000 mL.
5. 10 mM $ZnCl_2$: Dissolve 1.3632 g $ZnCl_2$ in H_2O to a total volume of 1000 mL.

6. ACE2 reaction buffer: Mix 500 mL 2 M NaCl, 150 ml 500 mM Tris–HCl pH 6.5, 50 mL 10 mM $ZnCl_2$, and 300 mL deionized H_2O. Store protected from light at room temperature.
7. ACE2 extraction buffer: Add 50 μL Triton X-100 to 9.95 mL ACE2 extraction buffer. Mix well by vortexing vigorously.
8. 4 mM Mca-APK(Dnp): Mca-APK(Dnp) can be purchased from Enzo Life Sciences (Plymouth Meeting, PA). Dissolve 1 mg Mca-APK(Dnp) in 358 μL dimethyl sulfoxide (DMSO). Store at −20 °C protected from light.
9. 400 μM Mca-APK(Dnp): Mix 100 μL 4 mM Mca-APK(Dnp) and 900 μL DMSO. Store at −20 °C protected from light.
10. 260 μM DX600: DX600 can be purchased from Phoenix Pharmaceuticals (Burlingame, CA). Dissolve 100 μg DX600 in 125 μL ultrapure H_2O. Store unused DX600 solution at −80 °C (*see* **Note 2**).
11. Artificial cerebrospinal fluid (aCSF): 10× stock solution is prepared by adding 0.161 g $Na_2HPO_4{\cdot}7H_2O$ (12 mM final), 0.102 g $MgCl_2{\cdot}6H_2O$ (10 mM final), 0.189 g $CaCl_2{\cdot}2H_2O$ (26 mM final), 0.112 g KCl (30 mM final), and 4.09 g NaCl (1.45 M final) to H_2O to a final volume of 50 mL. Filter-sterilize with a 0.22 μm filter. Adjust to pH 7.4 with 1 N NaOH or phosphoric acid. Store at 4 °C for up to 1 month. Dilute the stock solution to 1× prior to use with H_2O.
12. Ketamine/xylazine mix: 2 mL of 50 mg/mL ketamine and 0.5 mL of 20 mg/mL xylazine are added to 7.5 mL sterile 0.9% saline.

2.2 Equipment

1. Glass pestle tissue grinders or other tissue homogenization equipment.
2. Sonicator with microtip capable of sonicating samples in microcentrifuge tubes.
3. Commercial protein assay kit and spectrophotometer for determination of protein concentrations.
4. Black flat-bottomed 96-well microtiter plates useful for fluorescence measurements
5. Fluorometer capable of measuring fluorescence in 96-well microtiter plates with excitation at 320 nm and emission at 405 nm at 37 °C.
6. For CSF collection from mice: intracerebroventricular (ICV) cannula guide and microdialysis probes with membrane molecular weight cutoff ≥100 kDa (e.g., CMA 12 Guide Cannula and CMA12 MD High Cut-Off Probe 2 mm from CMA Microdialysis, Sweden), stereotaxic instrument for mouse, microdialysis system for rodents, low flow rate microdialysis pump, container for freely moving animals, refrigerated fraction collector, and freeze-dryer.

3 Methods

3.1 Preparation of Brain Tissue Extract

1. Following anesthesia, euthanize laboratory animals according to a method consistent with the recommendation of the Panel on Euthanasia of the American Veterinary Medical Association.
2. Dissect the whole brain or brain region of interest from the animal. Snap-freeze the tissue in liquid nitrogen or on dry ice and keep the frozen tissue at −80 °C until homogenization.
3. Homogenize the brain tissue in ACE2 extraction buffer with at least 1000 μL ACE2 extraction buffer per 100 mg tissue using a glass pestle or a tissue grinder on ice. Transfer the homogenate to 1.5 mL microcentrifuge tubes.
4. Sonicate the homogenate for 5 s, four times, on ice.
5. Perform centrifugation at 20,000 × *g* for 5 min at 4 °C.
6. Recover supernatants in fresh microcentrifuge tubes (*see* **Note 3**). These are the brain tissue extracts.
7. Take 10 μL aliquots of the extracts for determination of the protein concentration.
8. Following protein concentration determination, dilute samples in ACE2 extraction buffer to a protein concentration of 1 μg/μL (*see* **Note 4**).
9. Store the brain tissue extracts at −80 °C.

3.2 Generation of a Positive Control

1. Make an extract of the whole kidney of a wild-type or control animal similar to the protocol for brain tissue extracts (*see* **Note 5**).
2. Determine the protein concentration of the kidney extract.
3. Dilute the kidney extract in ACE2 extraction buffer to a protein concentration of 200 ng/μL (*see* **Note 4**).
4. Store 50 μL aliquots in microcentrifuge tubes at −80 °C.

3.3 Collection of CSF

The CSF can be collected by appropriate methods. Here we describe collection of CSF from mice using a microdialysis system [19].

1. Mice are anesthetized with a ketamine/xylazine mix (0.1 mL/10 g body weight, 100 mg/kg/10 mg/kg, injected intraperitoneally) and placed on a stereotaxic instrument (*see* **Note 6**).
2. Cannula guide is implanted intracerebroventricularly (1.0 mm lateral, 2.7 mm ventral, 0.3 mm caudal).
3. After at least 5 days of recovery, a probe with a 100 kDa molecular weight cutoff membrane is inserted into the cannula guide and microdialysis is performed in conscious freely moving mice.
4. Mice are perfused continuously with aCSF at a rate of 1 μL/min and the dialyzed CSF collected using a refrigerated fraction collector.

5. 250 μL of dialyzed CSF are concentrated with a freeze-dryer until completely dried and stored at −80 °C until use. The freeze-dried CSF is resuspended in 50 μL ACE2 reaction buffer before ACE2 activity assay.

3.4 ACE2 Activity Assay for Brain Tissue Extracts

1. Thaw samples on ice, vortex them briefly, and keep them on ice.
2. Make a master mix of reagents for hydrolysis of Mca-APK(Dnp) in the absence of DX600: 3.85 μL H_2O, 2.5 μL 400 μM Mca-APK(Dnp), and 83.65 μL ACE2 reaction buffer per measurement.
3. Make a master mix of reagents for hydrolysis of Mca-APK(Dnp) in the presence of DX 600: 3.85 μL 260 μM DX600, 2.5 μL 400 μM Mca-APK(Dnp), 83.65 μL ACE2 reaction buffer per measurement (*see* **Note 7**).
4. For each sample, dispense 10 μL aliquots into two wells of a black 96-well microtiter plate.
5. For each sample, add 90 μL of the hydrolysis reagent without DX600 to one of the wells and 90 μL of the hydrolysis reagent with DX600 to the other well.
6. Inspect wells for presence of floating bubbles. If any are present, puncture them with a fine pipette tip or sterile needle (do not use the same needle between wells).
7. Insert the microtiter plate into a fluorometer equilibrated to 37 °C. Measure fluorescence emitted at 405 nm after excitation at 320 nm every 10 min for 1 h.
8. Inspect the time courses of fluorescence development, i.e., curves of fluorescence versus time. It should approximate a straight line, at least from the 10 min time point as illustrated in Fig. 1b. Time courses that curve substantially toward a plateau are due to samples with ACE2 activities that are too high for the dynamic range of the assay. Such samples need to be further diluted.
9. Calculate the slope of the time courses of fluorescence development between time points 10 and 60 min (*see* **Note 8**).
10. For the positive control, calculate the slope for the well with DX600 in percentage of the slope for the well without DX600. This should be lower than 10%. If this is not the case, DX600 did not effectively inhibit ACE2, and the values for ACE2 activity will therefore be underestimated.
11. Subtract the slope in the presence of DX600 from the activity in the absence of DX600. Divide this parameter with the protein concentration of the sample. The resulting value expressed in fluorescence units/min/μg protein is the ACE2 activity of the sample (*see* **Note 9**).

3.5 ACE2 Activity Assay for CSF

The assay is conducted as for brain tissue extracts with the following modifications:

1. Make a master mix of reagents for hydrolysis of Mca-APK(Dnp) in the absence of DX600: 3.85 μL H_2O, 2.5 μL 400 μM Mca-APK(Dnp) and 73.65 μL ACE2 reaction buffer per measurement.
2. Make a master mix of reagents for hydrolysis of Mca-APK(Dnp) in the presence of DX 600: 3.85 μL 260 μM DX600, 2.5 μL 400 μM Mca-APK(Dnp), 73.65 μL ACE2 reaction buffer per measurement (*see* **Note 7**).
3. Dispense 20 μL aliquots of the concentrated CSF into two wells of a black 96-well microtiter plate.
4. For each sample, add 80 μL of the hydrolysis reagent without DX600 to one of the wells and 80 μL of the hydrolysis reagent with DX600 to the other well.
5. Measure fluorescence emitted at 405 nm after excitation at 320 nm every 10 min for 90 min.
6. Calculate the slope of the time courses of fluorescence development between time points 10 and 90 min.

4 Notes

1. It is important that pH is maintained at 6.5, as higher pH values lead to decreased hydrolysis rates of the fluorogenic substrate and inefficient inhibition of rodent ACE2 with DX600 [10].
2. The supplier of DX600 (Phoenix Pharmaceuticals) recommends that DX600 should be dissolved just before use. However, we have been able to effectively inhibit ACE2 with dissolved DX600 that has been stored at −80 °C for several months.
3. The supernatants are generally turbid to varying degrees. Except for the pellet, the whole of the supernatant should be recovered as the extract.
4. The protein concentrations listed are appropriate for whole brain and kidney extracts from C57BL/6J mice. For other types of samples, the investigator may need to adjust the protein concentration in order to ensure that the ACE2 content of the samples are within the dynamic range of the assay.
5. The mouse kidney ACE2 extract is useful as a positive control, as more than 95 % of the enzymatic activity hydrolyzing Mca-APK(Dnp) is due to ACE2 rather than other hydrolases. Alternative positive controls are extracts of Neuro-2a cells transfected with a plasmid for expression of ACE2 [10] or purified ACE2 protein from commercial vendors diluted in ACE2 extraction buffer.

6. Most of the mouse stereotaxic instruments come with a standard rat/mouse mouth piece that is not convenient for mice. We recommend using a Kopf nose-tooth assembly to prevent lateral movements of the head.
7. The final concentration of DX600 is 10 μM, which is sufficient to inhibit mouse and rat ACE2 more than 95%. However, 1 μM DX600 is sufficient for inhibition of human ACE2 [10]. For ACE2 from other species, the investigators should verify that DX600 effectively inhibits the enzyme.
8. The reaction rate of Mca-APK(Dnp) hydrolysis increases within the first 10 min, as the temperature of the reaction mixtures increases from room temperature to 37 °C. The 0 min time point is therefore excluded from the calculation of the slope.
9. The ACE2 activity values of fluorescence units/min/μg protein are useful for comparing the ACE2 activities of samples measured on the same 96-well microtiter plate. To minimize effects of plate to plate variation, the activities can be normalized relative to the activity of the positive control. An alternative unit for ACE2 activity is picomoles of Mca-APK(Dnp) cleaved per minute. The conversion from fluorescence units to picomoles Mca-APK(Dnp) is done with standard curves generated from different concentrations of 7-methoxycoumarin-3-carboxylic acid [20].

Acknowledgments

This work was supported by research grants from the American Heart Association (Established Investigator Award: 12EIA8030004) and National Institutes of Health, National Institute of General Medical Sciences (8 P20 GM103514-10), National Institute of Diabetes and Digestive and Kidney Diseases (DK084466), and National Heart, Lung, and Blood Institute (HL093178) to Dr. Eric Lazartigues.

References

1. Xia H, Lazartigues E (2010) Angiotensin-converting enzyme 2: central regulator for cardiovascular function. Curr Hypertens Rep 12:170–175
2. Xu P, Sriramula S, Lazartigues E (2011) ACE2/ANG-(1-7)/Mas pathway in the brain: the axis of good. Am J Physiol Regul Integr Comp Physiol 300:R804–R817
3. Vickers C, Hales P, Kaushik V, Dick L, Gavin J et al (2002) Hydrolysis of biological peptides by human angiotensin-converting enzyme-related carboxypeptidase. J Biol Chem 277:14838–14843
4. Tipnis SR, Hooper NM, Hyde R, Karran E, Christie G et al (2000) A human homolog of angiotensin-converting enzyme. Cloning and functional expression as a captopril-insensitive carboxypeptidase. J Biol Chem 275:33238–33243
5. Doobay MF, Talman LS, Obr TD, Tian X, Davisson RL et al (2007) Differential expression of neuronal ACE2 in transgenic mice with overexpression of the brain renin-angiotensin

system. Am J Physiol Regul Integr Comp Physiol 292:R373–R381

6. Warner FJ, Lew RA, Smith AI, Lambert DW, Hooper NM et al (2005) Angiotensin-converting enzyme 2 (ACE2), but not ACE, is preferentially localized to the apical surface of polarized kidney cells. J Biol Chem 280:39353–39362
7. Lambert DW, Yarski M, Warner FJ, Thornhill P, Parkin ET et al (2005) Tumor necrosis factor-alpha convertase (ADAM17) mediates regulated ectodomain shedding of the severe-acute respiratory syndrome-coronavirus (SARS-CoV) receptor, angiotensin-converting enzyme-2 (ACE2). J Biol Chem 280:30113–30119
8. Epelman S, Tang WH, Chen SY, Van Lente F, Francis GS et al (2008) Detection of soluble angiotensin-converting enzyme 2 in heart failure: insights into the endogenous counter-regulatory pathway of the renin-angiotensin-aldosterone system. J Am Coll Cardiol 52:750–754
9. Kawajiri M, Mogi M, Higaki N, Matsuoka T, Ohyagi Y et al (2009) Angiotensin-converting enzyme (ACE) and ACE2 levels in the cerebrospinal fluid of patients with multiple sclerosis. Mult Scler 15:262–265
10. Pedersen KB, Sriramula S, Chhabra KH, Xia H, Lazartigues E (2011) Species-specific inhibitor sensitivity of angiotensin-converting enzyme 2 (ACE2) and its implication for ACE2 activity assays. Am J Physiol Regul Integr Comp Physiol 301:R1293–R1299
11. Sriramula S, Cardinale JP, Lazartigues E, Francis J (2011) ACE2 overexpression in the paraventricular nucleus attenuates angiotensin II-induced hypertension. Cardiovasc Res 92:401–408
12. Wysocki J, Ye M, Soler MJ, Gurley SB, Xiao HD et al (2006) ACE and ACE2 activity in diabetic mice. Diabetes 55:2132–2139
13. Ferrario CM, Jessup J, Chappell MC, Averill DB, Brosnihan KB et al (2005) Effect of angiotensin-converting enzyme inhibition and angiotensin II receptor blockers on cardiac angiotensin-converting enzyme 2. Circulation 111:2605–2610
14. Poglitsch M, Domenig O, Schwager C, Stranner S, Peball B et al (2012) Recombinant expression and characterization of human and murine ACE2: species-specific activation of the alternative renin-angiotensin-system. Int J Hypertens 2012:428950
15. Enari M, Talanian RV, Wong WW, Nagata S (1996) Sequential activation of ICE-like and CPP32-like proteases during Fas-mediated apoptosis. Nature 380:723–726
16. Douglas GC, O'Bryan MK, Hedger MP, Lee DK, Yarski MA et al (2004) The novel angiotensin-converting enzyme (ACE) homolog, ACE2, is selectively expressed by adult Leydig cells of the testis. Endocrinology 145:4703–4711
17. Huang L, Sexton DJ, Skogerson K, Devlin M, Smith R et al (2003) Novel peptide inhibitors of angiotensin-converting enzyme 2. J Biol Chem 278:15532–15540
18. Feng Y, Xia H, Cai Y, Halabi CM, Becker LK et al (2010) Brain-selective overexpression of human Angiotensin-converting enzyme type 2 attenuates neurogenic hypertension. Circ Res 106:373–382
19. Zapata A, Chefer VI, Shippenberg TS (2009) Microdialysis in rodents. Curr Protoc Neurosci Chapter 7:Unit 7.2
20. Huentelman MJ, Zubcevic J, Katovich MJ, Raizada MK (2004) Cloning and characterization of a secreted form of angiotensin-converting enzyme 2. Regul Pept 122:61–67

Chapter 10

Measurement of Cardiac Angiotensin II by Immunoassays, HPLC-Chip/Mass Spectrometry, and Functional Assays

Walmor C. De Mello and Yamil Gerena

Abstract

The molecular mechanisms related to the effect of angiotensin II, its level on cardiac tissues, as well as its overexpression represent an important aspect of cardiovascular pharmacology and pathology. Severe alterations of cardiac functions are induced by hypertension including activation of circulating and local cardiac renin angiotensin systems. In this chapter, we are providing the methods and materials necessary for further investigation of this important topic.

Key words Heart, Cardiomyocytes, Angiotensin II, AT1 receptor, Intracellular, HPLC-MS, ELISA, Flow cytometry, Overexpression, Visualization

1 Introduction

The systemic renin angiotensin system (RAS) basically depends upon its rate-limiting enzyme renin which is produced in the juxtaglomerular (JG) apparatus of the kidney and is released under conditions of intravascular volume contraction, reduced arterial pressure, and hypokalemia. Renin released from the JG apparatus acts on angiotensinogen (synthesized by the liver) to generate the decapeptide angiotensin I which is converted to angiotensin II by ACE. Angiotensin II promotes vasoconstriction and stimulation of the adrenal cortex to restore intravascular volume and arterial pressure through its intrinsic negative feedback mechanism.

Independently of the canonic RAS, there is substantial evidence that local RAS is present in different tissues including the heart [1] and that components of the renin angiotensin system are taken up by different tissues [2] thereby influencing the synthesis of Ang II locally. Previous studies performed in pigs, indicated that as much as 75% of cardiac Ang II is synthesized at tissue sites [3]. Ang II and type 1 (AT1) and type 2 (AT2) receptors, for instance, are rapidly internalized contributing to the downregulation of renin expression in cardiomyocytes.

Rhian M. Touyz and Ernesto L. Schiffrin (eds.), *Hypertension: Methods and Protocols*, Methods in Molecular Biology, vol. 1527, DOI 10.1007/978-1-4939-6625-7_10, © Springer Science+Business Media LLC 2017

Mazzolai et al. [4] generated various transgenic mouse lines overexpressing angiotensinogen in the heart. In this reliable model, ventricular hypertrophy was developed while no change in blood pressure was seen. The ventricular hypertrophy generated was abolished by ACE inhibitors or AT1 blockers providing support to the view that there is a local cardiac renin angiotensin system. In further studies performed in patients with heart failure (HF) (New York Heart Association [NYHA] classes I through IV) and in 15 control subjects [5], several components of the RAS were found and angiotensinogen and ACE mRNA levels were increased. Moreover, Ang II was immunohistochemically detectable both on myocytes and interstitial cells. Furthermore, cardiac angiotensin levels increased with progression of heart failure [5].

Other studies showed that the intracellular administration of angiotensin II in isolated cardiomyocytes showed a decline in cell communication [6] and a significance change of inward calcium current [7]. Despite these findings, several molecular aspects of the role of angiotensin II on heart function during hypertension need further investigation. In this chapter, we are providing the methods and materials necessary for further investigation of this important topic including isolation of cardiomyocytes, enzyme immunoassay for measuring intracellular Ang II, HPLC-chip/mass spectrometric analysis of intracellular Ang II, and how overexpression of Ang II influences cardiac cell function.

2 Materials for the Experiment

2.1 Materials for Isolation Cardiomyocytes

1. Normal Krebs solution containing (mM)—136.5 NaCl, 5.4 KCl, 1.8 $CaCl_2$, 0.53 $MgCl_2$, 0.3 NaH_2PO_4, 11.9 $NaHCO_3$, 5.5 glucose, and 5 HEPES, with pH adjusted to 7.3.
2. Collagenase (0.4%) diluted in Ca^{2+}-free Krebs solution (Worthington Biochemicals).
3. Recovery solution (mM): taurine 10, oxalic acid 70, glutamic acid 25, KCl 10, KH_2PO_4, 11 glucose, and 0.5 EGTA, with pH adjusted to 7.4.
4. The discontinuous gradient of Percoll (Sigma) consisting of 40.5 and 58.5% will be prepared in the balanced salt solution (116 mM NaCl, 20 mM HEPES, 12.5 mM NaH_2PO_4, 5.6 mM glucose, 5.4 mM KCl, 0.8 mM $MgSO_4$, pH 7.35).

2.2 Angiotensin II Enzyme Immunoassay Components

1. Cell lysis buffer: Prepare lysis buffer containing 50 mM Tris/hydrochloride (HCl) pH 7.5, 5 mM ethylenediaminetetraacetic acid (EDTA), 250 mM NaCl, 0.1% Triton × 100, and 1 μl of a protease inhibitor cocktail (Sigma).
2. EIA buffer 1× (Peninsula Laboratories): Dilute the EIA buffer concentrate to 1000 ml with water and mix well.

3. Ang II standard (Peninsula Laboratories): Add 1 ml of standard diluent buffer to the vial of lyophilized standard peptide (1 μg) and vortex (*see* **Note 1**).
4. Antiserum (Peninsula Laboratories): Add 5 ml of EIA buffer and vortex.
5. Biotinylated tracer (Peninsula Laboratories): Add 5 ml of EIA buffer to the vial of lyophilized biotinylated peptide and vortex.
6. Streptavidin-HRP (Peninsula Laboratories): Dilute 1/200 in EIA buffer and vortex (*see* **Note 2**).
7. TMB substrate solution (Peninsula Laboratories).
8. 2 N HCl (Peninsula Laboratories).
9. 96-well immunoplate for Ang II quantitation (Peninsula Laboratories).
10. 1 mg/ml BSA: Dissolve 10 mg of BSA (Sigma) in 10 ml. Aliquot and store at 4 °C.
11. PBS 1×.
12. 96-well microplate for total protein quantitation (Fisher).
13. Protein detection reagents (solution A and solution B, Pierce).

2.3 HPLC/Mass Spectro-validation of ELISA

1. Agarose bead-coupled monoclonal anti-Ang II antibody (Biogenesis).
2. Microton-3K filter.
3. 3% acetonitrile: Prepare 100 ml of acetonitrile (3%) containing 3 ml of acetonitrile and 97 ml of water.
4. Solvent A (water with 0.1% formic acid) and 3% solvent B (acetonitrile with 0.1% formic acid).
5. Column with 97% solvent A (water with 0.1% formic acid) and 3% solvent B (acetonitrile with 0.1% formic acid).
6. Solvent (acetonitrile with 0.1% formic acid).

2.4 Flow Cytometry Components for AT1 Receptor Expression

1. AT1 receptor antibody (Abcam): Dilute antibody 1:1000 with PBS 1×. Store at 4 °C.
2. FITC-secondary antibody (Abcam): Dilute antibody 1:200 with PBS 1×. Store at 4 °C, wrapped with aluminum foil.
3. BD Cytofix/Cytoperm solution (BD Biosciences): store at 4 °C.
4. 0.5% paraformaldehyde (Sigma): Prepare a stock of 2% paraformaldehyde (Sigma P-6148). Weigh 10.0 g paraformaldehyde and dissolve in 500 ml water at 60–70 °C (*see* **Note 3**). Adjust pH to 7.3, filter, aliquot into tubes, and freeze. To prepare working dilution of 0.5% paraformaldehyde, thaw an aliquot of 2% paraformaldehyde and dilute 1 part to 3 parts in PBS (e.g., 60 μl + 180 μl to yield 0.5% final concentration).

5. BD Falcon round-bottom polystyrene tubes 12×75 mm (Fisher 14-959-6) (*see* **Note 4**).
6. Isoton II diluent (Fisher NC9681422).
7. FITC-calibration standard medium level (Bangs Laboratories 885) (*see* **Note 5**).

2.5 Overexpression of Intracellular Ang II Components

1. Intracellular Ang II expression vector (iAngII): Prepare iAngII expression vector containing the coding sequence for the eight amino acids of Ang II according to Baker and Kumar 2006 [8] (*see* **Note 6**).
2. Control Ang II expression vector (cAngII): Prepare cAngII expression vector containing the scrambled Ang II peptide coding sequence according to Baker and Kumar 2006 [8].
3. Effectene reagent (Qiagen).
4. Enhancer (Qiagen).
5. Buffer EC (Qiagen).
6. H9c2 cardiac cells (ATCC).
7. IMDM culture medium with 10% FBS: Prepare 100 ml of Iscove's Modified Dulbecco's Medium containing 89 ml of IMDM medium (ATCC), 10 ml fetal bovine serum, and 1 ml penicillin/streptomycin solution. Filter and store at 4 °C.

2.6 Angiotensin II Endocytosis Components

1. Angiotensin II-fluorescein conjugate (Life technologies): Prepare a stock solution of 50 μM Ang II-fluorescein in buffer 50 mM potassium phosphate (pH 9). Store solution at −20 °C, protected from light (*see* **Note 7**).
2. Alexa Fluor 594-labeled transferrin (Life Technologies): Reconstitute in 1 ml of deionized water to obtain a 5 mg/ml solution in PBS 1×. Store solution at 2–6 °C, protected from light, and with the addition of sodium azide at a final concentration of 2 mM. Do not freeze the solutions.
3. DAPI (Life Technologies): Prepare a 5 mg/ml DAPI stock solution. Dissolve the contents of one vial (10 mg) in 2 ml of deionized water or dimethylformamide. For long-term storage, the stock solution can be aliquoted and stored at ≤−20 °C. For short-term storage, the solution can be kept at 2–6 °C, protected from light. DAPI solutions are stable for at least 6 months.
4. Nunc chamber slides for cell culture (Fisher 125655).

3 Methods

3.1 Isolation of Cardiomyocytes

1. Animals will be kept at the animal house on a normal laboratory diet and tap water ad libitum.

2. Cells will be obtained by enzymatic dispersion of rat ventricle after the method of Powell and Twist [9].
3. After deep anesthesia, the heart will be removed and perfused immediately with normal Krebs solution. After 20 min, a calcium-free solution containing 0.4 % collagenase (Worthington Biochemicals) will be recirculated through the heart for 1 h.
4. The collagenase solution will be washed out with 100 ml of recovery solution.
5. Ventricles and auricles will be minced (1- to 2-mm-thick slices), and the resulting solution will be agitated gently with a Pasteur pipette.
6. Suspension will be filtered through a nylon gauze and the filtrate centrifuged 4 min at 22 ×*g*.
7. Add the Percoll solution to suspension of cells. The ventricular cells will be suspended in the layer of 58.5 % Percoll.
8. After centrifugation at 900 ×*g* for 30 min at 25 °C, the cardiomyocytes selectively migrated to the interface of the discontinuous layers [10].
9. The cell pellets will be then resuspended in normal Krebs solution.

3.2 Angiotensin II Enzyme Immunoassay

1. For determination of intracellular angiotensin II concentration, resuspend isolated cardiomyocytes (1×10^6 cells) in 150–210 μl of lysis buffer and centrifuge at 20,000 ×*g* for 8–10 min at 4 °C. Collect supernatant and store at −20 °C.
2. Prepare Ang II standard curve in 1.5 ml microfuge tubes. For example:

Buffer μl (diluent)	10 ng/ml Ang II (μl)	Final [Ang II] (ng/ml)
0	500	10
375	125	2.5
468.75	31.25	0.625
492.19	7.81	0.156
498.05	1.95	0.039
499.5	0.5	0.010

3. Add 50 μl standard or sample and 25 μl antiserum (in EIA buffer) into each well of the immunoplate for angiotensin II quantitation.
4. Add also 50 μl diluent and 25 μl EIA buffer to blank wells and incubate the plate at room temperature for 1 h.

5. Add 25 μl/well of rehydrated biotinylated tracer and incubate at room temperature for 2 h.
6. Wash immunoplate five times with 200 μl/well of EIA buffer using a multichannel pipette (*see* **Note 8**).
7. Add 100 μl/well of streptavidin-HRP and incubate at room temperature for 1 h (*see* **Note 9**).
8. Wash immunoplate five times with EIA buffer.
9. Add 100 μl/well of TMB solution to all wells, including the blank, and incubate at room temperature for 30 min (*see* **Note 10**).
10. Add 100 μl 2 N HCl to each well to terminate the reaction.
11. Read absorbance at 450 nm within 10 min.
12. Plot a standard curve on a semilog scale and calculate the unknown concentrations (*see* **Note 11**).
13. Quantify the intracellular total protein content using the BCA protein assay reagents, solutions A and B.
14. Prepare a solution of 1 mg/ml BSA in the buffer which the protein samples to be assayed and stored in.
15. Prepare BSA dilutions ranging from 1 to 1000 μg/ml final BSA concentration. Use 1× PBS as diluent.
16. Pipette 10 μl of each BSA concentration in duplicate into a microplate.
17. Pipette samples, diluting if necessary, using a total of 10 μl/well. Do in duplicate if enough sample can be spared.
18. Prepare reagent for detection by mixing 50 parts of solution A with 1 part of solution B.
19. Pipette 200 μl reagent into each sample-containing well, and incubate at 37 °C for 30 min or at room temperature for 2 h.
20. Meanwhile, warm up plate reader (15 min) and enter settings for analysis. Select 555 nm filter for the BCA.
21. Insert plate into reader, read samples, and print out data.
22. Plot a standard curve of absorbance vs. concentration to calculate the unknown sample concentrations.

3.3 HPLC-Chip/Mass Spectrometric Analysis

1. To validate the results of ELISA, Ang II content in cell lysates will be analyzed by tandem mass spectrometry (MS).
2. Ang II will be immunoprecipitated using an agarose bead-coupled monoclonal anti-Ang II antibody (Biogenesis), and coeluting proteins will be removed by passage through a Microcon-3K filter.
3. Samples will be dried in a Speedvac and redissolved in 3% acetonitrile _ 0.1% trifluoroacetic acid. A 0.1-_l aliquot of each sample will be injected into an ion trap mass spectrometer

(1100 series HPLC-Chip-LC/MSD Trap XCT Ultra, Agilent Technologies).

4. Peptides will be loaded onto the enrichment column with 97% solvent A (water with 0.1 % formic acid) and 3 % solvent B (acetonitrile with 0.1 % formic acid) at 4 ml/min.
5. Elution will be performed with a gradient of solvent B (3–80 % in 7 min) at a flow rate of 0.3 ml/min.
6. Data-dependent MS/MS analysis will be performed on the six most intense peaks in each full-scan spectrum, as reported previously [11].
7. Spectrum Mill Server software (revision A.03.02) will be used to search tandem MS spectra against a custom peptide database that contained angiotensin peptides [11].

3.4 Flow Cytometry Quantification of Membrane-Bound and Intracellular AT1 Receptor Expression

1. For determination of membrane-bound angiotensin type 1 receptors, resuspend isolated cardiomyocytes (1×10^6 cells) in 100 μl of PBS, and then incubate with an anti-angiotensin type I receptor primary antibody (1:1000) solution for 1 h at 4 °C.
2. Wash the cells two times with PBS (1×) by allowing cells to settle down, and then incubate with FITC-secondary antibody (1:200) solution for 1 h at 4 °C.
3. Wash the cells two times with PBS (1×) and then fix with 0.5 % paraformaldehyde.
4. Analyze the samples using a flow cytometer equipped with a 488 nm laser and quantify using specific FITC-calibration standards (*see* **Note 12**).
5. For determination of intracellular AT1 receptors, resuspend isolated cardiomyocytes (1×10^6 cells) in 300 μl BD Cytofix\Cytoperm solution for 20 min at 4 °C (*see* **Note 13**).
6. Incubate the cells then incubated with anti-angiotensin type I receptor primary antibody (1:1000) solution for 1 h at 4 °C.
7. Repeat **step 2**.
8. Analyze the samples by flow cytometry and determine the MESF units of each unknown sample using the FITC standards and QuickCal® software (BD Biosciences) (*see* **Note 14**).

3.5 Overexpression of Intracellular Ang II in Cardiac Cells

1. The day before transfection, culture H9c2 cardiac cells in small flasks at a density of 2.5×10^4 cells in 5 ml of growth medium at 37 °C and 5 % CO_2 until they reach 70 % confluence.
2. The day of transfection, dilute 3 μg of plasmid containing the cytomegalovirus (CMV) promoter driving expression of angiotensin II dissolved in TE buffer, pH 7 to pH 8 (minimum DNA concentration: 0.1 μg/μl) with the DNA-condensation buffer, buffer EC, to a total volume of 150 μl. Add 24 μl enhancer and mix by vortexing for 1 s (*see* **Note 15**).

3. Incubate at room temperature for 2–5 min and then add 25 μl Effectene reagent to the DNA-enhancer mixture. Mix by pipetting up and down five times.
4. Incubate the samples for 5–10 min at room temperature (15–25 °C) to allow transfection-complex formation.
5. Add 1 ml growth medium (can contain serum and antibiotics) to the tube containing the transfection complexes. Mix by pipetting up and down twice, and immediately add the transfection complexes dropwise onto the cells with fresh growth medium. Gently swirl the dish to ensure uniform distribution of the transfection complexes.
6. Incubate for 48 h to allow for gene expression (*see* **Note 16**).
7. For transient transfections, cells transfected are typically incubated for 24–48 h post-transfection to obtain maximal levels of gene expression. For stable transfections, passage cells to the appropriate selective medium 48 h after transfection. Maintain cells in selective medium until colonies appear (*see* **Note 17**).

3.6 Angiotensin II Endocytosis Visualization

1. Culture isolated cardiomyocytes or H9c2 cardiac cells in Nunc chamber slides with 1 ml growth medium until they reach 70% confluence.
2. Incubate cells for 30 min with 1 μM Ang II-fluorescein conjugate, 15 nM Texas-Red transferring to visualize endosomal trafficking, and 500 ng/ml 4,6-diamidino-2-phenylindole (DAPI, blue) to stain nucleus.
3. Wash two times with PBS 1×.
4. Visualize fluorescence of each color by confocal laser scanning microscopy using a Zeiss Axioscope microscope (Carl Zeiss Microimaging, Thornwood, NY) and an objective with a magnitude of 63×. Merge images to visualize Ang II co-localization.

4 Notes

1. If samples are to be extracted and resuspended in EIA buffer, use EIA buffer as a diluent. Otherwise, use your own diluent such that standards and samples will be treated equally.
2. Tap or centrifuge the SA-HRP vial to collect all liquid contents on the bottom of the vial.
3. Weigh 10.0 g PFA in fume hood. Dissolve in 475 ml distilled water in 60–70 °C water bath on hot plate in fume hood. Do not allow water bath to go over 70 °C (formaldehyde will vaporize!). While dissolving, label 100×4 ml and 7×12 ml tubes (or other combinations of useful aliquots) with 2% PFA and the date. After 1 h add one or two drops of 5 M

NaOH. Cloudy suspension will then turn clear. Allow to cool to room temperature. Add 25 ml 20× PBS and adjust pH to 7.3. Filter, aliquot into tubes, and freeze. Aliquots are good for at least 5 years.

4. Use tubes with cap if necessary.
5. Use low-, medium-, or high-level standards depending on the fluorescence intensity of your samples with antibodies. Do not use a set of standards far from the fluorescence intensity of your unknown samples.
6. The iAng II expression cassette (pcDNA/TO-iAng II) was similar to that which has been previously described for adenoviral expression of iAng II [12]. Briefly, two complimentary oligonucleotides containing the coding sequence for the eight amino acids of Ang II, start and stop codons, flanked by BamHI and XbaI sites (sense strand: 5′-GATCCATGGACCGCGT ATACATCCACCCCTTTTAAT-3′), were annealed and cloned into the pcDNA4/TO vector (Invitrogen). The coding sequence was flanked on the 5′-side by a complete cytomegalovirus enhancer-promoter sequence, containing two copies of the tetracycline operator TetO 2 sequence, and by a 225 bp bovine growth hormone polyadenylation sequence on the 3′-side. A control vector was similarly generated, containing the scrambled Ang II peptide coding sequence (sense strand: 5′-GATCCATGTACGACCACCGCGTATTTCCCATCT AG-3′).
7. It is a good practice to centrifuge the protein conjugate solution briefly in a microcentrifuge before use; only the supernatant should then be added to the experiment. This step will eliminate any protein aggregates that may have formed in solution, thereby reducing nonspecific background staining.
8. Be very careful not to cross contaminate between wells in the first wash/dispensing cycle. In each wash cycle, empty plate contents with a rapid flicking motion of the wrist, then gently blot dry the top of plate on paper towels. Dispense 300 μl of EIA buffer into each well and gently shake for at least a few seconds. Thorough washing is essential.
9. Tap or centrifuge the streptavidin-HRP vial to collect all liquid contents in the bottom of the vial. Dilute 1/200 in EIA buffer and vortex. Add 100 μl to all wells including blanks.
10. In this step, you may read the developing blue color at 650 nm and use the data for your calculations.
11. Use the y axis for the average of the OD readings (minus the blank average) and the *x* axis for the standard concentrations in ng/ml. Use the "constant" y intercept and "x coefficient" (slope) from the regression output to calculate Ang II concentration of the unknown samples.

12. Do not forget to run an unstained sample of cells to determine the background. FITC emission is measured in the FL1 channel (band-pass filter 530/30 nm). Data on scatter parameters and histograms are acquired in log mode. At least, count twenty thousand events for each sample.
13. BD Cytofix/Cytoperm solution can be used for the simultaneous fixation and permeabilization of cells prior to intracellular staining [12].
14. Obtain the median peak channel of each sample and FITC standards from the flow cytometric histograms data. Subtract the background on each stained sample using the median peak value detected from the autofluorescence of unstained cells. Enter the corresponding median peak channel number of the FITC standards into the QuickCal® program (Bangs Laboratories) to generate a calibration plot of MESF vs. median peak channel. Determine the MESF units of each unknown sample using the FITC standard calibration plot.
15. Always keep the ratio of DNA to enhancer constant. Plasmid DNA quality strongly influences efficiency, reproducibility, and toxicity. Use plasmid DNA of the highest purity.
16. If cytotoxicity is observed, remove the Effectene-DNA complexes after 6–18 h, wash the cells once with PBS, and add 5 ml fresh growth medium.
17. It is highly recommended to establish a kill curve (dose-response curve) with each combination of cell line and antibiotic used.

References

1. De Mello WC, Frohlich ED (2011) On the local cardiac renin angiotensin system. Basic and clinical implications. Peptides 32(8):1774–1779, Epub 2011 Jun 25
2. Kurdi M, De Mello WC, Booz GW (2005) Working outside the system: an update on the unconventional behavior of the renin-angiotensin system components. Int J Biochem Cell Biol 37(7):1357–1367
3. van Kats JP, Danser AH, van Meegen JR, Sassen LM, Verdouw PD, Schalekamp MA (1998) Angiotensin production by the heart: a quantitative study in pigs with the use of radiolabeled angiotensin infusions. Circulation 98(1):73–81
4. Mazzolai L, Nussberger J, Aubert JF, Brunner DB, Gabbiani G, Brunner HR, Pedrazzini T (1998) Blood pressure-independent cardiac hypertrophy induced by locally activated renin-angiotensin system. Hypertension 31(6):1324–1330
5. Serneri GG, Boddi M, Cecioni I, Vanni S, Coppo M, Papa ML, Bandinelli B, Bertolozzi I, Polidori G, Toscano T, Maccherini M, Modesti PA (2001) Cardiac angiotensin II formation in the clinical course of heart failure and its relationship with left ventricular function. Circ Res 88(9):961–968
6. De Mello WC (1996) Renin-angiotensin system and cell communication in the failing heart. Hypertension 27(6):1267–1272
7. De Mello WC (1998) Intracellular angiotensin II regulates the inward calcium current in cardiac myocytes. Hypertension 32(6):976–982
8. Baker KM, Kumar R (2006) Intracellular angiotensin II induces cell proliferation independent of AT1 receptor. Am J Physiol Cell Physiol 291:C995–C1001
9. Powell T, Twist VW (1976) A rapid technique for the isolation and purification of adult cardiac muscle cells having respiratory control

and a tolerance to calcium. Biochem Biophys Res Commun 72(1):327–333

10. Harada M, Itoh H, Nakagawa O, Ogawa Y et al (1997) Significance of ventricular myocytes and nonmyocytes during cardiac hypertrophy: evidence for endothelin-1 as a paracrine hypertrophic factor from cardiac nonmyocytes. Circulation 96: 3737–3744
11. Singh VP, Le B, Bhat VB, Baker KM, Kumar R (2007) High-glucose-induced regulation of intracellular ANG II synthesis and nuclear redistribution in cardiac myocytes. Am J Physiol Heart Circ Physiol 293:H939–H948
12. Prussin C, Metcalfe DD (1995) Detection of intracellular cytokine using flow cytometry and directly conjugated anti-cytokine antibodies. J Immunol 188:117–128

Chapter 11

Analysis of the Aldosterone Synthase (*CYP11B2*) and 11β-Hydroxylase (*CYP11B1*) Genes

Scott M. MacKenzie, Eleanor Davies, and Samantha Alvarez-Madrazo

Abstract

The aldosterone synthase (CYP11B2) and 11β-hydroxylase (CYP11B1) enzymes are known to be important players in the development of hypertension. Sequencing of the *CYP11B2* and *CYP11B1* genes and quantification of their respective mRNAs is greatly complicated by their high degree of sequence similarity. The need to ensure gene specificity during such analysis has required the development of particular methods for the detection of key polymorphisms at these loci, which are detailed in this chapter.

Key words Aldosterone synthase, 11β-Hydroxylase, *CYP11B1*, *CYP11B2*, Polymorphisms, Genotyping, PCR, RT-PCR

1 Introduction

The enzymes responsible for the terminal stages of aldosterone and cortisol production are encoded by the *CYP11B2* and *CYP11B1* genes. The human *CYP11B1* and *CYP11B2* genes are located in tandem on chromosome 8 and share 90–95 % sequence identity in their coding regions and introns. These genes, their enzyme products, and the steroids they produce have each been implicated in the pathogenesis of hypertension and other cardiovascular disorders, and therefore, robust methodology is required to adequately differentiate between the two genes. The high degree of sequence identity between the two genes presents unique challenges for researchers who wish to genotype or measure expression levels as specific amplification is difficult and many high-throughput methodologies are therefore not appropriate. Here we describe our rigorous protocols for genotyping the *CYP11B1* and *CYP11B2* genes for common polymorphisms, which we have used extensively in our studies [1, 2]. We also provide a protocol for monitoring expression of these genes through specific real-time RT-PCR quantitation of *CYP11B1* and *CYP11B2* mRNA.

Rhian M. Touyz and Ernesto L. Schiffrin (eds.), *Hypertension: Methods and Protocols*, Methods in Molecular Biology, vol. 1527, DOI 10.1007/978-1-4939-6625-7_11, © Springer Science+Business Media LLC 2017

2 Materials

2.1 Genotyping of CYP11B2 rs1799998 (-344 C/T) SNP

2.1.1 PCR of Genomic DNA

1. dNTP mix: To 960 μl of Nuclease-Free (NF) water, add 10 μl of each of the four stock dNTPs (Promega) for a final concentration of 200 μM.
2. Mastermix for a 96-well plate: mix 250 μl of Thermo-Start buffer (10×; ABGene, Surrey UK), 150 μl of $MgCl_2$ (25 mM), 500 μl of the aforementioned dNTP mix, 25 μl of Thermo-Start DNA Polymerase (1.25 U/reaction), 130 μl SF1F primer (10 μM), 130 μl SF1R primer (10 μM; Table 1), and 815 μl of NF water. The total volume of the mastermix is 2000 μl.
3. Genomic DNA at a concentration of 5 ng/μl.

2.1.2 Determination of PCR Product

1. Tris Borate EDTA (TBE) buffer (Fisher Scientific, UK). Prepare 1 l by diluting stock buffer 1:10 with distilled water. It can be stored at room temperature.
2. 1% agarose gel: Weigh 1 g of agarose and add to 100 ml of TBE buffer. Heat in a 950 W microwave oven for 1 min at full power until the solution is clear and agarose melted.
3. Ethidium bromide solution. Store in the fume hood (*see* **Note 1**).
4. 1 kb DNA ladder (Promega).
5. Loading dye: Weigh 12.5 mg of bromophenol blue and 12.5 mg of xylene cyanol into a tube and add 35 ml of water.

Table 1
Primer sequences

Primer	Method	Sequence 5′–3′
SF1F	PCR & sequencing	GTG TCA GGG CAG GGG GTA
SF1R	PCR	AGG CGT GGG GTC TGG ACT
ICTAQMANF	PCR	GAT GGC ATG AAG CAC AAA GCT
ICTAQMANR	PCR	CCT TGG GCG ACA GCA CA
B1 5′UTR	PCR	TCC TTC GCA TCC CTT GTA AGT T
B1Prom260	PCR	CTT GGA TTA TTC ATC TCC TTG CAA GG
B1 5′7-32	PCR	GCA TCC CTT GTA AGT TGG ATT CCT AA
B1 369-393	PCR	AAG CAT TCC CTT TGA AAA CTG GTA C
INTCONR(B1B2)	Sequencing	GTG TTC GAG CTG CAG CCT TTT C
B1PROM 250-229AS	Sequencing	AAG TCA AAT TGT CTC TGT TTG

Weigh 7.5 g of Ficoll (*see* **Note 2**) and add little by little to the solution previously prepared. Let it soak slowly and do not agitate vigorously, as lumps can be formed. Top up the volume to 50 ml with water and vortex the solution once all the Ficoll has dissolved.

2.1.3 PCR Product Cleanup

1. AMPure (Agencourt, USA): vortex before using in order to resuspend the magnetic beads.
2. 70% ethanol: In a container mix 35 ml of 100% ethanol with 15 ml NF water.
3. NF water.
4. 96-well SPRI (solid phase reversible immobilization) magnet (Agencourt, USA).

2.1.4 Direct Sequencing

1. ABI PRISM BigDye v3.1 Sequencing Buffer.
2. ABI PRISM BigDye Termination v3.1 Ready Reaction Mix.
3. Sequencing reaction mix (for a 96-well plate): Mix 500 μl NF water, 350 μl ABI PRISM BigDye v3.1 Sequencing Buffer (5×), 100 μl of sequencing primer (i.e., SF1F primer at 3.2 pmol/μl stock concentration; Table 1), and 50 μl of ABI PRISM BigDye Termination v3.1 Ready Reaction Mix.

2.1.5 Sequencing Product Cleanup

1. CLEANSEQ (Agencourt, USA).
2. 85% ethanol: Mix 34 ml of 100% ethanol with 6 ml of NF water.
3. NF water.

2.1.6 Sequencing Hardware and Software

1. 3730 DNA Analyzer (ABI, USA).
2. SeqScape software (version 2.1.1).

2.2 Genotyping of CYP11B2 Intron Conversion Polymorphism

2.2.1 PCR of Genomic DNA

1. dNTP mix: To 960 μl of nuclease-free (NF) water, add 10 μl of each of the four stock dNTPs (Promega) for a final concentration of 200 μM.
2. Mastermix for a 96-well plate: mix 250 μl of Thermo-Start buffer (10×; ABGene, Surrey UK), 200 μl of $MgCl_2$ (25 mM), 500 μl of the aforementioned dNTP mix, 12.5 μl of Thermo-Start DNA Polymerase (0.625 U/reaction), 50 μl ICTAQMANF primer (10 μM), 50 μl ICTAQMANR primer (10 μM; Table 1), and 437.5 μl of NF water. The total volume of the mastermix is 1500 μl.
3. Genomic DNA at a concentration of 5 ng/μl.

2.3 Genotyping of CYP11B1 rs142570922 (-1889 A/C) and rs149845727 (-1859 C/T) SNPS

2.3.1 PCR of Genomic DNA

1st PCR reaction

1. dNTP mix: To 960 μl of nuclease-free (NF) water, add 10 μl of each of the four stock dNTPs (Promega) for a final concentration of 200 μM.
2. Mastermix for a 96-well plate: mix 250 μl of Thermo-Start buffer (10×; ABGene, Surrey UK), 150 μl of $MgCl_2$ (25 mM), 500 μl of the aforementioned dNTP mix, 25 μl of Thermo-Start DNA Polymerase (1.25 U/reaction), 100 μl B1 5′UTR primer (10 μM), 100 μl B1prom-260 primer (10 μM; Table 1), and 875 μl of NF water. The total volume of the mastermix is 2000 μl.
3. Genomic DNA at a concentration of 5 ng/μl.

2nd PCR reaction

1. dNTP mix: To 960 μl of nuclease-free (NF) water, add 10 μl of each of the four stock dNTPs (Promega) for a final concentration of 200 μM.
2. Mastermix for a 96-well plate: mix 250 μl of Thermo-Start buffer (10×; ABGene, Surrey UK), 150 μl of $MgCl_2$ (25 mM), 500 μl of the aforementioned dNTP mix, 12.5 μl of Thermo-Start DNA Polymerase (0.625 U/reaction), 100 μl B1 5′7-32 primer (10 μM), 100 μl B1 369–393 primer (10 μM; Table 1), and 1287.5 μl of NF water. The total volume of the mastermix is 2400 μl.

2.4 Quantification of CYP11B1 and CYP11B2 Gene Expression

2.4.1 RT-PCR

1. ImProm-II Reverse Transcription System (Promega, Madison, Wisconsin, USA).

2.4.2 Quantitative RT-PCR

1. ABsolute QPCR ROX Mix (ABgene, Epsom, UK).
2. ABI 7900 HT Prism Sequence Detection System (Applied Biosystems, Foster City, CA, USA).
3. Custom Primers (Eurofins MWG Operon, Ebersberg, Germany).
4. Oligonucleotide Probes (Universal Human Probe Library (UPL, Roche Diagnostics, Burgess Hill, UK; Table 2).

3 Methods

3.1 Genotyping of CYP11B2 rs1799998 (-344 C/T) SNP

This protocol enables the amplification and sequencing of a 232 bp fragment located in the 5′ region of the *CYP11B2* gene. The primers used for the PCR reaction and sequencing are shown in Table 1.

Table 2
Primer sequences for RT-PCR

Gene	Sequence primer 5′–3′	UPL probe
CYP11B2	(F) GCACCTGCACCTGGAGATG (R) CACACACCATGCGTGGTCC	#57
CYP11B1	(F) ACTAGGGCCCATTTTCAGGT (R) GGCAGCATCACACACACC	#68
β-ACTIN	(F) CCA ACC GCG AGA AGA TGA (R) CCA GAG GCG TAC AGG GAT AG	#64

3.1.1 PCR of Genomic DNA

Prepare and store dNTP mix and mastermix on ice. Genomic DNA can be kept at room temperature for short periods during preparation.

1. In a 96-well plate, add 20 μl of the mastermix to each well.
2. To each well, add 5 μl of genomic DNA.
3. Seal the plate.
4. Perform the amplification reaction with the cycling parameters as follows:

Program	
1. 94 °C	15 min
2. 94 °C	30 s
3. 68 °C	30 s
4. 72 °C	1 min
5. Cycle to **step 2** for 29 more times	
6. 72 °C	7 min
7. Incubate at 10 °C forever	

5. Once the amplification reaction has finished the product can be stored at 4 °C.

3.1.2 Determination of PCR Product

Steps 1–5 are performed in the fume hood

1. Assemble the gel-casting tray and comb.
2. Add 1 μl of ethidium bromide solution to the 1 % agarose gel. Swirl with a pipette tip to mix.
3. Pour agarose solution into the gel-casting tray. Remove any bubbles with the aid of a pipette tip.
4. Leave to set for approximately 30 min.

5. Once set, transfer to the electrophoresis chamber and remove the comb. Check that the TBE buffer is covering the gel.
6. Transfer 10 μl of PCR reaction to a clean 96-well plate and add 5 μl of loading dye to each sample.
7. Load 5 μl of 1 kb DNA ladder to the first well of the gel. Load samples mixed with the loading dye in the remaining wells. Avoid air bubbles in the pipette tip as these cause the sample to be displaced from the well, contaminating adjacent wells.
8. Electrophorese at a constant voltage of 90 V for 30 min.
9. Remove gel carefully from the tank.
10. Visualize the DNA under UV light. The expected length of the PCR fragment is 232 bp, verifiable by comparison with the DNA ladder.

3.1.3 PCR Product Cleanup

The AMPure purification method is used to remove PCR reagents from PCR product prior to the sequencing reaction. Alternative PCR product cleanup methodology can be used.

1. Carefully remove the PCR plate seal.
2. To each 25 μl PCR reaction, add 36 μl of AMPure.
3. Seal the plate again, vortex, and centrifuge at 210 × *g* for 30 s.
4. Leave the plate for 3 min at room temperature, then place it on the 96-well SPRI (solid phase reversible immobilization) magnet for 10 min.
5. While still on the magnet, wrap the plate in tissue and invert it to remove supernatant. This step can be repeated until there is no supernatant left.
6. Add 150 μl of freshly prepared 70% ethanol to each well.
7. Incubate for 30 s at room temperature.
8. Discard ethanol by wrapping the plate in tissue and inverting it, as before.
9. Centrifuge the plate, inverted and on tissue, at 76 × *g* for 30 s.
10. Remove the plate from the magnet and air-dry at room temperature for at least 20 min. Elute the sample by adding 40 μl of NF water to each well.
11. Vortex and centrifuge the plate at 210 × *g* for 30 s.
12. Place the plate on the magnet for 5 min. Transfer 10 μl of the clear PCR product to a clean plate for the sequencing reaction (*see* **Note 3**).

3.1.4 Direct Sequencing

Keep all reagents on ice.

1. In a 96-well plate, add 10 μl of the sequencing reaction mix.
2. Then transfer, with a multichannel pipette, 10 μl of the clear PCR product obtained from the PCR product cleanup.

3. Subject the plate to the following conditions:

Program
1. Incubate at 96 °C for 45 s
2. Incubate at 50 °C for 25 s
3. Incubate at 60 °C for 4 min
4. Cycle to **step 1** for 24 more times
5. Incubate at 12 °C for 5 min

3.1.5 Sequencing Product Cleanup

1. Carefully remove the seal from the PCR plate.
2. To a 20 μl sequencing reaction, add 10 μl of CLEANSEQ to each well, followed by 62 μl of freshly prepared 85 % ethanol.
3. Seal the plate again, vortex, and centrifuge at 210 × *g* for 30 s.
4. Place the plate on an SPRI magnet for 5 min.
5. While still on the magnet, once the solution is clear, remove seal, wrap the plate in tissue and invert it to remove supernatant. This step can be repeated until there is no supernatant left.
6. Add 150 μl of freshly prepared 85 % ethanol to each well.
7. Incubate for 30 s at room temperature.
8. Discard ethanol by wrapping plate in tissue and inverting it.
9. Centrifuge the plate, inverted and on tissue, at 76 × *g* for 30 s.
10. Remove the plate from the magnet and air-dry at room temperature for at least 20 min. Elute the sample by adding 40 μl of NF water.
11. Vortex and centrifuge at 210 × *g* for 30 s. Place the plate on the magnet for 5 min. Transfer 20 μl of cleaned sequence product to a barcoded plate (*see* **Note 4**).
12. DNA sequences can be analyzed using a 3730 DNA Analyzer and visualized using SeqScape software.

3.2 Genotyping of CYP11B2 Intron Conversion Polymorphism

This is the amplification and sequencing of a 600 bp fragment located in intron 2 of *CYP11B2*, encompassing the Intron2 polymorphism. This polymorphism is called on the basis of the sequence in positions 143996983-82 (according to Genome Build Assembly GRCh37p5, Genome Build 37.3 reference assembly). Wild-type individuals homozygous for this polymorphism (intron 2 of *CYP11B2*) have only T and G at these positions. Those homozygous for the conversion (presence of intron 2 of *CYP11B1*) are characterized by two C alleles at these positions, while T and G alleles in one strand and two C alleles on the other correspond to heterozygotes.

3.2.1 PCR of Genomic DNA

Prepare and store the dNTP mix and mastermix on ice. Genomic DNA can be kept at room temperature for short periods during sample preparation.

1. To a 96-well plate, add 15 μl of the mastermix.
2. Add to each well 10 μl of genomic DNA.
3. Seal the plate.
4. Perform the amplification reaction with the cycling parameters as follows:
   Program:

1. 95 °C	15 min
2. 95 °C	15 s
3. 62 °C	30 s
4. 72 °C	2 min
5. Cycle to **step 2** for 44 more times	
6. 72 °C	7 min

3.2.2 Determination of PCR Product

The same steps as for rs1799998(-344 C/T) are followed. The expected length of the PCR fragment is 600 bp.

Clean up the products using AMPure, as described previously, then transfer 10 μl of the cleaned PCR product to a new 96-well plate. Sequencing reactions are performed as in the previous section, with the sequencing primer INTCONR(B1B2) (for more details, *see* Table 1). The reaction is performed with the following conditions:

Program
1. Incubate at 96 °C for 45 s
2. Incubate at 60 °C for 4 min
3. Cycle to **step 1** for 24 more times
4. Incubate at 10 °C forever

Clean up the products using CLEANSEQ, as described in the previous section. DNA sequences can be analyzed as before.

3.3 Genotyping of CYP11B1 rs142570922 (-1889 A/C) and rs149845727 (-1859 C/T) SNPs

This method uses two sequential PCRs to achieve specificity in the amplification of the *CYP11B1* promoter fragment, encompassing SNPs rs142570922 and rs149845727.

3.3.1 PCR of Genomic DNA

1st PCR reaction

Prepare and store the dNTP mix and mastermix on ice. Genomic DNA can be kept at room temperature for short periods during reaction preparation.

1. Add 20 μl of the mastermix to the wells of a 96-well plate.
2. To each well, add 5 μl of genomic DNA.
3. Seal the plate.
4. Perform the amplification reaction with the cycling parameters as follows:

Program	
1. 95 °C	15 min
2. 95 °C	30 s
3. 60 °C	30 s
4. 72 °C	3 min
5. Cycle to **step 2** for 34 more times	
6. 72 °C	7 min

5. Make a 1:10 dilution of the PCR products with NF water and use 1 μl of this as a template for the second PCR reaction.
   2nd PCR reaction

Prepare and store dNTP mix and mastermix on ice. Genomic DNA can be kept at room temperature for short periods during preparation.

1. To a 96-well plate, add 24 μl of the mastermix.
2. Add to each well 1 μl of the 1:10 dilution of the 1st PCR product.
3. Seal the plate.
4. Perform the amplification reaction with the cycling parameters as follows:

Program	
1. 95 °C	15 min
2. 95 °C	30 s
3. 60 °C	30 s
4. 72 °C	3 min
5. Cycle to **step 2** for 19 more times	
6. 72 °C	7 min

3.3.2 Determination of PCR Product

The same steps are followed as for rs1799998 (-344 C/T), the only difference being that the gel is resolved at 100 V for 40 min. The expected length of the 2nd PCR fragment is 387 bp.

Products are cleaned up using AMPure, as described previously. For sequencing, transfer 10 μl of the resulting cleaned PCR product to a new PCR plate. Sequencing reactions are performed as described in the previous section, using the sequencing primer B1PROM 259-229AS (for more details *see* Table 1). The reactions are performed using the same conditions as for the intron conversion, described in the previous section. Clean up the products using CLEANSEQ, as described in previous section. DNA sequences can be analyzed as before.

3.4 Quantification of *CYP11B1* and *CYP11B2* Gene Expression

3.4.1 RT-PCR

200 ng of total RNA is reverse transcribed to cDNA using the ImProm-II Reverse Transcription System on a 96-well plate according to the standard protocol, with a reaction volume of 20 μl. Every sample has an equivalent negative control (-RT control), omitting reverse transcriptase. For blank controls water is substituted for RNA.

Denature

Reagent	Volume per reaction (μl)
RNA	2
Random primers (0.5 μg/reaction)	1
Nuclease free water	2
Total	5

Heat to 70 °C for 5 min and then immediately chill on ice for 5 min.

Reverse transcription

Reagent	Volume per reaction (μl)	Final concentration
Nuclease free water	3.7	
ImProm-II 5× reaction buffer	4.0	
$MgCl_2$	4.8	6 mM
dNTPs	1.0	0.5 mM each dNTP
Inhibitor	0.5	20 U
RT/Water	1.0	
Total	15	

Table 3
qRT-PCR master mix

Reagent	Volume per reaction (μl)	Final concentration (nM)
Nuclease free water	2.1	
ABsolute QPCR ROX mix	5.0	
Forward primer (10 μM)	0.4	400
Reverse primer (10 μM)	0.4	400
Probe	0.1	100
Total	8	

The reverse transcription conditions are as follows:

1. 25 °C for 5 min.
2. 42 °C for 1 h.
3. 70 °C for 15 min.

The resulting cDNA sample is diluted to a final volume of 100 μL with NF water.

Store at 4 °C until required.

3.4.2 Quantitative RT-PCR

To measure levels of *CYP11B1* and *CYP11B2* mRNA, the β-actin gene (ACTINB) is used as a housekeeping gene. 8 μl of master-mix, containing ABsolute QPCR ROX Mix, is added to the well of a 384-well plate (*see* Table 3 for the reagents and volume per reaction), followed by 2 μl of each corresponding cDNA. All reactions are performed on an ABI 7900 HT Prism Sequence Detection System. The sequence of the primers and probes used from the Universal Human Probe Library are shown in Table 2 (*see* **Note 5**).

4 Notes

1. Ethidium bromide is toxic. Always use in a fume hood, while wearing gloves. Dispose of waste materials in a specified container.
2. Ficoll is very light so must be weighed in a suitable container.
3. Avoid touching the sides of the wells as this increases the risk of transferring beads and reducing the efficiency of subsequent reactions.
4. In this step, it is crucial to avoid transferring beads to the barcoded plate, as they can damage the capillaries of the sequencing apparatus.

5. The absolute specificity of primers designed to amplify coding regions of *CYP11B1* or *CYP11B2* can be verified using expression plasmids containing cDNA for either *CYP11B1* or *CYP11B2*.

References

1. Barr M, MacKenzie SM, Friel EC, Holloway CD, Wilkinson DM, Brain NJ, Ingram MC, Fraser R, Brown M, Samani NJ, Caulfield M, Munroe PB, Farrall M, Webster J, Clayton D, Dominiczak AF, Connell JM, Davies E (2007) Polymorphic variation in the 11beta-hydroxylase gene associates with reduced 11-hydroxylase efficiency. Hypertension 49(1):113–119
2. Alvarez-Madrazo S, Mackenzie SM, Davies E, Fraser R, Lee WK, Brown M, Caulfield MJ, Dominiczak AF, Farrall M, Lathrop M, Hedner T, Melander O, Munroe PB, Samani N, Stewart PM, Wahlstrand B, Webster J, Palmer CN, Padmanabhan S, Connell JM (2013) Common polymorphisms in the CYP11B1 and CYP11B2 genes: evidence for a digenic influence on hypertension. Hypertension 61(1):232–239

Chapter 12

Dopaminergic Immunofluorescence Studies in Kidney Tissue

J.J. Gildea, R.E. Van Sciver, H.E. McGrath, B.A. Kemp, P.A. Jose, R.M. Carey, and R.A. Felder

Abstract

The kidney is a highly integrated system of specialized differentiated cells that are responsible for fluid and electrolyte balance in the body. While much of today's research focuses on isolated nephron segments or cells from nephron segments grown in tissue culture, an often overlooked technique that can provide a unique view of many cell types in the kidney is slice culture. Here, we describe techniques that use freshly excised kidney tissue from rats to perform a variety of experiments shortly after isolating the tissue. By slicing the rat kidney in a "bread loaf" format, multiple studies can be performed on slices from the same tissue in parallel. Cryosectioning and staining of the tissue allow for the evaluation of physiological or biochemical responses in a wide variety of specific nephron segments. The procedures described within this chapter can also be extended to human or mouse kidney tissue.

Key words Proximal tubule, Human renal epithelial cells, Tissue staining

1 Introduction

In the last 30 years, the study of renal proximal tubule cells has proven to be important in the study of hypertension. While cell culture experiments have been used in a majority of these studies, there is debate on whether or not cell cultures accurately reflect their in vivo counterparts. Slice culture techniques using freshly excised tissue have been performed since the mid-twentieth century, when Forster studied the transport of phenol red into the tubular lumen of kidney slices [1]. The slice culture model allows for experiments on cells that maintain their in vivo configurations such as polarity and tubule shape and communication with surrounding cells. Various durations of slice viability have been reported from 11 h to over 24 h [2, 3]. Studies have also shown that human renal cortical slices that have been cryopreserved remain viable for experiments after thawing [4]. Performing experiments on cells in a slice culture format within the first 30 min of

Rhian M. Touyz and Ernesto L. Schiffrin (eds.), *Hypertension: Methods and Protocols*, Methods in Molecular Biology, vol. 1527, DOI 10.1007/978-1-4939-6625-7_12, © Springer Science+Business Media LLC 2017

their isolation allows for the study of signal transduction. However, caution must be observed in the interpretation of some physiological responses because slicing can stimulate tissue deterioration. For example, one study highlights deterioration of brush border membrane following 15-min incubation [5]. Slice culture allows the researcher to study kidneys in animals exposed to dietary variations, such as high or low salt, high or low fat diets, etc. Slice culture also allows a unique opportunity to study tissues from the same animal before and after an induced disease. For example, this can be accomplished by performing a uninephrectomy on a spontaneously hypertensive rat (SHR) before the development of hypertension. The other kidney could then be removed and studied following the onset of hypertension. Inherent in the technique itself, immunofluorescent staining of precision-cut renal slices allows the study of multiple sections of the kidney as well as multiple nephron segments in the same tissue. In the following experiments, we validated in vivo translocation events with slice culture and compared them with control/vehicle-treated slices.

A rat kidney slice culture experiment is depicted in Fig. 1. In this example, freshly isolated rat kidneys are precision cut, placed in temperature and CO_2 pre-equilibrated media, and then incubated with the D_1-like receptor agonist fenoldopam (FEN, 1 μmol/L), with and without the D_1-like receptor antagonist 6,7,8,9,14,15-hexahydro-7-methyl-5*H*-indolo[3,2-*f*][3]benzazecine (LE300, 1 μmol/L). Using immunofluorescent microscopy, a 30-min FEN incubation led to a dramatic decrease in angiotensin type-1 receptor (AT_1R) abundance, which is partially blocked when LE300 is added just prior to FEN. This result has been shown previously in cultured human [6, 7] and rat [8] proximal tubule cells, as well as in mouse kidney [7], but not using rat slice culture. Also shown in Fig. 1 is the dramatic change in localization of the AT_1R when incubated with angiotensin II (Ang II). In vehicle-treated slices, AT_1R localizes to both the apical brush border membrane and cytoplasm but Ang II dramatically alters the staining to a punctate vesicular pattern. This change in localization is partially blocked when the AT_1R antagonist losartan (LOS, 1 μmol/L) is added just prior to Ang II. This effect of Ang II in renal slice culture mimics Ang II-induced AT_1R internalization and desensitization shown previously in cell culture experiments [9], but this data has not previously been shown using rat slice culture. Thus, these experiments demonstrate the utility of the slice culture technique for measuring short time-frame dopaminergic D_1-like and AT_1R cell signaling events ex vivo prior to confirmation in cell culture and in vivo experiments.

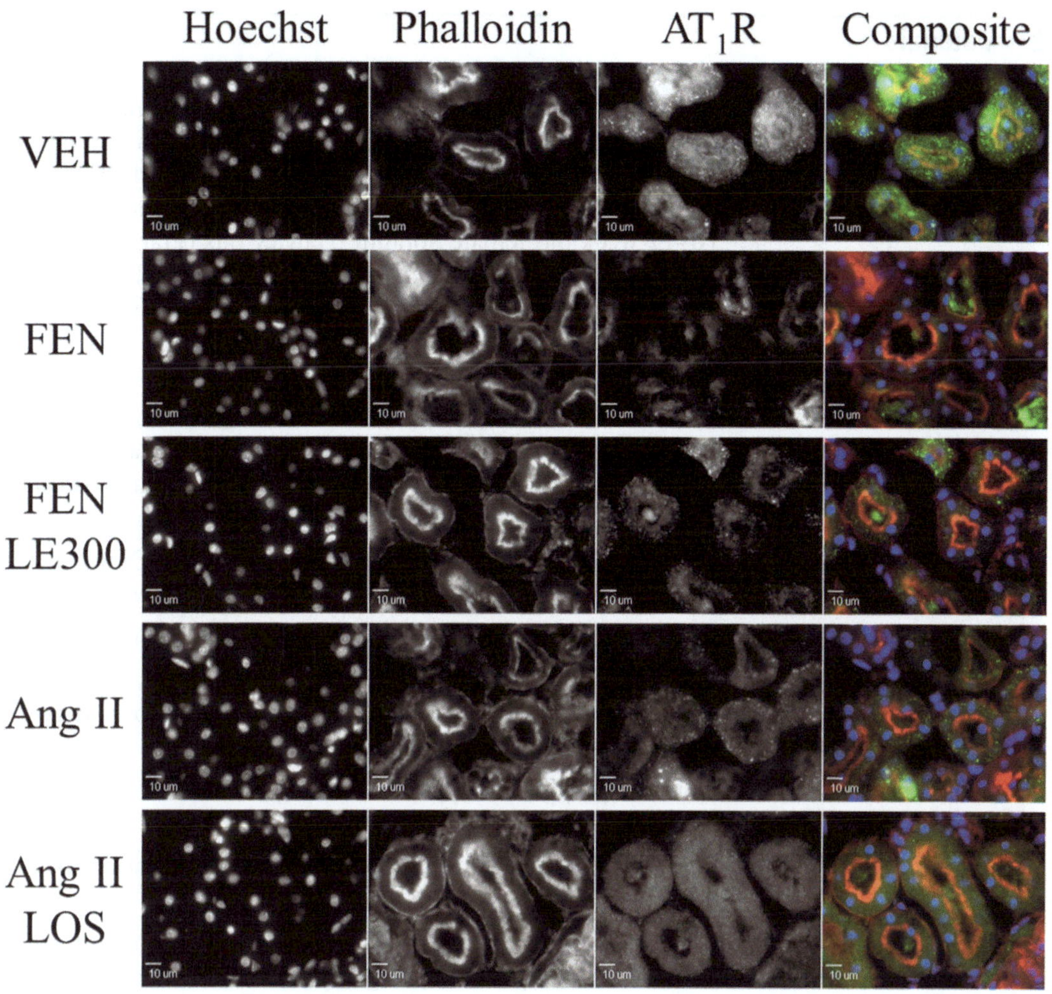

Fig. 1 Angiotensin type 1 receptor (AT_1R) immunofluorescent microscopy from rat renal slice cultures. Addition of either the D_1-like receptor agonist fenoldopam (FEN, 1 μmol/L), or the AT_1R ligand, angiotensin II (Ang II, 10 nM) causes dramatic changes in AT_1R abundance or localization, respectively. The first column on the left shows Hoechst staining, which labels nuclei. The second column is Alexa Fluor® 594 phalloidin staining, which labels the brush border membrane of the renal proximal tubule. The third column is Alexa Fluor® 647 AT_1R immunofluorescent staining. The fourth (far right) column is a composite image of all stains, pseudocolored, so that *green* is AT_1R, red is phalloidin, and blue is Hoechst. An overlap of the AT_1R stain with the phalloidin stain shows up as an orange to yellow color. 30-min incubation with FEN leads to a dramatic decrease in AT_1R abundance that is partially blocked by LE300 (1 μmol/L), a D_1-like receptor antagonist. 30-min incubation with Ang II leads to a dramatic localization change into punctate staining of intracellular vesicles; this localization is partially blocked by the AT_1R antagonist, losartan (LOS, 1 μmol/L). Magnification is at 600×, the scale bar is 10 μm

2 Materials

2.1 Animal Preparation and Kidney Isolation

1. The experimental protocols were approved by the Animal Care and Use Committee at the University of Virginia and were performed in accordance with the NIH Guide on the Care and Use of Laboratory Animals. The studies were conducted on 10–12 week old female Sprague-Dawley rats (Harlan, Teklad) that were housed in a vivarium under controlled conditions (temperature 21 ± 1 °C; humidity 60 ± 10%; light 8:00 a.m. to 8:00 p.m.). The rats were fed normal rat chow (0.3% Na^+; Harlan, Teklad).
2. Anesthesia: 0.2 mL of ketamine (Ketaset®) at a concentration of 100 mg/mL and 0.2 mL of xylazine (AnaSed®) at a concentration of 20 mg/mL are administered via an intraperitoneal (IP) injection for short-term anesthesia.
3. Petrolatum ophthalmic ointment (Paralube® Vet Ointment) is used to prevent the eyes from drying during surgery.
4. 70% Isopropyl alcohol is used for cleaning and disinfection the rat abdominal region following shaving.
5. Topical microbicide solution (Betadine®) is used for additional disinfection of the rat abdominal region following shaving.
6. Cotton tip applicators (MediChoice®) are used to isolate the kidney.
7. 2.0 Silk sutures (Deknatel® Teleflex® Medical) are used to stop renal blood flow by constricting the renal artery.
8. Rat teeth forceps, operating sharp surgical scissors, full curve hemostatic forceps, and spring loaded abdominal retractor are used during surgery (Roboz Surgical Instrument Company, Inc). Surgical instrument information (technical name, supplier if specified).
9. Opti-MEM® (Invitrogen™) at 4 °C.

2.2 Preparation of Kidney Slices

1. RPMI-1640 (Invitrogen™) is used to incubate the slices.
2. McIlwain Tissue Chopper MTC/2 (The Mickle Laboratory Engineering Co. Ltd.) is used to chop 1-mm-thick coronal sections (*see* **Note 1**).
3. Blunt curved forceps.
4. 12-Well tissue culture plate.
5. Tissue slices are incubated on a rocking platform at an oscillation of 1 Hz at an inclination of 10°.

2.3 Short-Term Tissue Incubation with Agonists and Antagonists

1. The diluent for the agonists is Dulbecco's phosphate buffered saline without calcium and magnesium (DPBS, Invitrogen™). Each is prepared at a 1000× concentration of its working dilution.

2. Fenoldopam monohydrobromide (FEN, Sigma-Aldrich®) is a D_1-like receptor agonist but cannot distinguish between the two D_1-like receptors (D_1R and D_5R). For these experiments, FEN is prepared at a concentration of 1 mmol/L for a working concentration of 1 μmol/L.
3. Angiotensin II peptide (Ang II, Sigma-Aldrich®) is the natural ligand for AT_1R. Ang II is prepared at the concentration of 10 μmol/L and subsequently diluted to approximate its renal proximal tubule fluid concentration of 10 nmol/L [10, 11].
4. The diluent for the antagonists is dimethyl sulfoxide (DMSO, Sigma-Aldrich®). Each is prepared at a 1000× concentration of its working concentration.
5. Losartan potassium (LOS, Sigma-Aldrich®) is used as an AT_1R antagonist. LOS is prepared at a concentration of 1 mmol/L with a working concentration of 1 μmol/L.
6. LE300 (Tocris Bioscience) is used as a D_1-like receptor-specific antagonist; it cannot distinguish D_1R from the other D_1-like receptor D_5R. It is prepared at a concentration of 1 mmol/L, with a working concentration of 1 μmol/L.

2.4 Tissue Fixation and Sectioning

1. Fixing of cells is achieved with 4% paraformaldehyde (Electron Microscopy Sciences) in DPBS, diluted 1:8 from 32% stock, and made fresh for each use.
2. Fixative is stopped by washing with Tris buffer (100 mmol/L Tris with an adjusted pH of 7.4).
3. OCT Compound (Tissue-Tek®) is an embedding medium for frozen tissue specimens to ensure Optimal Cutting Temperature (OCT).
4. Cryomold® standard (Tissue-Tek®) disposable vinyl specimen molds (25×20×5mm) are used for embedding the frozen tissue specimens.
5. 25×75×1.0 mm Superfrost®/Plus Microscope Slides (Fisherbrand®) are used to capture the tissue slices from the microtome.
6. A HM505E microtome cryostat (Leica Biosystems) is used to cut 8 μm slices of the fixed frozen tissue.

2.5 Permeabilization and Immunofluorescent Staining

1. ImmEdge™ pen (Vector Laboratories, Inc.) is used to draw a hydrophobic ring around the tissue slices.
2. A plastic microscope slide storage box with cover (Fisherbrand®) is used to create a humidity chamber for antibody incubations.
3. Kimwipes® (KimTech Science®) are used to maintain humidity in the slide storage box.

4. 0.2% Triton-X100 in Tris-Buffered Saline (TBS, 10 mmol/L Tris, 150 mmol/L NaCl with pH adjusted to 7.4) is used to permeabilize the tissue slices.
5. Washing of slices is done with TBS-T (TBS with 0.02% Tween).
6. Blocking solution is 2% milk in TBS-T. A 5× stock is made by dissolving 10 g of nonfat dry milk into 100 mL TBS-T, heated to 60 °C for 10 min, sonicated for 1 min, and centrifuged at 9000×g for 30 min at room temperature. This 5× stock may be frozen at −20 °C for storage. The 5× stock is diluted to a 1× working concentration to make a 2% milk blocking solution. All primary and secondary antibodies are diluted in this blocking solution.
7. The primary antibody used in these experiments is AT_1R antibody N-10 (Santa Cruz Biotechnology, Inc.), a rabbit polyclonal antibody to the AT_1R, diluted 1:200 in blocking solution.
8. The secondary antibody used in the experiments shown in the figure is Alexa Fluor® 647 (Molecular Probes®) anti-rabbit antibody, diluted 1:500 in blocking solution (*see* **Note 2**).
9. Alexa Fluor® 594 Phalloidin (Molecular Probes®, 1:200 dilution) is added along with the secondary antibody to selectively label F-actin. Using phalloidin at 594 nm allows the visualization of the brush border membrane distinct from the antibody staining.
10. Hoechst 33342 (Molecular Probes®, 1:2000 dilution) is also added along with the secondary antibody as a nucleic acid stain used to visualize nuclei.
11. A coverslip (Corning) number 1.5, 24×55-mm size is used to cover the entire slide with sections of tissue.
12. Fluoromount-G™ (Electron Microscopy Sciences) is an aqueous mounting medium used to mount the coverglass over the fixed tissue slices.
13. Clear nail polish.

3 Methods

Although rat kidneys are used for the purposes of the techniques explained in this chapter, these techniques can easily be extended to mouse and human kidneys. Human kidneys may be obtained from a variety of sources. The freshest and most convenient source is normal kidney tissue surgically removed from patients with renal cell carcinoma or Wilms' tumors, which usually affect only one pole of the kidney cortex. Another source may be transplant tissue that cannot be used, or fresh cadaveric tissue. All tissues should be obtained and used under institutional review board approval. The methods described below investigate the dopaminergic system of the rat renal proximal tubule. These methods can be extended to study any nephron segments within the kidney by identifying the segment or cell type by costaining with a cell-type or segment-specific marker. In the case of the renal proximal tubule, the thick brush border is stained with phalloidin as a segment-specific marker [12].

3.1 Animal Preparation and Kidney Isolation

1. Rats are placed under short-term anesthesia with 0.2 mL of ketamine (100 mg/mL) and 0.2 mL of xylazine (20 mg/mL) via an IP injection.
2. Rats are placed in a dorsal position on a hot water circulating heating pad (Gaymar, Braintree Scientific) to maintain body temperature at 37 °C.
3. The abdominal region of the rat is shaved and disinfected with multiple applications of 70% isopropyl alcohol and Betadine® topical solution.
4. Using sterile technique, a midline laparotomy is performed with surgical scissors and a curved hemostat is inserted into the IP cavity to bluntly dissect the connecting tissue. An abdominal spring-loaded retractor is then inserted into the IP cavity to visualize the abdominal contents. Cotton tip applicators are used to isolate the left kidney and separate it from the surrounding adipose tissue.
5. Two pieces of 2.0 silk suture spaced a few mm apart are tied around the renal artery.
6. The kidney is removed by cutting between the sutures with surgical scissors.
7. The kidney is subsequently decapsulated and sagittally cut to remove the pelvis and inferior lobes of the kidney.
8. The freshly excised kidney tissue is then immersed in cold (4 °C) Opti-MEM® media.
9. This process is repeated on the right kidney if more tissue is desired for experimentation.
10. After tissue collection, the rat is euthanized with a 0.3 mL injection of pentobarbital sodium (Virbach, Animal Health Industries; 390 mg/mL) into the IP cavity, followed by a thoracic incision cutting through the sternum.

3.2 Preparation of Kidney Slices

1. Pre-warm RPMI-1640 media by adding 1 mL to each well of a 12-well plate and rock in a 37 °C CO_2 incubator for 10 min.
2. Set the tissue chopper slice thickness for 1 mm and maximum blade force. Set up the tissue chopper with a new blade and three filter papers securely fastened to the stage.

3. Place the kidney on the filter paper and slice along the width with the coronal cut on the far side of the blade where there is more space.
4. Using the tissue chopper, 1 mm thick coronal sections are cut, yielding 12–14 slices per kidney.
5. Using blunt forceps, each slice is quickly placed into a single well of a 12-well plate with 1 mL pre-warmed media per well. The slices should be allowed to move freely in suspension as movement is important to renal slice viability [2].
6. The slices are then equilibrated by rocking for 30 min in a 37 °C 5 % CO_2 incubator.

3.3 Short-Term Tissue Incubation with Agonists and Antagonists

1. 1 μL of the prepared solutions of agonists and antagonists are then added to the desired wells of the 12-well plate. In the case of a blocking antagonist co-incubating with an agonist, the antagonists are always added first.
2. The D_1-like receptor agonist fenoldopam (FEN) is used either alone or with the D_1-like receptor antagonist LE300.
3. The AT_1R ligand, Ang II, is used either alone or with the AT_1R antagonist losartan (LOS).
4. The slices are incubated with rocking at 37 °C for another 30 min in the CO_2 incubator.

3.4 Tissue Fixation and Sectioning

1. Slices are washed by gentle ice-cold DPBS replacement three times.
2. Slices are then fixed in 4 % paraformaldehyde at room temperature for 4 h.
3. Slices are then rinsed twice in TBS.
4. Slices are then immersed in 1 mL TBS with 30 % sucrose per well overnight at 4 °C.
5. The following day, slices are embedded in OCT compound in a Cryomold® specimen mold. The specimen mold well is filled ¾ full with OCT compound. A tissue slice is placed in the OCT compound as flat and centered as possible, and the rest of the well is filled with OCT (*see* **Notes 3** and **4**).
6. The slices in the frozen specimen molds are then placed in a plastic box and frozen at −30 °C for at least 1 h. This preparation can be kept indefinitely at −80 °C until ready to cut sections.
7. Tissue should be transported to a cryostat microtome on dry ice, along with OCT compound, new blades, and Superfrost®/ Plus microscope slides.

8. Remove the frozen OCT compound block from the specimen mold and adhere to the cryostat microtome stage using a dab of fresh OCT compound as an adhesive.
9. 8 μm frozen sections are prepared with the cryostat microtome according to the instrument instructions (*see* **Note 5**).
10. Look at each slide under the microscope to ensure that the slices look normal and flat and not folded onto themselves. Three sections can be added to a single slide.
11. It is best to use the slides on the day of cutting for the lowest background autofluorescence levels. If storage is required, place the slides in a slide box at −80 °C for up to 6 months. Thaw only the slides to be used on the day of each experiment. Multiple freeze/thaw cycles of the slides cause increased background signals.
12. Slides are then prepared for immunofluorescent staining and imaging.

3.5 Permeabilization and Immunofluorescent Staining

1. When the slide is dry, an ImmEdge™ pen (Vector Laboratories, Inc.) is used to draw a hydrophobic ring around the sections to allow the use of very small volumes of antibodies.
2. Allow the ImmEdge™ reagent to dry on the slide before proceeding.
3. Add Kimwipes® to the bottom of a slide box with tight fitting lid and saturate with deionized water to make a humidity chamber.
4. The tissue sections are permeabilized for 5 min in TBS and 0.2% Triton-X100 (*see* **Note 6**).
5. Use a pipet tip with a vacuum to suction off excess liquid between each step and rinses, being careful not to touch the slice.
6. Rinse three times for 5 min in TBS-T (TBS with 0.02% Tween).
7. The tissue is blocked for 1 h with 2% milk in TBS-T.
8. Primary antibodies are incubated with the tissue for 1 h at room temperature or at 4 °C overnight. One kidney slice section with no primary antibodies and only blocking solution is incubated as a background control. For the data presented here, the primary rabbit polyclonal AT_1R antibody N-10 is added for 1 h at room temperature in the humid slide box.
9. The sections are washed three times for 5 min in TBS-T.
10. The secondary antibody used for the data presented here is Alexa Fluor® 647 (Molecular Probes®) anti-rabbit antibody. This antibody is prepared with Alexa Fluor® 594 Phalloidin, a filamentous actin-binding mushroom toxin, and Hoechst

DNA stain. The tissue slices are incubated in this mixture for 1 h at room temperature.

11. The sections are then washed three times for 5 min in TBS-T. After the last wash, remove as much liquid as possible from the slide.
12. If unable to image slides on the same day, a post-fixing step is recommended (*see* **Note 7**).
13. Add a small amount of fluoromount-G™ onto the kidney section, cover it with a coverslip, and then seal with clear nail polish.
14. Confocal microscopy is performed on the sections and intensity line profiling is calculated to quantify the observed changes in staining (*see* **Note 8**).

4 Notes

1. Many studies cite the use of smaller sections of tissue. When we investigated the use of sizes smaller than 1-mm, we found that more tubules could be visualized and available for measurements with a thicker slice. We did not find differences in agonist-induced AT_1R degradation events among various sizes, indicating adequate access to agonist and antagonist by the renal tissues internal to the section.
2. Care must be taken to match the secondary antibody to the species used to generate the primary antibody. The fluorophore that the secondary antibody is conjugated to must also be chosen with careful consideration. For low abundance staining, choosing a wavelength with low autofluorescence prevents masking of the desired signal. Fluorescein is not advised for kidney tissue due to the kidney having high autofluorescence near 480 nm excitation and 510 nm emission wavelengths.
3. When filling the well with OCT compound, the well is filled ¾ full with OCT compound. The tissue slice is then placed on the top of the OCT compound as flat and centered in the well as possible. The rest of the well is filled with OCT compound until a slight bulge is visible (overfilling). Avoid bubbles. If bubbles are present, they can be carefully aspirated out with a pipet or moved to the edge of the well.
4. The slices may be reassembled to form their original configuration following separation and incubation. These reassembled kidney slices may then be placed into the cryomold before adding OCT compound. The advantage here is that a single slice from the microtome will include all conditions tested.

5. Keeping the cryostat and samples cold is essential to cutting clean and unfolded sections.
6. An alternative to permeabilization with Triton-X 100 may be required for some antibodies. Some antibody stains only work with 1 % SDS for permeabilization.
7. To post-fix the tissue slices, treat with 2 % paraformaldehyde for 5 min following the last wash. Rinse once with 100 mmol/L Tris–HCl, pH 7.4 and proceed to the next step.
8. Confocal microscopic examination of the tissues on slides must be performed that day unless the slide has been post-fixed. The antibody staining will not last more than 24 h without the post-fix step. Take numerous pictures to assure capturing a valid representative image of the tissue and staining.

References

1. Forster RP (1948) Use of thin kidney slices and isolated renal tubules for direct study of cellular transport kinetics. Science 108:65–67
2. Dogterom P (1993) Development of a simple incubation system for metabolism studies with precision-cut liver slices. Drug Metab Dispos 21:699–704
3. Ruegg CE (1994) Preparation of precision-cut renal slices and renal proximal tubular fragments for evaluating segment-specific nephrotoxicity. J Pharmacol Toxicol Methods 31:125–133
4. Vittorelli A, Gauthier C, Michoudet C, Baverel G (2004) Metabolic viability and pharmacotoxicological reactivity of cryopreserved human precision-cut renal cortical slices. Toxicol In Vitro 18:285–292
5. Crljen V, Sabolić I, Susac J, Appenroth D, Herak-Kramberger CM, Ljubojević M, Anzai N, Antolović R, Burckhardt G, Fleck C (2005) Immunocytochemical characterization of the incubated rat renal cortical slices. Pflugers Arch 450:269–279
6. Gildea JJ, Wang X, Jose PA, Felder RA (2008) Differential D1 and D5 receptor regulation and degradation of the angiotensin type 1 receptor. Hypertension 51:360–366
7. Li H, Armando I, Yu P, Escano C, Mueller SC, Asico L, Pascua A, Lu Q, Wang X, Villar VA, Jones JE, Wang Z, Periasamy A, Lau YS, Soares-da-Silva P, Creswell K, Guillemette G, Sibley DR, Eisner G, Gildea JJ, Felder RA, Jose PA (2008) Dopamine 5 receptor mediates Ang II type 1 receptor degradation via a ubiquitin-proteasome pathway in mice and human cells. J Clin Invest 118:2180–2189
8. Zeng C, Luo Y, Asico LD, Hopfer U, Eisner GM, Felder RA, Jose PA (2003) Perturbation of D1 dopamine and AT1 receptor interaction in spontaneously hypertensive rats. Hypertension 42:787–792
9. Hein L, Meinel L, Pratt RE, Dzau VJ, Kobilka BK (1997) Intracellular trafficking of angiotensin II and its AT1 and AT2 receptors: evidence for selective sorting of receptor and ligand. Mol Endocrinol 11:1266–1277
10. Seikaly MG, Arant BS, Seney FD (1990) Endogenous angiotensin concentrations in specific intrarenal fluid compartments of the rat. J Clin Invest 86:1352–1357
11. Navar LG, Lewis L, Hymel A, Braam B, Mitchell KD (1994) Tubular fluid concentrations and kidney contents of angiotensins I and II in anesthetized rats. J Am Soc Nephrol 5:1153–1158
12. Gildea JJ, Shah I, Weiss R, Casscells ND, McGrath HE, Zhang J, Jones JE, Felder RA (2010) HK-2 human renal proximal tubule cells as a model for G protein-coupled receptor kinase type 4-mediated dopamine 1 receptor uncoupling. Hypertension 56:505–511

Chapter 13

Techniques for the Evaluation of the Genetic Expression, Intracellular Storage, and Secretion of Polypeptide Hormones with Special Reference to the Natriuretic Peptides (NPs)

Adolfo J. de Bold and Mercedes L. de Bold

Abstract

Techniques developed over the years in our laboratory for the study of tissue expression, storage, and secretion of the cardiac hormones ANF, BNP, and CNP are described below. They have proven highly reliable in our hands when the steps outlined are followed as described. Given the generic nature of the procedures, these should be applicable to other polypeptides.

Key words Natriuretic peptides, Peptide isolation, HPLC, Radioimmunoassay, Immunocytochemistry, In situ hybridization, PCR

1 Introduction

The vast majority of techniques described below, although referenced to cardiac natriuretic peptides (NP), are largely applicable to the study of polypeptide hormones in general.

2 Extraction of NP from Tissues and Plasma (Modified from [1])

Since polypeptide hormones are present at relatively low concentrations in both tissues and blood and in other biological fluids, it is of the utmost importance that once obtained, these are rapidly processed using the extracting techniques described below or rapidly frozen in liquid nitrogen and kept in a −80 °C freezer until processed in order to avoid proteolytic degradation.

Dissection of tissues once removed should be carried out under ice-cold saline.

The best way to freeze tissues for later processing is to place them in cryovials with enough saline or extracting fluid to prevent

Rhian M. Touyz and Ernesto L. Schiffrin (eds.), *Hypertension: Methods and Protocols*, Methods in Molecular Biology, vol. 1527, DOI 10.1007/978-1-4939-6625-7_13, © Springer Science+Business Media LLC 2017

desiccation and placing them in liquid nitrogen followed by freezer storage at −80 °C or lower.

The extracting fluid used consists of a strongly acidic aqueous mixture. to prevent enzymatic action, acetic acid that is a good peptide solvent, and NaCl that help prevents protein associations.

Extracting fluid: 0.1 N HCl/1.0 M acetic acid/1 % NaCl.

Use a ratio of tissue to extractant of 1:10. For small tissue pieces (e.g., 100 mg), use 3.0 mL extractant in order to have enough volume to homogenize.

Procedure:

1. Place the frozen sample in a round bottom 50 mL centrifuge tube and homogenize for 15 s using a Polytron® fitted with a toothed probe and set at 80 % power.
2. Leave the tube in ice for about 30 min and then centrifuge at 10,000 × *g* for 30 min at 4 °C. Keep the supernatant.
3. Re-homogenize the pellet with half the amount of extractant and centrifuge as above. Combine supernatants and freeze at −80 °C for later processing.

Blood samples are drawn into EDTA-containing tubes gently mixing with the anticoagulant and placed immediately in ice. The plasma is separated as soon as possible by centrifugation in a refrigerated centrifuge for 30 min at 3000 × *g* and frozen at −80 °C until used. Hemolyzed plasma specimens are just about useless for most subsequent uses.

2.1 Batch Isolation of Peptides from Tissue Extracts and Plasma

Batch adsorption onto octadecylsilyl silica (ODS) (C_{18}) of NPs and other polypeptide hormones from tissue extracts or plasma allows for rapid desalting, pre-purification, and reduction in volume of the sample necessary to take it to purification by high-performance liquid chromatography (HPLC) or quantitation by radioimmunoassay or other high-sensitivity detection techniques. Water's Sep-Paks (C_{18}) (http://www.waters.com/waters/partDetail.htm?partNumber=WAT051910) may be used for this purpose.

Sep-Paks must be pre-wetted (activated) just before use by passing 5 mL of 80 % acetonitrile (ACN) in 0.1 % trifluoroacetic acid (TFA). The cartridge is then washed with 20 mL of 0.1 % TFA and it is ready to receive the sample. We use glass syringes for these steps.

To process plasma, 1–3 mL is acidified with 100 μL/mL of 1.0 N HCl and passed three times through a previously activated Sep-Pak C_{18} cartridge.

In order to minimize handling of the plasma, we fit a disposable pipette tip to the outlet of the cartridge. In turn, the inlet of the cartridge is attached to the Luer lock tip of a disposable syringe. The plasma sample is aspirated, expelled, and then aspirated again. The material now in the syringe is discarded and the cartridge is rinsed with 20 mL of 0.1 % TFA. A small glass syringe is next used to deliver 3 mL of 80 % ACN in 0.1 % TFA through the cartridge, hence eluting the adsorbed material. We normally use siliconized Vacutainer® tubes (www.bd.com) to receive the eluate which is frozen in liquid nitrogen for several hours in the −80 °C. Prior to freezing the Vacutainer tubes are covered with a small piece of tissue paper, which is secured with a rubber band to the neck of the tube. Following freezing, the tubes are rapidly transferred to a freeze-dryer.

A well-functioning freeze-dryer (i.e., one producing a vacuum of less than 10 mmHg) will produce a fluffy desiccated material in each tube at the end of about 24 h of operation. The procedure followed to process tissue extracts through Sep-Paks is virtually identical to that described above for blood plasma except that considerable lager volumes of tissue extracts (e.g., ~10 mL) can be treated with a Sep-Pak.

Because both the TFA and the ACN are volatile, the sediment in the tubes after freeze-drying consists solely of the extracted material, which is readily soluble in water, assay buffers, or 0.1 % TFA if the latter is the vehicle used for HPLC analysis. Any small sediment can be removed by spinning for a minute or so in a microcentrifuge.

3 HPLC of NP

Few tools have been developed for the isolation, purification, and analysis of proteins and peptides that are as useful as HPLC in terms of efficiency and speed. Of the various modalities that this type of chromatography can be performed in, reverse phase chromatography using ODS columns provided by several manufacturers and of various particles, pore sizes, and capacity can be employed to accommodate the particular composition of the sample. For analytical purposes we use the Vydac 218TP54 column (www.chem.agilent.com) for analytical purposes and the Vydac 218TP510 for semi-preparative purposes.

The samples obtained from Sep-Pak cartridges need not be dried to reduce volume prior to injecting in the HPLC as long as it is diluted sufficiently to reduce the ACN concentration to or below the concentration of ACN at which the column is equilibrated (in most cases 15 % of and 80 % ACN in 0.1 % TFA). In cases where large volumes are pumped into the column, an online filter must be used. Water, TFA, and ACN must be HPLC grade. Otherwise non-specific interference will be obtained while UV monitoring the effluent. The volume resulting from such dilution is generally larger that the injector volume so that it is best to pump the sample in.

The mobile phase is commonly a linear gradient using two solutions: 0.1 % TFA (solution A) and 80 % ACN in 0.1 % TFA (solution B) over 1 h. The starting and end mobile phase concentrations are 15 and 80 % B, respectively, at a flow rate of 1.5 mL/min for the analytical column and 3.0 mL/min for the semi-preparative column. UV monitoring is done at 260 nm. Sample collection is normally done at 2 min intervals. Changing the counterion from TFA to heptafluorobutyric acid (HFBA, 12 % ACN/0.13 % HFBA) often changes in a dissimilar manner the hydrophobicity of peptides in a mixture, resulting in improved separations.

We use siliconized Vacutainer® tubes for sample collection that are capped and freeze-dried as described above for tissue or plasma extracts.

4 Radioimmunoassay (RIA) of NPs (Modified from [2])

Many commercial kits are available to determine concentration of NPs. We have continued to use our originally developed RIA because of its unparalleled sensitivity not only for NPs but many other polypeptide hormones. Essential for a well-performing RIA are of course a "good" antibody defined in terms of specificity and ED_{50} and an appropriately labeled tracer peptide, the latter defined as one with high specific activity. We have found that for NPs our iodination method yields a radiolabeled peptide with superior specific activities than those commercially available. For a successful RIA, a purified bovine serum albumin is essential, and although RIA quality albumin is commercially available, we continue to prepare our own. The techniques for iodination of NPs and preparation of albumin are given below.

4.1 Iodination of Peptide

The technique that follows illustrates the iodination of $ANF_{99\text{-}126}$ to high specific activity. Key to obtaining a good specific activity is the purification of the iodinated peptide by HPLC using the analytical column mentioned above. This type of purification eliminates non-radiolabeled peptide and di-iodinated peptide that adversely affects the purity of the mono-iodinated ^{125}I-ANF. It is almost essential to have a dedicated HPLC system and column for radioiodination given the residual radioactivity in the column and instrument after the procedure.

The steps below, up to HPLC purification of the radioiodinated peptide, are carried out in rapid succession so that all elements and solutions needed must be prepared in advance of the actual iodination. This procedure must be done in a fume hood certified for use with radioisotopes.

5 Materials

1. 0.05 M sodium phosphate buffer pH 7.4 (20 mL) in a 50 mL falcon tube.
2. 80% ACN/0.1% TFA and 0.1% TFA in 50 mL beakers.
3. Set an Eppendorf P10 pipette or equivalent to 10 μL, set the P100 pipette to 50 μL, and set the P1000 pipette to 500 μL.
4. A timer to be set for 15 s.
5. Set one 10 mL siliconized Vacutainer 10 (with the lid off) in a rack.
6. Pre-wet the Sep-Pak with 3 mL 80% ACN/0.1% TFA and 10 mL of 0.1% TFA as described previously.
7. Label two sets of 72 RIA tubes from 1 to 72. One set is used to collect 1 min fractions from HPLC and another set to receive 10 μL of each fraction for determination of the radioactivity profile eluted from the column.

6 Iodination Procedure

1. Centrifuge I^{125} in its container for ~30 s at about 200 rpm (to get the I^{125} to the bottom of the vial from supplier).
2. Thaw solution of 10 μg/μL $ANF_{99\text{-}126}$ (www.phoenixpeptide.com) peptide in water from −80 °C freezer.
3. Freshly prepare Chloramine T: 10 mg Chloramine T (www.sigmaaldrich.com) to 10 mL of 0.05 M sodium phosphate buffer.
4. Add 10 μL of the 10 μg/μL ANF peptide to the I^{125} vial.
5. Add 50 μL of stock 0.5 M sodium phosphate buffer to the vial containing the I^{125}.
6. Add 10 μL of chloramine T to the I^{125} vial.
7. Start the timer (15 s) and shake the mixture gently.
8. Stop reaction by adding 500 μL of 0.1% TFA to the mixture.
9. Aspirate the entire mixture into the pre-wetted Sep-Pak (Fig. 1).
10. Aspirate ~10 mL of 0.1% TFA.
11. Disassemble the syringe/Sep-Pak apparatus. Put the needle and tubing into the sharps radioactive waste and the 20 mL syringe into the solid radioactive waste container.
12. Load 3 mL of 80% ACN/0.1% TFA into a 5 mL glass syringe and then attach it to the Sep-Pak.

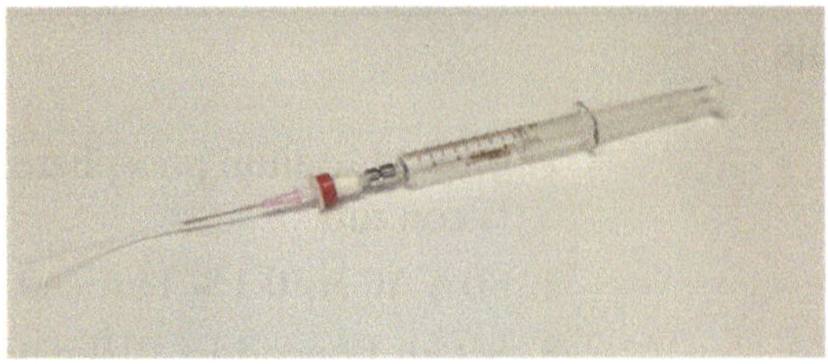

Fig. 1 Sep-Pak purification of iodinated peptide. The iodination reaction diluted with 0.1 % TFA is aspirated through the cartridge followed by 20 mL of 0.1 %. The content of the syringe is discarded and the radioiodinated peptide is now eluted with 3 mL of 80 % ACN in 0.1 % TFA previously loaded in a glass syringe (shown)

13. Slowly elute the Sep-Pak into a 10 mL Vacutainer® (you should have approximately 3 mL). Throw the Sep-Pak into the solid radioactive waste container.
14. Evaporate the mixture down using the nitrogen stream set on low flow (test this out on your hand before you put the Vacutainer© under the stream so as not to have any mixture splashing out). Mixture needs to evaporate down to 1 mL (takes ~30–60 min).
15. Aspirate the concentrated mixtured into a 1 mL plastic syringe with an injection needle suitable for the HCPLC injector.
16. 16 The HPLC should be at baseline condition: 15 % of 80 % ACN and 1.5 mL/min. Be extremely careful with the injection in order to avoid leaks.
17. Start gradient program elution from baseline to 100 % of the solution containing 80 % ACN.
18. Collect the first 72 fractions at 1 min intervals into the pre-labeled RIA tubes.
19. Once all of the fractions have been collected, put a waste container under the HPLC machine to collect the rest of the flow through the column.
20. Take 10 μL of each fraction and put it into a new set of tubes.
21. Set up the gamma counter for 60 s counts and count the 10 μL fractions.

    The peak of interest will be the one containing the most radioactivity followed by a smaller peak representing di-iodinated peptide, which should be discarded. The "cold" peptide elutes before the peak of interest so that only the fraction with the most activity should be retained and diluted with RIA buffer for assay.

7 Preparation of RIA Grade Bovine Serum Albumin (BSA)

1. Weigh 200 g BSA (Fraction V Powder, Catalogue # A 7888, www.sigmaaldrich.com) and stir gently until dissolved in 1 L of 0.05 M Na_2HPO_4/0.15 M NaCl.

   pH should be more than 6.0; if not, add a few drops of 1 N NaOH while stirring.
2. Place in water bath of 56 °C and shake gently to prevent bubbles from forming. When solution gets to 56 °C, incubate for 2 h longer.
3. Cool on ice while stirring.
4. After cooling, add 1 mL penicillin/streptomycin (GIBCO catalogue #15070-063, www.invitrogen.com).
5. Cut six lengths of Spectra/Por membrane tubing (45 mm standard cellulose dialysis tubing: vol./cm: 6.4 mL, MW cutoff: 12,000–14,000).
6. Wet the tubing in distilled water overnight.
7. Tie a double knot in the base of each piece of tubing and fill them up to 40 cm from the top.
8. Wrap the top of the tubing around a glass rod several times, finally making a double knot (there should be about 30 cm space between the knot and the top of the albumin solution).
9. Dialyze in large cylinder containing distilled water at 4 °C and a magnetic stirring bar and stir at medium speed. Add a few drops of chloroform.
10. Change the water two times a day for 2 days (*do not* forget to add chloroform each time the water is changed).
11. Break the dialyzing tubing into a 2000 mL Erlenmeyer flask. Use the Pellicon (Millipore XX80EL001) peristaltic pump to filter the BSA. Vacuum should be avoided due to foam. Connect one end of the pump tubing with the Erlenmeyer containing the BSA (using a 10 mL pipette). The other end of the tubing is connected to the Swinnex (Millipore) filter housing (Fig. 2).
12. Filter the BSA with the disc filter holder fitted with an AP2504700 prefilter and a SMWP04700 MF spacer mesh filter followed by a SMWP04700 5 μ filter, another spacer and 5 μ filters, and finally a spacer filter followed by a 0.8 μ AAWP04700 filter.
13. The above filters are replaced with a 45 μ filter (HVLP04700) for a final filtration.
14. Collect the albumin in freeze-drying flasks and freeze-dry until BSA is completely dry.

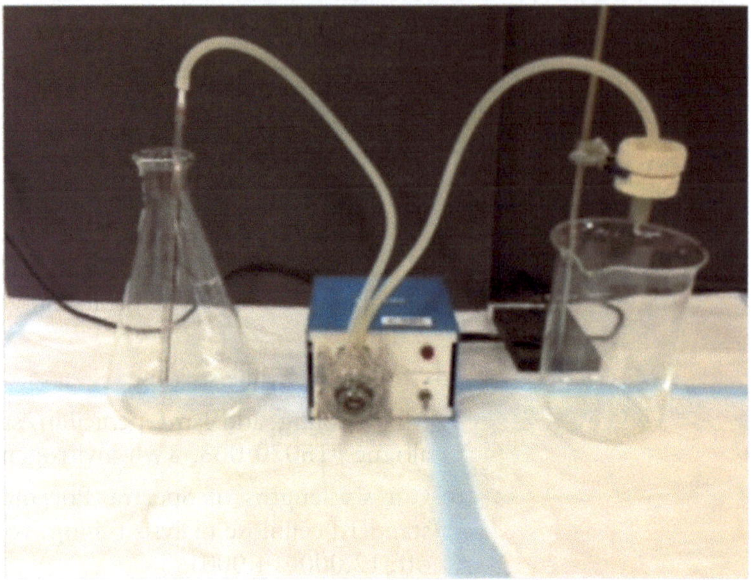

Fig. 2 Filtration setup used in the preparation of heat-treated BSA. The filter makeup is described in the text

8 RIA Procedure

8.1 Reagents

RIA buffer: Dibasic sodium phosphates 81 and 19 mM of monobasic (pH: 7.4), 0,05 M NaCl, 0.1 % of heat-treated BSA, 0.1 % Triton X-100, and 0.01 % NaN_3.

ANF_{99-126} (or ANP, rat, mouse) (www.Phoenixpeptide.com) 200 µg.

Rabbit, antimouse, human, and rat ANF $_{99-126}$ (www.Phoenixpeptide.com) diluted following manufacturer's instructions.

^{125} I-ANF available commercially, which is also available commercially with a somewhat lower specific activity than that obtained with the iodination procedure described above.

5 % normal rabbit serum (www.lifetechnologies.com) in RIA buffer.

6.5 % polyethylenglycol (PEG) (www.fishersci.ca) in water.

8.2 Preparation of ANF Dilutions for Standard Curve

Solution A: Add 150–180 µL of 10 mM HCL to the ANF $_{99-126}$ vial (200 µg), the volume of acid depends on the purity of ANF. Stock: 100 µg/0.1 mL.

Solution B: Make 1:10 dilutions, e.g., 100 µL of A plus 900 µL of RIA buffer.

Concentration: 10 µg/0.1 mL.

Aliquot 120 µL of B into eight cryovials, freeze-dry, and store at −80 °C.

Solution C: Take 100 µL of B (10 µg/0.1 mL) plus 900 µL of RIA buffer.

Concentration: 1 μg/0.1 mL.

Aliquot 120 μL of C into eight cryovials, freeze-dry, and store at −80 °C.

Solution D: Take 100 μL of C (1 μg/0.1 mL) plus 900 μL of RIA buffer.

Concentration: 100 ng/0.1 mL.

Aliquot 120 μL of D into eight cryovials, freeze-dry, and store at −80 °C.

Solution E: Take 100 μL of D (100 ng/0.1 mL) plus 9900 μL of RIA buffer.

Concentration: 1 ng/0.1 mL.

Aliquot 1250 μL of E into seven Vacutainer® tubes (www.bd.com), freeze-dry, and store at −80 °C.

Standard curve

Reconstitute an aliquot of E by adding 1250 μL of Milli-Q water.

Solution F: Take 1 mL of E (1 ng/0.1 mL) plus 1 mL of RIA buffer.

Concentration: 500 pg/0.1 mL.

Standard Curve

Add the following to make standards:

Concentration (pg/0.1 mL)	Solution F (mL)	RIA buffer (mL)
100	0.2	0.8
50	0.1	0.9
25	0.1	1.9
12.5	0.1	3.9
6.25	0.05	3.950
3.125	0.025	3.975

- For RIA, rehydrate the lyophilized samples with 1.0 mL RIA buffer on ice for 1 h. Clear the supernatant if necessary by centrifuging
- Remove the supernatant and transfer to labeled cryovial
  Pipetting of samples and standards

Tubes	Buffer (mL)	Standard/sample (mL)	Primary antibody (antihuman ANF mL)	I^{125} ANF (mL)	Normal rabbit serum 2.5% (mL)	Secondary antibody (goat antihuman IgG mL)
T	None	None	None	0.1	None	None
B	0.2	None	None	0.1	0.1	0.1
O	0.1	None	0.1	0.1	0.1	0.1

(continued)

Tubes	Buffer (mL)	Standard/sample (mL)	Primary antibody (antihuman ANF mL)	I^{125} ANF (mL)	Normal rabbit serum 2.5% (mL)	Secondary antibody (goat antihuman IgG mL)
3.125	None	0.1	0.1	0.1	0.1	0.1
6.250	None	0.1	0.1	0.1	0.1	0.1
12.50	None	0.1	0.1	0.1	0.1	0.1
25.00	None	0.1	0.1	0.1	0.1	0.1
50.00	None	0.1	0.1	0.1	0.1	0.1
100.00	None	0.1	0.1	0.1	0.1	0.1
Samples	None	0.1	0.1	0.1	0.1	0.1
Quality control	None	0.1	0.1	0.1	0.1	0.1

Note: All the tubes will contain 0.5 mL except the total counts ("T") tube which only has 0.1 mL of I^{125} ANF and doesn't undergo any treatment with PEG or need centrifugation.

- Add 0.1 mL of primary antibody and buffer/sample to the proper tubes, shake, and incubate all samples for 4 h at 4 °C. The racks should be covered with Parafilm and then wrapped in aluminum foil.
- This is followed by the addition of I^{125} $ANF_{99\text{-}126}$, shake the rack, cover the tubes, and incubate for 18–24 h at 4 °C.
- Next day add the second antibody shaking the tubes followed by normal rabbit serum, cover, shake, and incubate for 2 h at 20 °C.
- Add 1.5 mL of PEG to every tube except T.
- Centrifuge at 2700 rpm centrifuge for 45 min at 4 °C.
- Discard the supernatant and place tubes in a gamma counter.

9 Immunocytochemistry [3, 4] (Fig. 3)

9.1 Light Microscopy Immunocytochemistry

Tissue samples are fixed in 4% buffered paraformaldehyde (see below) overnight at 4 °C and embedded in paraffin using routine procedures.

(a) Five micron sections are deparaffinized, incubated with 3% hydrogen peroxide to quench endogenous peroxidase activity for 30 min at room temperature (RT).

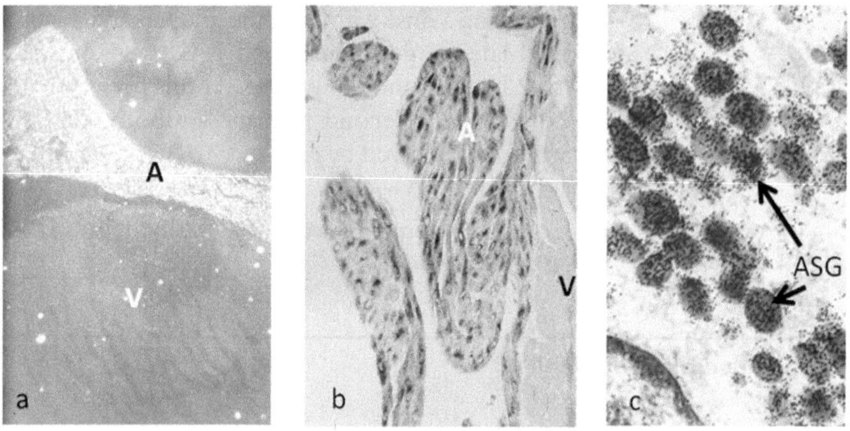

Fig. 3 ANF mRNA by in situ hybridization (dark-field microscopy) (**a**) and peptide by immunocytochemistry at the light (bright field) (**b**) and electron microscopic levels (**c**). *A* atrium, *V* ventricle, *ASG* atrial specific granules

(b) The sections are incubated for 20 min at RT with 20 μL of 10% normal goat serum (NGA, blocking serum). Do not wash the slides.

(c) Primary antibody incubation is done for 12 h at 4 °C.

(d) After rinsing twice with phosphate-buffered saline (PBS), the sections are incubated with biotinylated goat anti-rabbit IgG (www.vectorlabs.com) for 60 min at RT.

(e) The sections are rinsed with PBS followed by incubation with Avidin Texas Red following the manufacturer's instructions (www.vectorlabs.com).

(f) Controls: (1) Antibodies used are pre-adsorbed with 1 μg/mL with authentic peptides. (2) Sections are incubated with nonimmune serum instead of primary antibody. (3) Sections known to be positive for the antibodies in use are used as positive controls.

(g) Sections can be now exposed to another primary antibody, after a previous exposure for 1 h to citric phosphate buffer pH 2.2.

9.2 Electron Microscopy Immunocytochemistry

(a) Atrial and/or ventricular samples are fixed in 4% paraformaldehyde (www.sigmaaldrich.com) overnight at 4 °C.

(b) Epon-embedded sections are mounted on nickel grids and etched with 4–8% aqueous sodium metaperiodate at for 1 h at RT.

(c) Rinse five times with water and incubate with polyclonal rabbit anti-rat $ANF_{99\text{-}126}$ (R_5 B_{11}) produced in our laboratory at 1:1000 dilution for 24–48 h at 4 °C. Antibodies from Phoenix work as well (www.Phoenixpeptide.com).

(d) Following a rinse with PBS, the grids are incubated with 5 nm gold-labeled goat anti-rabbit IgG (www.emsdiasum.com) for 2 h at RT and jet washed. At this point the grids can be exposed to a second primary antibody, e.g., anti-BNP_{45} antibody followed by exposure to 25 nm gold-labeled goat anti-rabbit IgG.

(e) Controls should be run as described in *see* Subheading 9.1(f) above.

10 Buffered 4% Paraformaldehyde

Materials needed:

Fume hood, stirring hot plate, stirring magnetic bar, 100 mL beaker, thermometer, 100 mL volumetric flask.

Paraformaldehyde (www.sigmaaldrich.com) 4.0 g.

Water at 40 °C ~40.0 mL.

Preparation:

Place a stirring hot plate in a fume hood and heat the water in a 100 mL beaker with a stirring bar until it reaches 40 °C. Add the paraformaldehyde with constant stirring and bring the water temperature to 60–70 °C. Add 1.0 N NaOH drop-wise (~2–3 drops) until a clear solution is obtained. Cool under running cold tap water. Once cool bring to 50 mL, transfer to a 100 mL volumetric flask and bring up to 100 mL with 0.2 M sodium phosphate buffer pH 7.2–7.4.

11 In Situ Hybridization

In studies of tissue expression of NPs and their receptors in human coronary arteries, we visualized mRNA expression for $ANF_{99\text{-}126}$, BNP_{45}, CNP, and the NP receptors A, B, and C using synthetic riboprobes. The general experimental strategy consisted in the generation of PCR-derived riboprobe self-templates using four overlapping oligonucleotides corresponding to human portions of the gene-coding region of each peptide or receptor flanked by restriction sites and T3 or T7 phage RNA polymerase promoters used in PCR reactions as a self-priming template. After generation of free 3′ and 5′ ends by restriction endonucleases, the riboprobes, which in all cases were 161 bp long and were isolated and purified. Detailed procedures for rehydration and blocking, probe generation, transcription, and hybridization have been previously described [5].

12 Total RNA Extraction and Real-Time RT-PCR

Homogenization of tissues for RNA extraction is carried out in TRIzol© (www.invitrogen.com) according to manufacturer's instructions and observing the precautions discussed above for the extraction of NPs from tissues. The quality of the RNA extracted is assessed using an Agilent 2100 Bioanalyzer (www.agilrnt.com) (*Agilent Technologies*) with the Agilent RNA 6000 Nano Kit (www.agilrnt.com). First strand cDNA synthesis is carried out using the Transcriptor First Strand cDNA Synthesis Kit (www.roche-applied-sciende.com).

RT-PCR is performed using LightCycler 480 SYBR Green I Master Mix and analyzed on the LightCycler 480 SW 1.5 relative quantification software (www.roche-applied-sciende.com) according to manufacturer's instructions.

Primer nucleotide sequences are generally obtained from literature but are validated using Primer3 Input Version 0.4.0 (http://frodo.wi.mit.edu). Glucose-6-phosphate dehydrogenase (G6PD) is used as the reference gene, and concentration ratios are normalized to the calibrator and corrected using primer efficiency. Each primer pair is validated by conducting a standard curve in triplicate. Primers are commercially synthesized by Operon (http://www.operon.com/).

Prime sequences for human are given below.

Gene	Human primer sequences (5′ → 3′) (sense (+), antisense (−))	PCR product size (bp)
ANF	(+)CCAGAGGGGAGACAGAGC (−)ATGGGGTGGGGAGAGGCGAGG	726
BNP	(+)CAGCAGCAGCCTCCGCAGTC (−)CCTCCCAAAGCAGCCAGACC	376
CNP	(+)CTCTCCCAGCTGCTGGCCTG (−)GCTCATGGAGCCGATTCGGTC	394
NPR-A	(+)CATCCTGGACAACCTGC (−)TAGGTCCGAACCTTGCC	714
NPR-B	(+)GTGGGGCTGCTGCTTTATCC (−)CCTGGCTCTCGGGCATACAC	645
NPR-C	(+)GGACTGGGAGGCGGCTTCTG (−)TGATGCTCCGGATGGTGTCA	552

13 Western Blotting

Tissues are homogenized in RIPA buffer (150 mM NaCl, 50 mM Tris–HCl pH 7.4, 1 mM EDTA pH 8.0, 1 % Nonidet P-40, 0.5 % sodium deoxycholate) containing a 1:100 dilution of protease inhibitor cocktail (P8340, www.sigmaaldrich.com), using a Polytron®. The homogenate is centrifuged at 10,000 rpm for 10 min at 4 °C. The protein concentration in the supernatants is determined using the Pierce® BCA Protein Assay Kit (www.pierce.net.com).

Samples are prepared by adding 7 μg of protein to 3× Blue loading dye (7722, www.cellsignal.com) and 10 % DTT and boiled for 2 min at 95 °C. Thirty microliters of proteins were loaded onto a 4–20 % Mini-PROTEAN® TGX™ precast gel (www.bio-rad.com) and run at 200 V for 45 min, along with a biotinylated Precision-Plus Protein™ WesternC ladder (161-0399, www.bio-rad.com). The gel is transferred to a 0.45 μm PVDF membrane (www.millipore.com) at 100 V for 1 h (hour) and blocked for 1 h (blocking buffer: 5 % fat-free milk in TBST (tris-buffered saline, 0.1 % Tween 20)). Membranes are rinsed three times with TBST and incubated overnight at 4 °C with the desired antibodies diluted in blocking buffer. Membranes are rinsed three times with TBST and incubated for 1 h at room temperature with secondary antibodies conjugated to HRP diluted in blocking buffer. Membranes are rinsed three times with TBST and visualized using the FluorChem Alpha Ease ECL imaging system (wwwalphainnotech.com) following enhancement with Luminata™ Forte chemiluminescence (www.millipore.com).

References

1. Ogawa T, Linz W, Stevenson M, Bruneau BG, Kuroski de Bold ML, Chen JH, Eid H, Scholkens BA, de Bold AJ (1996) Evidence for load-dependant and load-independant determinants of cardiac natriuretic peptide production. Circulation 93:2059–2067
2. Sarda IR, de Bold ML, de Bold AJ (1989) Optimization of atrial natriuretic factor radioimmunoassay. Clin Biochem 22:11–15
3. Bensimon M, Chang A, Kuroski-de Bold ML, Ponce A, Carreras D, de Bold AJ (2004) Participation of G proteins in natriuretic peptide hormone secretion from heart atria. Endocrinology 145:5313–5321
4. de Bold ML, de Bold AJ (1985) Immunocytochemical demonstration of cardionatrins in human atrial myocardium. In: Russo J (ed) Immunocytochemistry in tumor diagnosis. Martinus Nijhoss Publishing, Boston
5. Casco VH, Veinot JP, Kuroski de Bold ML, Masters RG, Stevenson MM, de Bold AJ (2002) Natriuretic peptide system gene expression in human coronary arteries. J Histochem Cytochem 50:799–809

Chapter 14

Intracellular Free Calcium Measurement Using Confocal Imaging

Ghassan Bkaily, Johny Al-Khoury, Yanick Simon, and Danielle Jacques

Abstract

Confocal microscopy, coupled to high-performance hardware and software systems, has provided scientists with the capability of overcoming some of the limitations of standard microscopic imaging measurements of intracellular ions. The technique for loading of ion fluorescent probes is easily achieved; however, the quality of calcium measurements depends on the way of using the confocal system. In order to optimize this technique, scientists need to be familiar with the basic approaches and limitations of confocal microscopy. In this chapter, we will describe sample preparation, fluorescent probe loading, labeling of intracellular compartments, and the setting of parameters as well as protocols for measurements and limitations of the technique.

Key words Confocal microscopy, Calcium probe, Fluo-3, Indo-1, Fluo-4, Intracellular calcium, Nuclear calcium

1 Introduction

Progress in confocal microscopy permitted opening of a new field of intracellular ion measurement. This progress led to measurement of intracellular ions at the nuclear level [1–11]. Measurement of intracellular ions using confocal microscopy and real 3D reconstruction of the ion distribution and level in the cell became a routine technique in many laboratories across the world. However, any misuse of this outstanding technique due to insufficient knowledge in the field of biological confocal microscopy, image processing, and biophysical properties of the ion fluorescent probes may bring forth invalid results. Therefore, it is highly important that a scientist who desires to use the technique of confocal microscopy and real 3D image analysis of ion measurement should be aware of the loading technique of fluorescent probes and the conditions and settings of the confocal needed to obtain the best reliable and reproducible results in the field. Our technique of loading and

Rhian M. Touyz and Ernesto L. Schiffrin (eds.), *Hypertension: Methods and Protocols*, Methods in Molecular Biology, vol. 1527, DOI 10.1007/978-1-4939-6625-7_14, © Springer Science+Business Media LLC 2017

confocal setting as well as the quantitative real 3D measurements permitted us to overcome many problems related to ion fluorescent measurements such as photobleaching and/or leak of the fluorescent probe with excellent accuracy. In this chapter, we will describe the loading technique of the fluorescent ion probe, and we will discuss basic approaches and limitations of confocal microscopy.

2 Materials

2.1 Choice of Cell Types for Confocal Microscopy

To date, several cell types have been used for ion measurement using confocal microscopy [1–13]. Most of the work has been performed using freshly isolated and/or cultured single cells either in primary culture or from cell lines. There is no doubt that the choice of the cell type is crucial for obtaining satisfactory results. In order to obtain sufficient loading with the ion fluorescent probe and accurate details from 3D reconstructions, the following criteria should be taken into account:

1. Isolated cells should be plated on 25 mm diameter sterile glass coverslips (plastic should be avoided) which permits insertion of the coverslip in a bath designed for confocal microscopy. Furthermore, this permits a better contact with the oil objective of the microscope. The small thickness of the coverslip permits more space for laser scanning of the whole cell.
2. Cells should be attached in order to avoid displacement during serial sectioning. This ensures that, with repeated sectioning, laser scanning will always start and end at the same positions.
3. Serial sectioning should be taken at rest or when the steady-state effect of a compound is reached unless the goal is to measure calcium transient frequency including puffs and sparks using single line scanning of the confocal.
4. In order to eliminate electrical and chemical coupling between cells, they should be grown at low density.
5. Cells should be relatively thick and not flattened in order to allow a minimum of 75–150 serial sections (according to the cell type). This could be done by using the cells as soon as they are attached and/or by lowering serum concentration.
6. When cell lines or proliferative cells are used, it is recommended to replace the culture medium overnight with a medium free of serum and growth factors before starting the experiments. This will allow the cells to settle in a latent phase of mitosis and will increase the accessibility of receptors and channels for agonist and antagonist actions, by washing out the effects of compounds present in the culture medium.
7. Using specific fluorescent markers, the origin, purity, and phenotype of the cells should be checked continually.

8. Since ions and other free functional components of the cells are not homogeneously distributed, and since the increase or decrease of the probed free component seems to be faster than computer sampling and acquisition, it is difficult to assess these fast-occurring phenomena at the quantitative 3D level. Hence, large rapid scans of the area under interest should be done.

2.2 Ion Probe Intracellular Loading

All solutions are prepared using sterile water for irrigation, USP (Baxter, Toronto, Ontario, Canada) which ensures a stable quality and resistivity as well as sterility. The osmolarity of all solutions is adjusted with sucrose to 310 mOsm using an osmometer.

1. The calcium probe Fluo-3/AM (or Fluo-4/AM or the ratiometric probe Indo-1/AM) is purchased already reconstituted in DMSO at a concentration of 1 mM (Molecular Probes).
2. The probe is aliquoted in the dark under red light at 10.6 μl per 1.5 ml amber Eppendorf tube and stored at −20 °C till it is used. Before the start of cell loading, the content of the Eppendorf is diluted to a final concentration of 13.6 μM with 800 μl of Tyrode-BSS buffer containing 5 mM Hepes, 136 mM NaCl, 2.7 mM KCl, 1 mM $MgCl_2$, 1.9 mM $CaCl_2$, and 5.6 mM glucose, buffered to pH 7.4 with Tris base and supplemented with 0.1 % bovine serum albumin (BSA).
3. The working buffer solution is the Tyrode-BSS buffer described above without BSA.
4. The nuclear fluorescent probe Syto-11 is purchased in a 1 mM DMSO solution (Molecular Probes) and is aliquoted at 5 μl per 0.5 ml amber Eppendorf. Before starting the experiment, the Syto-11 working solution is prepared by adding 495 μl of Tyrode-BSS experimental solution.
5. Ca^{2+} calibration buffer kits No. 2 (0–40 μM free Ca^{2+}) and No. 3 (1 μM to 1 mM free Ca^{2+}) (Molecular Probes).
6. 0.1 % Triton X-100 solution (Sigma).

2.3 Confocal Settings

There is no doubt that one of the major elements in confocal microscopy is the setting of optimal parameter conditions [3, 4]. These should be determined in the confocal before starting to use the machine [3, 4]. Once these settings are determined, they should not be changed throughout the life of the confocal system. This will allow a realistic comparison between results obtained using the same fluorescent probe year after year. The following parameters and conditions of the confocal should be set:

1. Using different types of cultured cells, the autofluorescence of the cell should be determined by adjusting the photomultiplier tube (PMT) and laser intensity of the confocal. Once this is achieved, the value of PMT as well as the laser intensity should

be decreased below the values at which cell autofluorescence was observed. This prevents any possible contamination of the fluorescence of the calcium probe with the autofluorescence of the cell's proteins. For example, the settings for PMT and laser intensity for a Molecular Dynamics Multiprobe 2001 confocal krypton/argon laser scanning microscopy (CSLM) system equipped with a Nikon Diaphot epifluorescence inverted microscope and a X60 (1.4 NA) Nikon Oil Plan achromat objective are 700 and 9.0 mV, respectively. The photometric gain should be set at 2×. However, for the Bio-Rad MRC1024 Krypton/Argon and UV laser confocal system equipped with an inverse phase epifluorescence microscope and 60× Nikon Oil Plan achromat objective, these settings are 900 and 15 mV, respectively. These optical settings are also valid with other confocal microscopes.

2. For Fluo-3/AM and Fluo-4/AM, when the krypton/argon laser is used, the 488 nm (9.0–12.0 mV) or 514 nm laser line (15–20 mV) should be directed to the sample via a 510 nm or 535 nm primary dichroic filter and attenuated with 1–3 % neutral density filter to reduce photobleaching of the fluorescent probe.
3. Pinhole size should be set at 100 μm for ion-specific dyes. In most cases, the image size is set at 512 × 512 pixels with pixel size of 0.08 μm for small ovoid-shaped cells and 0.034 μm for elongated cells.

3 Methods

3.1 Loading with Calcium Fluorescent Probes Using the Inverted Coverslip Method

The inverted coverslip method offers considerable time and money savings. More importantly, the use of smaller aliquots of concentrated stock solution needed to prepare the final probe concentration reduces the percentage of DMSO in the incubation medium. We have found that cell blebbing and photobleaching were commonly encountered with final DMSO concentrations greater than 0.6 %. Loading should also be performed at room temperature in a humidified environment when inverting coverslips on less than 100 μl of solution in order to avoid evaporation problems.

1. Culture single cells from the heart, aortic vascular smooth muscle, endothelium, or T lymphocytes or osteoblasts on coverslips or glass-bottom culture dishes.
2. Wash the cells three times with 2 ml of the Tyrode-BSA solution.
3. Place the glass coverslip cell side down on a 100 μl drop of the Fluo-3 solution (Tyrode-BSA), on a sheet of Parafilm stretched over a glass plate, and incubate for 45–60 min in the dark at room temperature.

4. After the loading period, carefully recover or the coverslip and wash the cells three times with Tyrode-BSS buffer.
5. Leave the loaded cells for an additional 15 min period to ensure complete hydrolysis of acetoxymethyl ester groups.

3.2 Acquisition of Intracellular Calcium Whole-Cell Images

1. After cleaning the objective lens, a drop of nonfluorescent oil is applied and then the chamber containing the loaded cells is placed in contact with the objective lens. Using the lowest possible intensity of the mercury lamp of the microscope, we choose a cell that presents a stable fluorescence level and that does not have a flat appearance. This should be done without exposing the chosen cell for a long period of time to mercury lamp light in order to avoid photobleaching.
2. The mercury lamp is turned off and the shutter of the microscope is set in the position allowing the passage of the laser excitation waves.
3. At first, a continuous section scanning is done in order to estimate the basal level of cytosolic and nuclear calcium. The cytosolic level should be between 50 and 100 nM, and the nuclear level should be all the time higher than that of the cytosol (near 300 nM) according to the calibration curve already determined for the calcium fluorescent dye. This permits all the cells used to have nearly the same starting normal calcium. During this process, the focus should be adjusted with the fine adjustment knob.
4. When the continuous sectioning is terminated, we proceed to the determination of the thickness of the cell by performing a vertical scan which allows the determination of the starting section (just above the cell) and the number of sections needed to scan the whole cell. The step size should be kept at the minimum value.
5. Serial *Z*-axis optical scans (section series) taken for the intracellular calcium of the cell are captured by a photodetector, digitalized, and saved (Fig. 1a). The captured section series can then be presented either as 2D or real quantitative 3D reconstructions using various angles of rotation and inclination as well as a variety of cutting planes. These real quantitative 3D reconstructions of cells (Fig. 1b, c) are then used for the measurement of basal level fluorescence intensity and/or the cellular response after the addition of different agents [1–5].
6. At the end of each experiment, the nucleus is stained with 100 nM of the live nucleic acid stain Syto-11 (Fig. 1c) (Molecular Probes, OR, USA) [1–5]. Serial *Z*-axis optical scans are taken after development of the stain (3–5 min) while maintaining positioning, number of sections, and step size identical to those used throughout the experiment. Nuclear labeling is

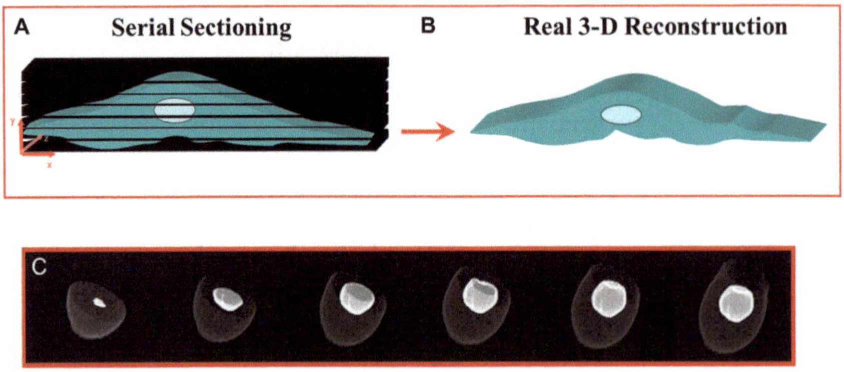

Fig. 1 Serial sectioning and real 3D reconstruction. (**a**) Using confocal microscopy, cells (and nuclei) are subjected to sequential serial scans, which permits the recording of fluorescence from conjugated antibodies and/or probes which target intracellular proteins (receptors and ligands), membranes, organelles, and ions. (**b**, **c**) Serial sections captured by confocal microscopy are reconstructed in real quantitative 3D using the ImageSpace software. The real quantitative 3D reconstruction allows measuring the total fluorescence (per μm^3) of a given target in volume. It also allows to designate the locations of organelles in the cell (**c**: 10-day-old single embryonic chick ventricular myocyte) and the specific fluorescence related to them

important because it permits the isolation or extraction of the nucleus from the cytoplasm by setting a lower-intensity threshold filter to confine relevant pixels [1–5]. Fluorescence intensities of the calcium probe can then be measured in the entire volume of each compartment (cytosol and nucleus) separately to provide quantitative 3D information (Fig. 1).

3.3 Rapid Scan of Intracellular Calcium

The confocal setting can be changed to the rapid-scan feature. This rapid-scan technique permits measurements of temporal rapid changes of intracellular calcium (Fig. 2). It is employed to visualize transitory variations of calcium (Fig. 2) which cannot be otherwise visualized by the real quantitative 3D scan given the fact that the duration of image acquisition in 3D can surpass that of the studied phenomenon. The rapid scan generates consecutive images of the section at the focal plane of the sample, with a speed of 0.320 s/image in the case of the Molecular Dynamics Multiprobe 2001 confocal microscope and 1.61 s/image for the MRC1024 Bio-Rad confocal microscope. With these speeds, even the smallest changes in fluorescence intensity, which would otherwise be undetected with conventional fluorescence microscopy tools, can be captured (Fig. 2). Up to 200 frames can be recorded. Each frame consists of 32 lines/scan, with a 512×512 pixel resolution. Graph tracings of fluorescence variations in the cytosol and the nucleus give the corresponding exact pattern of registered Ca^{2+} variations that occur spontaneously or as a consequence of pharmacological interventions (Fig. 2). Since the rapid scan is a result of 2D section image (Fig. 2), it cannot be used for measuring the level of calcium. However, it is an excellent tool to measure the kinetics of intracellular calcium variations as well as the frequency and relative amplitude of spontaneous calcium waves (Fig. 2).

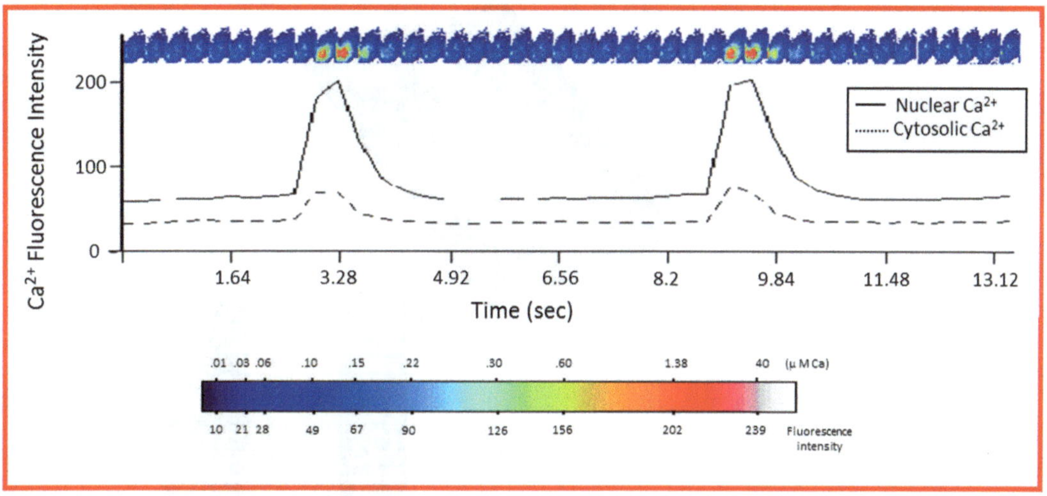

Fig. 2 Rapid scan of spontaneous cytosolic and nuclear calcium waves. Representative figure illustrating a continuous rapid scan of a section of heart cells contracting spontaneously and the corresponding graphic representation of the variation of cytosolic (discontinuous line) and nuclear (continuous line) using confocal microscopy. Images are generated continuously at the speed of 0.320 s/image at a resolution of 256 × 256 pixels of 0.7 μm each. At the end of the experiment, the nucleus is labeled with Syto-11. The pseudocolor bar represents the intensity of Ca^{2+} fluorescence and the absolute concentration of Ca^{2+} measured using the calcium calibration method described in Subheading 3.6

3.4 Intracellular Calcium Sparks and Puff Measurements Using Line-Scan Technique

The line scan is a versatile technique on the MRC1024 confocal microscope which allows to capture and visualize transient ion movements such as calcium sparks, puffs [14, 15], and waves occurring locally at a certain subcellular location in a cell.

1. After the right sample is chosen and set in focus, the scan line is placed at the desired location of the sample (e.g., in the cytosol, the perinuclear area, or the nucleoplasm) (Fig. 3). Upon execution, the system excites and scans the sample only along the designated scan line in the focal plane (Fig. 3). Up to 3000 line scans can be recorded in around 6 s, with a speed of 2 ms/line.
2. The images of the scan lines are stacked to generate an xt frame, where x is the scan line and t is time. Any change of fluorescence intensity along the line, in this case as a result of increase or decrease of Ca^{2+}, and any passage of Ca^{2+} transients through the line are therefore recorded and presented in the xt frame.
3. Using an appropriate image treatment software such as the ImageSpace software, the xt frames can be presented topographically, as a surface plot of fluorescence intensities, which allows a better appreciation of small Ca^{2+} signals (sparks and puffs). The frequency, amplitude, and kinetics of calcium sparks and puffs could be determined.

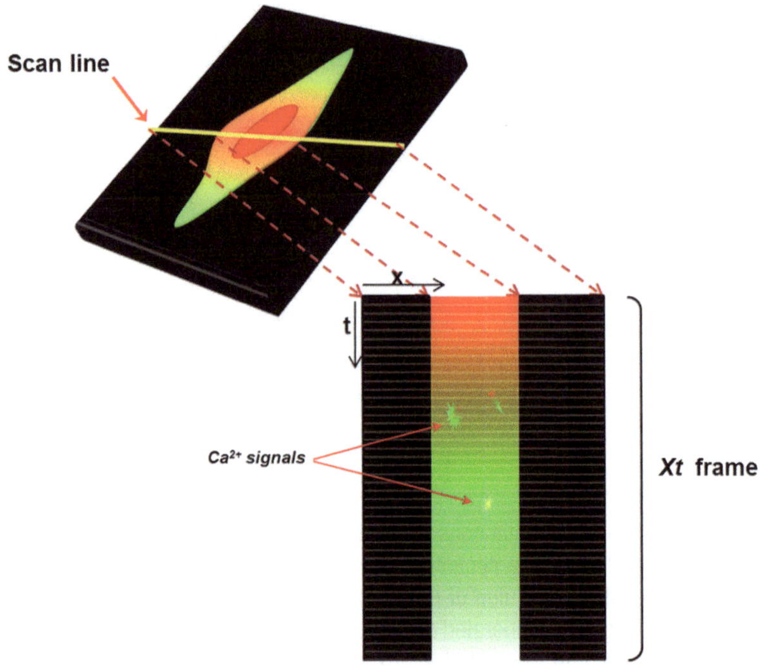

Fig. 3 Principle of line-scan technique for spontaneous Ca^{2+} sparks and puffs. Ca^{2+} probe-loaded cells are mounted on the metallic chamber of the confocal microscope, and after a sample cell is chosen, the scan line is positioned in the desired area of the cell (*red arrow*). Upon execution, up to 3000 scans can be performed at the line position, and the images of the recorded lines are stacked adjacently next to each other. The resultant is an xt frame, which depicts any temporal changes of fluorescence (sparks, puffs, waves) occurring at the line position or crossing through it

3.5 Volume Rendering for Cytosolic and Nuclear Calcium Measurements

1. Scanned images are transformed onto a Silicon Graphics O2 analysis station equipped with Molecular Dynamics Imagespace 3.2 analysis and volume workbench software modules. Reconstruction of quantitative real 3D images is performed on unfiltered serial sections (Fig. 1). All quantitative 3D reconstructions are presented using the "maximum intensity" top-view image format which produces high-contrast images and is sensitive to noise. It is worth noting that images are presented as pseudocolored representations according to an intensity scale of 0–255, with 0 intensity in black indicating the absence of fluorescence and 255 in white indicating the maximal fluorescence intensity [4].
2. The quantitative 3D reconstructions (section series) of cells are used for the measurement of whole-cell fluorescence intensities (per μm^3) where cells are simply delimited.
3. When the quantitative measurement of the nuclear and cytosolic fluorescence intensities is needed to be done separately, the nuclear area (following Syto-11 staining) is isolated from

the rest of the cell by setting a lower-intensity threshold filter to confine relevant pixels.

4. A 3D binary image series of the nuclear volume is generated for each cell, using the exact same x, y, and z set planes. Thus, by applying these binary image patterns, which now serve as a cookie cutter, to their corresponding cells (but labeled for calcium), two new real 3D projections are created depicting fluorescence intensity levels in the nucleus and cytosol separately [1–5].
5. Intensities are measured in the entire volume of sections for each compartment (cytosol and nucleus) to provide quantitative real 3D information. Since the measurements are done over the whole volume of the cell (per μm^3), and not in one or a few sections (per μm^3) for the entire cell volume, they eliminate any possible problem concerning drifting of the Z line.

3.6 Calcium Calibration Curve for Fluo-3

1. For each concentration of Ca^{2+} of kits No. 2 and No. 3, a final concentration of 13.5 μM Fluo-3 acid is added.
2. The cell membranes are perforated by exposing the cell to the 0.1% Triton solution for 10 min and then washed with the zero Ca^{2+} buffer of kit No. 2.
3. The confocal system is set for measuring Fluo-3 Ca^{2+} fluorescence as described before.
4. The perforated cells are then exposed to each different concentration of Ca^{2+} buffer containing 13.5 μM Fluo-3 acid, and the fluorescence intensity is recorded in the whole area under the field of the microscope.
5. At the end of the experiment, the fluorescence intensity of the last sample (1 mM free Ca^{2+}) is recorded and then Syto-11 is added to delimit the nuclear regions.
6. The calibration curve is plotted on intensity vs. concentration axes, and the results are fitted to the pseudocolor fluorescence intensity bar of the calcium dye (Fluo-3) (Fig. 3).

4 Notes

In order to overcome the limitation of using fluorescence imaging for the detection of intracellular calcium distribution and measurement in the cytosol and nucleus, the following should be taken into consideration:

1. For ionic probes, optimal loading should be ensured by determining the relative concentration of the bound and non-bound probe by using ionomycin to perforate the cell membrane. This also could be used at the end of each experiment (in the absence of Syto-11) in order to determine if the probe is completely bound to calcium.

2. A minimum of 36 serial sections and preferentially near 75–150 serial sections of the cell (depending on the morphology) should be taken at rest for quantiative real 3D imaging.
3. In order to avoid measurement problems due to difference in volumes between cells or between organelles, the fluorescence intensity should be normalized and expressed per μm^3. Furthermore, intensity measurement in a single section of a cell is that of a surface (μm^2) and does not represent absolute levels of intensity.
4. It is recommended to verify the distribution of the Ca^{2+} probe when a new type of cell is used.
5. Fluo-3 and other Ca^{2+} probes such as Indo-1, Fluo-4, Ca^{2+} green, yellow cameleon, and Fura-2 are equally distributed in the cytosol and the nucleus of the heart, vascular smooth muscle cells (VSMCs), vascular endothelial cells (VECs), and endocardial endothelial cells (EECs) of human (h), rat, rabbit, hamster, and mouse origins [2, 3, 5, 10, 12, 13]. Thus, these fluorescent probes can be used safely in these cell types.
6. For experiments longer than 20 min, it is absolutely important to replace the medium in order to avoid the effect related to evaporation of the experimental solution. If a drug is already present in the experimental bath, the replacement solution should already contain this drug. At least 2 min is necessary before continuing the experiment.

All of these aspects in addition to others should be established in order to accurately determine the fluorescence distribution and density of a fluorescent probe.

Acknowledgments

This study was supported by grants from the Canadian Institutes of Health Research (CIHR), the Natural Sciences and Engineering Research Council of Canada (NSERC), and the Heart and Stroke Foundation of Quebec (HSFQ) (grants awarded to Drs. Ghassan Bkaily and Danielle Jacques).

References

1. Bkaily G (1994) Ionic channels in vascular smooth. In: G. Bkaily (ed) Molecular Biology Intelligence Unit, Austin
2. Bkaily G, Gros-Louis N, Naik R, Jaalouk D, Pothier P (1996) Implication of the nucleus in excitation contraction-coupling of heart cells. Mol Cell Biochem 154:113–121
3. Bkaily G, Pothier P, Orleans-Juste P, Simaan M, Jacques D, Jaalouk D, Belzile F, Hassan G, Boutin C, Haddad G, Neugebauer W (1997) The use of confocal microscopy in the investigation of cell structure and function in the heart, vascular endothelium and smooth muscle cells. Mol Cell Biochem 172:171–194

4. Bkaily G, Jacques D, Pothier P (1999) Use of confocal microscopy to investigate cell structure and function. Methods Enzymol 307:119–135
5. Bkaily G, Nader M, Avedanian L, Choufani S, Jacques D, D'Orléans-Juste P, Gobeil F, Chemtob S, Al-Khoury J (2006) G -protein-coupled receptors, channels, and Na^+-H^+ exchanger in nuclear membranes of heart, hepatic, vascular endothelial, and smooth muscle cells. Can J Physiol Pharmacol 84:431–441
6. Bkaily G, Avedanian L, Jacques D (2009) Nuclear membranes' receptors and channels as targets for drug development in cardiovascular diseases. Can J Physiol Pharmacol 87(2):108–119
7. Bkaily G, Avedanian L, Al-Khoury J, Provost C, Nader M, D'Orleans-Juste P, Jacques D (2011) Nuclear membrane receptors for ET-1 in cardiovascular function. Am J Physiol Integr Comp Physiol 300(2):R251–R263
8. Bkaily G, Avedanian L, Al-Khoury J, Ahmarani L, Perreault C, Jacques D (2012) Receptors and ionic transporters in nuclear membranes: new targets for therapeutical pharmacological interventions. Can J Physiol Pharmacol 90:953–965
9. Avedanian L, Jacques D, Bkaily G (2011) Presence of tubular and reticular structures in the nucleus of human vascular smooth muscle cells. J Mol Cell Cardiol 50(1):175–186
10. Jacques D, Abdel Malak NA, Sader S (2003) Angiotensin II and its receptors in human endothelial endothelial cells: role in modulating intracellular calcium. Can J Physiol Pharmacol 81:259–266
11. Abdel-Samad D, Perreault C, Ahmarani L, Avedanian L, Bkaily G, Magder S, D'Orléans-Juste P, Jacques D (2012) Differences in neuropeptide Y-induced secretion of endothelin-1 in left and right human endocardial endothelial cells. Neuropeptides 46:373–382
12. Abernica B, Gilchrist JS (2000) Nucleoplasmic Ca^{2+} loading is regulated by mobilization of perinuclear Ca^{2+}. Cell Calcium 28:127–136
13. Abernica B, Pierce GM, Gilchrist JS (2003) Nucleoplasmic calcium regulation in rabbit aortic vascular smooth muscle cells. Can J Physiol Pharmacol 81:301–310
14. Cheng H, Lederer WJ, Cannell MB (1993) Calcium sparks: elementary events underlying excitation-contraction coupling in heart muscle. Science 262:740–744
15. Yao Y, Choi J, Parker I (1995) Quantal puffs of intracellular Ca^{2+} evoked by inositol trisphosphate in Xenopus oocytes. J Physiol 482:533–553

Chapter 15

Measuring T-Type Calcium Channel Currents in Isolated Vascular Smooth Muscle Cells

Ivana Y. Kuo and Caryl E. Hill

Abstract

Patch clamp electrophysiology is a powerful tool that has been important in isolating and characterizing the ion channels that govern cellular excitability under physiological and pathophysiological conditions. The ability to enzymatically dissociate blood vessels and acutely isolate vascular smooth muscle cells has enabled the application of patch clamp electrophysiology to the identification of diverse voltage dependent ion channels that ultimately control vasoconstriction and vasodilation. Since intraluminal pressure results in depolarization of vascular smooth muscle, the channels that control the voltage dependent influx of extracellular calcium are of particular interest. This chapter describes methods for isolating smooth muscle cells from resistance vessels, and for recording, isolating, and characterizing voltage dependent calcium channel currents, using patch clamp electrophysiological and pharmacological protocols.

Key words Voltage dependent calcium channel, Patch clamp electrophysiology, Vascular smooth muscle cells

1 Introduction

Peripheral resistance vessels play an important role in the regulation of blood pressure and exist in a state of partial constriction known as vascular tone. The maintenance of vascular tone results from elevation of the intracellular calcium concentration of smooth muscle cells, following influx of extracellular calcium or release of calcium from intracellular calcium stores. The myogenic response is an important regulatory response, which links increases in intraluminal pressure to vasoconstriction through depolarization of vascular smooth muscle cells and influx of calcium through voltage dependent calcium channels (VDCCs) [1, 2]. As these channels inactivate at various rates, the ability of VDCCs to contribute to the myogenic response results from the persistent calcium influx that occurs over the range of voltages where the steady-state activation and inactivation curves overlap [3]. This is known as the window current.

Rhian M. Touyz and Ernesto L. Schiffrin (eds.), *Hypertension: Methods and Protocols*, Methods in Molecular Biology, vol. 1527, DOI 10.1007/978-1-4939-6625-7_15, © Springer Science+Business Media LLC 2017

The VDCC superfamily is comprised of five families; the L- (Ca_v1), N-, P/Q-, R- (Ca_v2), and T-type (Ca_v3) channels. Of the 10 molecular subtypes of VDCCs comprising these families, the L-type channel, $Ca_V1.2$, is the main contributor to vascular tone [4] and increased activity of these channels has been linked to hypertension and cerebrovascular disease [5]. The resting membrane potential of smooth muscle cells of pressurized arteries and arterioles in vivo and in vitro is relatively depolarized; lying in the range, −45 to −30 mV [4, 6–10]. This voltage range encompasses the window current of L-type channel splice variants isolated from small cerebral arteries [11, 12]. However, recent studies have provided evidence for the expression of other VDCCs, particularly the T-type channels, $Ca_v3.1$ and $Ca_v3.2$, in the vasculature (see [13]). Unfortunately, defining the contribution of T-type channels to vascular tone has been complicated by the inability of many of the commonly used T-type channel antagonists to clearly select between L- and T-type effects [13]. Nevertheless, patch clamp electrophysiology of isolated vascular smooth muscle cells provides a very useful technique to assist in identifying a role for T-type channels in physiological and pathological states, such as hypertension, since this technique enables investigation of the differing biophysical characteristics of the endogenous currents. Unlike the L-, N-, P/Q-, and R-type VDCCs, the T-type channels are low voltage activated, i.e., they are activated at more hyperpolarized potentials than the other VDCC superfamily members.

The patch clamp technique, developed by Sakmann, Neher, and colleagues in the late 1970s, is a powerful tool to measure currents produced by the opening of ion channels in cells [14]. In this technique, a tight seal is formed between a glass micropipette filled with solution and the membrane of a cell. To obtain the whole-cell configuration, the cell membrane at the mouth of the pipette is disrupted by suction and the membrane reseals around the mouth of the pipette, providing electrical access to the whole cell. Another configuration, which allows study of individual ion channels, involves isolation of a patch of the cell membrane in the mouth of the pipette. Through the single electrode, either current or voltage steps can be delivered to the cell or the membrane patch, and the resultant changes in voltage (current clamp) or current (voltage clamp) can be recorded. The reader is directed to the following resources for a review of the theory behind the patch clamp electrophysiological technique [15, 16].

In this chapter, we describe procedures for the isolation of vascular smooth muscle cells from cerebral arteries and application of the whole-cell patch clamp configuration in voltage clamp mode to measure and characterize the VDCCs of these cells. Several prominent laboratories have studied VDCCs and other ion channels expressed in vascular smooth muscle cells and references to some of these studies are provided in Table 1.

It should be noted that the protocols described here have been developed to study T-type calcium channel currents in cerebrovascular smooth muscle cells. Since T-type channels are low voltage activated, investigation of these channels involves the use of protocols that employ voltage steps from membrane potentials (holding potentials) that are more negative than those likely to be experienced by smooth muscle cells of pressurized vessels. We therefore also focus on the pharmacological tools that can be used to assist in the differentiation of L- and T-type calcium channels in smooth muscle cells [13].

Table 1
Examples of studies of ion channels in vascular smooth muscle cells

Reference (first author)	Year	Animal	Age/weight	Vessel	Channel
Droogmans [19]	1987	Rabbit	1–2 kg	Ear	VDCC
Wang [20]	1989	Rat	100–200 g	Tail	VDCC
Simard [21]	1991	Guinea pig	200–500 g	Basilar	VDCC
Worley [22]	1991	Rabbit	N/A	Basilar	Includes VDCC
Langton [23, 24]	1993	Rat	N/A	Basilar	VDCC
Quayle [25]	1993	Rat	16–25 Weeks	PCA	VDCC
Ohya [26]	1993	Rat	4–5, 16–18 Weeks	Mesenteric	VDCC
McHugh [27]	1996	Guinea pig	350–400 g	Basilar	VDCC
Yokoshiki [28]	1997	Rat	250–350 g	Mesenteric	VDCC
Petkov [29]	2001	Rat	Adult	Tail	VDCC
Matchkov [30]	2004	Rat	12–18 Weeks	Mesenteric	VDCC, Cl^-
Nikitina [31]	2007	Dog	Adult	Basilar	VDCC
Zhang [32]	2007	Mouse	12–18 Weeks	Mesenteric	VDCC
Criddle [33]	1994	Rat	150–200 g	Mesenteric	Potassium
Jackson [34]	1997	Rat Hamster	250–450 g rats 80–150 g hamster	Cremaster	Potassium
Park [35]	2007	Rabbit	1–2 kg	Basilar	Potassium
Wu [36]	2007	Rat	10–12 Weeks	Basilar	Potassium
Morita [37]	2007	Rat	10–12 Weeks	PCA, MCA	TRP
Welsh [38]	2000	Rat	12–16 Weeks	Cerebral, PCA	Cl^-
Berra Romani [18]	2005	Mouse, rats	3–4 Month mice 200–250 g rats	Mesenteric	Na_V

VDCC voltage dependent calcium channel, *TRP* transient receptor potential channel, Cl^- chloride channels, Na_v voltage dependent sodium channels, *PCA* posterior cerebral artery, *MCA* middle cerebral artery, *N/A* not available

2 Materials

All solutions should be prepared using MilliQ distilled water (18 MΩ at 25 °C). Solutions should be stored at 4 °C, unless otherwise stated.

2.1 Isolation of Cerebral Blood Vessels

1. Isoflurane vaporisor, or other suitable, approved short-acting anesthetic.
2. Surgical instruments: rongeurs, forceps, large and small scissors, scalpel handle and clean blade, iridectomy scissors, No. 5 watchmakers forceps.
3. Dissecting microscope.
4. Dissecting dishes (5 cm glass dishes) with a layer of sylgard polymer set in the base.
5. Fine pins, cut to size from a roll of tungsten wire (0.05 mm diameter).

2.2 Enzymatic Dissociation of Blood Vessels

1. Physiological Saline Solution: (PSS, mM): NaCl 140, KCl 5, $MgCl_2 \cdot 6H_2O$ 1, HEPES 10, Glucose 10 (*see* **Note 1**). Add 1 % albumin (endotoxin-free) and 0.01 mM $CaCl_2$. Adjust pH to 7.3 at room temperature with NaOH, filter at 0.22 μm. Check osmolarity (315–325 mOsmol).
2. Enzyme Solution A: Papain 0.5 mg/ml, dithioerythritol (DTE) 1.6 mg/ml, DNasel 5 U/ml in PSS. Adjust pH to 7.3 at room temperature with NaOH, filter at 0.22 μm. Make up fresh.
3. Enzyme Solution B: Collagenase 1.5 mg/ml (Type IV; Worthington), DNasel 5 U/ml in PSS (*see* **Notes 2** and **3**). Adjust pH to 7.3 at room temperature with NaOH, filter at 0.22 μm.
4. Acid washed coverslips for plating cells: Wash glass coverslips in 1 M HCl overnight with shaking. Rinse twice in distilled water over 30 min. Dry in oven. Coverslips can be cut into small pieces so that 4–6 pieces would fit in a single tissue culture dish (see below).
5. Tissue culture grade petri dishes (35 mm diameter) for plating cells.
6. Glass Pasteur pipettes for dissociation of blood vessels; tips are fire polished to prevent damage to tissues and cells during trituration.

2.3 Patch Clamp Electrophysiology

1. Electrodes: pulled from borosilicate glass (GC150 F-15, Clark Electromedical Instruments; outer diameter 1.5 mm, inner diameter 0.8 mm), tips are fire polished to facilitate high resistance seals. Tip resistance is 5–7 MΩ in bath solution and filled with Electrode solution (see below). Tips may be coated with sylgard to minimize noise, if necessary.

2. Vapor pressure osmometer (*see* **Note 4**).
3. Electrode solution (mM): CsCl 110, Na_2phosphocreatine 20, EGTA 10, Na_2ATP 5, $MgCl_2$ 5, NaGTP 0.2, HEPES 10, adjusted using CsOH to pH 7.3, 315–325 mOsmol. Filter at 0.22 μm.
4. Barium Extracellular Bath Solution (mM): NaCl 135, $BaCl_2$ 10, TEA-Cl 10, HEPES 10, CsCl 5, Glucose 10, pH 7.3, 315–325 mOsmol (*see* **Note 5**). Store at 4 °C. Filter before use.
5. Calcium Extracellular Bath Solution: as above, except 10 mM $BaCl_2$ is replaced with 2 mM $CaCl_2$ and 5 mM 4-aminopyridine.
6. Inverted phase contrast microscope with 10×, 20×, and 40× lenses; Faraday cage; perfusion system for fast exchange of solutions.
7. Electrode puller.
8. Axopatch or equivalent amplifier.
9. Analogue-to-digital converter.
10. Computer and software capable of delivering electrophysiological protocols (e.g., Axograph, pClamp).

2.4 Pharmacology

1. Nifedipine/nimodipine: Dissolved in DMSO (stock concentration 10 mM), store at −20 °C. As dihydropyridines undergo photodegeneration, these drugs were protected from light and fresh stocks made weekly. The final concentration of DMSO in bath solution not greater than 0.1 % v/v.
2. Mibefradil/NNC 55-0396/$NiCl_2$/diltiazem: Dissolved in water.
3. Efonidipine: Due to the limited solubility of the efonidipine enantiomer in aqueous solution, stock solutions of 400 μM efonidipine were made in DMSO; however, the final concentration was 5 % DMSO when used at 20 μM.
4. *See* Table 2 for suggested concentrations and comments for L-type and T-type channel antagonists.

3 Methods

3.1 Blood Vessel Dissection

1. Anesthetize and decapitate rat/mouse according to approved animal ethics protocols.
2. Remove skin from dorsal part of skull. Use rongeurs to remove the dorsal skull from the neck to the optical orbits. Use scalpel to cut through the brain anteriorly, remove brain from the skull by gently cutting through the cranial nerves as they exit the skull. Transfer brain into beaker of prechilled PSS.

Table 2
Pharmacological tools used to investigate VDCCs in smooth muscle cells

L-type channel antagonists	T-type channel antagonists
Nifedipine: use at 1 μM	Mibebradil: 1 μM blocks all currents including L-type
Nimodipine: use at 10 μM	NNC 55-0396: 1 μM blocks all currents including L-type
Diltazem: use at 10 μM	Efonidipine: 20 μM blocks all currents including L-type
Calciseptine: use at 500 nM	Nickel: 100 μM specifically targets the $Ca_v3.2$, without inhibiting the Ca_v 3.1 or Ca_v 3.3 channels

3. Transfer brain into dissecting dish and, under a dissecting microscope, carefully remove the pial membranes containing the cerebral vessels of interest. Transfer to a clean dissecting dish containing prechilled PSS.
4. Using the tungsten pins, immobilize the pia and carefully remove the vessels.
5. If the vessel is large enough, pin and cut open along the axial length.
6. Cut vessel into short segments and transfer into a 10 ml volumetric flask using a glass, fire polished Pasteur pipette.

3.2 Enzymatic Dissociation of Vessel Segments

1. Remove PSS and add 2 ml Enzyme Solution A (*see* **Note 6**).
2. Incubate with gentle agitation (gently shaking water bath) for ~15 min at 36 °C (*see* **Note 7**).
3. Remove supernatant gently with glass pasteur pipette.
4. Rinse once with 2 ml enzyme-free PSS (room temperature solution).
5. Add 2 ml Enzyme Solution B and incubate without shaking for 15 min at 36 °C.
6. Remove supernatant and rinse twice with 2 ml enzyme-free PSS (room temperature solution).
7. Triturate with fire polished wide bore pipette—usually between 20 and 40 times. The tissue should start to break up into little pieces.
8. Pipette total volume, onto acid washed glass coverslips in a 35 mm tissue culture dish.
9. Allow cells to settle for 20 min at room temperature. Check cell morphology under a microscope. Cells should be elongated in shape (Fig. 1).

3.3 Electrophysiological Measurements

1. Place coverslip with cells gently into the recording chamber filled with bath solution. Connect Ag-AgCl ground electrode to the bath using a 10% agar salt bridge containing 200 mM NaCl.

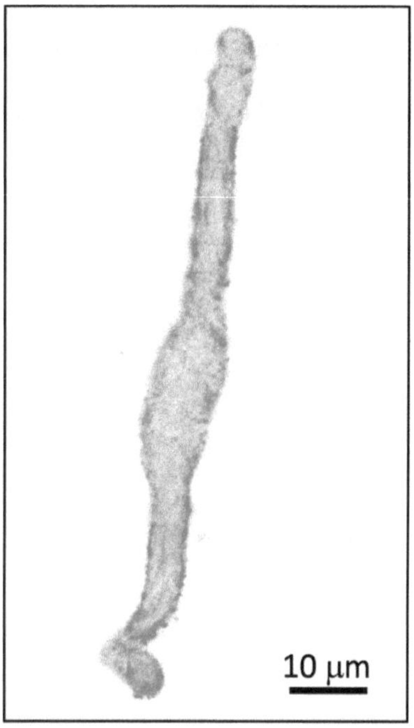

Fig. 1 Smooth muscle cells dissociated with papain should retain an elongated morphology

2. Fill electrode with electrode solution, mount in micromanipulator and lower electrode tip visually toward an isolated elongated cell.
3. Apply slight positive pressure to the patch pipette, to blow off any remaining debris, and to prevent clogging of the patch pipette (*see* **Note 8**).
4. Keep slowly lowering the pipette and when the pipette touches the cell, apply negative pressure to help the seal form. Sometimes, releasing the pressure aids in seal formation.
5. Once a gigaseal (1 GΩ) is reached, break through the cell membrane by applying increasing bursts of negative pressure.
6. The cell capacitance of these cells should be around 11.3 pF, with an input resistance of around 2 GΩ (*see* Table 3). Cells can be fixed and stained at this point to ensure that the VDCCs still remain in the membrane.

3.4 Protocols to Characterize Voltage Dependent Calcium Currents

1. Various protocols can be utilized to determine the biophysical characteristics of the voltage dependent calcium currents in smooth muscle cells. Differing holding potentials can be used to evoke low voltage activated (T-type channels) and high voltage activated (L-, N-, P/Q-, R-) VDCCs. For example, a holding potential of −100 mV will maximally activate T-type channels, while a holding potential of −50 mV will maximally

Table 3
Characteristics of smooth muscle cells from basilar artery

% of elongated smooth muscle cells	80–90 %
Cell capacitance (pF)	11.3 ± 0.7 (n = 27)
Input resistance (GΩ)	2.0 ± 0.2 (n = 27)

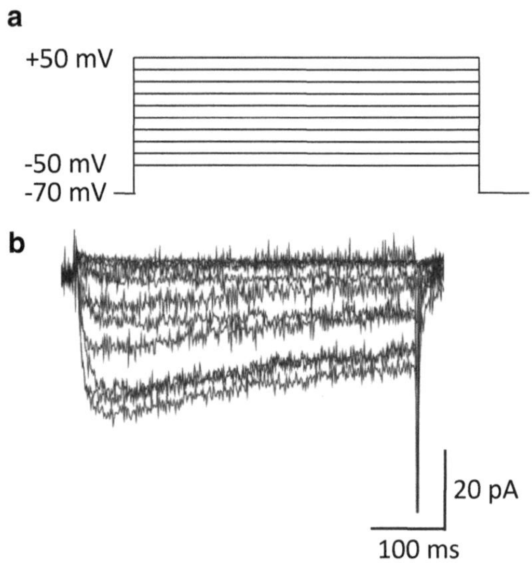

Fig. 2 Example of the voltage protocol for current activation from a holding potential of −70 mV (**a**). Corresponding calcium currents elicited by this series of depolarizing voltage steps (**b**)

activate the high voltage activated channels. In addition to −100 mV, we chose to use a holding potential of −70 mV, as it approximates the membrane potential of smooth muscle cells in fully relaxed arteries, and −50 mV, as it approximates the membrane potential of smooth muscle cells in pressurized arteries.

2. Current records can be low-pass filtered at 2 or 10 kHz. Leak currents can be subtracted online from all measurements by scaling a 10 mV hyperpolarizing pre-pulse, repeated four times, to the size of the test pulse.
3. Current/voltage (I/V) curve for current activation: Incremental 10 mV depolarizing voltage steps from holding potentials of −100, −70, or −50 mV to voltages between −50 and +50 mV for 100 ms every 5 s can be used to evoke voltage dependent calcium currents (*see* Fig. 2).

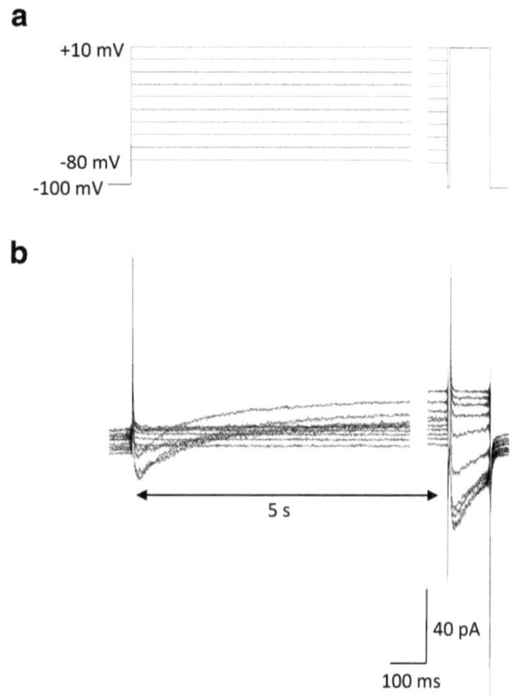

Fig. 3 Example of the voltage protocol for current inactivation from a holding potential of −100 mV (**a**). Corresponding calcium currents elicited during the 5 s inactivation step to voltages between −80 and +10 mV, and the currents activated during the test pulse to +10 mV (**b**)

4. *I*/*V* curve for current inactivation: Inactivation currents can be elicited by examining the currents after applying a 5 s conditioning pulse (sufficiently long to enable even slowly inactivating L-type channels to reach steady state conditions) from holding potentials of −100, −70, or −50 mV, to varying potentials from −80 to +10 mV, followed by a brief repolarizing step to close any open channels (10 ms), followed by a depolarizing test pulse to +10 mV (100 ms) to assess channel availability (*see* Fig. 3).
5. Channel deactivation (Tail currents): A hallmark of T-type channels is their slow deactivation; a measure of channel closure. Tail currents showing channel closure can be evoked following a voltage step from −100 to +10 mV for 20 ms, then rapid repolarization to −90 mV (*see* **Note 9**).

3.5 Analysis of Current Characteristics

1. *I*/*V* curves can either be fitted as a function of cell capacitance, or normalized to I_{max}. Normalization to cell capacitance takes into account any variation in cell size.
2. Window currents: Both activation and inactivation curves determined from the protocols described above can be fitted

with Boltzman equations and overlaid to obtain the window current. Typical parameters include the $V_{0.5}$ (voltage for half maximal activation), V_h (voltage for half maximal inactivation), V_{max} (voltage for maximum activation), the slope of the activation/inactivation curves (k), and the time constants (τ) for activation/inactivation (measure of the rate of increase/decrease in the current).

3. Tail currents: Time constants for deactivation can be calculated by fitting either double or single exponentials.

3.6 Pharmacological Analysis of Currents

1. There are no entirely selective antagonists of T-type channels available. Mibefradil, NNC 55-0396 (1 μM), efonidipine (20 μM) all block the L-type current (*see* Table 2).
2. To pharmacologically isolate T-type like currents, apply an L-type channel antagonist (*see* Table 2 for examples) or combination of L-, N-, P/Q-, and R-type antagonists (*see* **Note 10**).
3. Drug-sensitive and insensitive components can be analyzed for differences in several parameters, including $V_{0.5}$, k, and τ [17].

4 Notes

1. PSS can be made up as a 10× stock without BSA or $CaCl_2$ and frozen in appropriately sized aliquots.
2. Collagenase can be made as 10× stock in PSS, pH adjusted to 7.3, filter sterilized at 0.22 μm, and frozen in 200 μl aliquots.
3. RNase free DNase is added to prevent DNA released from dead cells causing aggregation of tissue pieces and cell damage during the trituration phase.
4. Use an osmometer to ensure that the osmolarity of the electrode and bath solutions is ~320 mOsmol. Check the osmolarity of solutions daily, as fluctuations greater than 10 mOsmol can impair currents. Correct pH of solutions is also critical.
5. The standard bath solution is designed to block potassium currents that contribute to outward leak current and an underestimation of inward calcium current.
6. Other investigators have utilized alternative enzymatic cocktails to dissociate smooth muscle cells (see references in Table 1; particularly [18]). In our experience, other enzymatic methods, for example, collagenase and elastase, produced cells that were more contractile and had lower cell capacitances (7.6 pF).
7. The optimal incubation time in the enzyme solution should be determined by the investigator, since it varies depending on the type of vessel used; for example, basilar artery 15 min, middle cerebral artery 11–12 min, branches of basilar artery 9 min. We prefer to use a water bath for incubations.

8. The slight positive pressure will also cause some internal solution to escape from the pipette. The ATP within the pipette will cause the cell to constrict slightly. If the cells do not immediately constrict to ATP, the metabotropic receptors, and thus, by extension, the membrane, may be damaged, rendering it unlikely that VDCCs currents will be obtained.
9. Tail currents are amplified during the rapid repolarization step due to the increase in driving force for calcium as the membrane potential moves rapidly away from the equilibrium potential for calcium.
10. The block by nifedipine is stable after 3 min of constant perfusion. Nifedipine can be washed out after 3 min perfusion of bath solution. Sometimes, facilitation of the current is observed after washout.
11. **Trouble Shooting:** Low cell yield. This usually occurs when the cells have not been sufficiently digested. Ensure that the temperature of the water bath is 36 °C. Check the papain, as it loses its activity quickly. If the papain bottle has been opened for 2–3 months, it may be necessary to raise the papain concentration. The DTE concentration can also be increased to 2 mg/ml.
12. **Trouble Shooting:** Cells are alive, but shrivel up in bath solution: Ensure the pH of all solutions is 7.3. Ensure the osmolarity of all solutions is 320 ± 10 mOsmol.
13. **Trouble Shooting:** Cells are tough to break into: Try increasing the concentration of the papain or the incubation time in papain.

References

1. Davis MJ, Hill MA (1999) Signaling mechanisms underlying the vascular myogenic response. Physiol Rev 79:387–423
2. Schubert R, Mulvany MJ (1999) The myogenic response: established facts and attractive hypotheses. Clin Sci (Lond) 96:313–326
3. Perez-Reyes E (2003) Molecular physiology of low-voltage-activated T-type calcium channels. Physiol Rev 83:117–161
4. Knot HJ, Nelson MT (1998) Regulation of arterial diameter and wall [Ca2+] in cerebral arteries of rat by membrane potential and intravascular pressure. J Physiol 508:199–209
5. Pesic A et al (2004) High blood pressure upregulates arterial L-type Ca2+ channels: is membrane depolarization the signal? Circ Res 94:e97–e104
6. Loutzenhiser R et al (1997) Membrane potential measurements in renal afferent and efferent arterioles: actions of angiotensin II. Am J Physiol 273:F307–F314
7. Welsh DG, Segal SS (1998) Endothelial and smooth muscle cell conduction in arterioles controlling blood flow. Am J Physiol 274: H178–H186
8. Siegl D et al (2005) Myoendothelial coupling is not prominent in arterioles within the mouse cremaster microcirculation in vivo. Circ Res 97:781–788
9. Kotecha N, Hill MA (2005) Myogenic contraction in rat skeletal muscle arterioles: smooth muscle membrane potential and Ca(2+) signaling. Am J Physiol Heart Circ Physiol 289:H1326–H1334
10. Wolfle SE et al (2011) Non-linear relationship between hyperpolarisation and relaxation enables long distance propagation of vasodilatation. J Physiol 589:2607–2623

11. Liao P et al (2007) A smooth muscle $Ca_V1.2$ calcium channel splice variant underlies hyperpolarized window current and enhanced state-dependent inhibition by nifedipine. J Biol Chem 282:35133–35142
12. Cheng X et al (2009) Alternative splicing of Cav1.2 channel exons in smooth muscle cells of resistance-size arteries generates currents with unique electrophysiological properties. Am J Physiol Heart Circ Physiol 297:H680–H688
13. Kuo IY et al (2011) T-type calcium channels and vascular function: the new kid on the block? J Physiol 589(Pt 4):783–795
14. Hamill OP et al (1981) Improved patch-clamp techniques for high-resolution current recording from cells and cell-free membrane patches. Pflugers Arch 391:85–100
15. Hille B (2001) Ion channels of excitable membranes, 3rd edn. Sinauer Associates Inc, Sunderland, MA
16. Sakmann B, Neher E (eds) (2009) Single-channel recording, 2nd edn. Springer Science + Business Media, LLC, New York
17. Kuo IY et al (2010) Dihydropyridine-insensitive calcium currents contribute to function of small cerebral arteries. J Cereb Blood Flow Metab 30:1226–1239
18. Berra-Romani R et al (2008) Ca2+ handling is altered when arterial myocytes progress from a contractile to a proliferative phenotype in culture. Am J Physiol 295:C779–C790
19. Droogmans G et al (1987) Effect of adrenergic agonists on Ca^{2+}-channel currents in single vascular smooth muscle cells. Pflugers Arch 409:7–12
20. Wang R et al (1989) Two types of calcium channels in isolated smooth muscle cells from rat tail artery. Am J Physiol 256:H1361–H1368
21. Simard JM (1991) Calcium channel currents in isolated smooth muscle cells from the basilar artery of the guinea pig. Pflugers Arch 417:528–536
22. Worley JF et al (1991) Regulation of single calcium channels in cerebral arteries by voltage, serotonin, and dihydropyridines. Am J Physiol 261:H1951–H1960
23. Langton PD (1993) Calcium channel currents recorded from isolated myocytes of rat basilar artery are stretch sensitive. J Physiol 471:1–11
24. Langton PD, Standen NB (1993) Calcium currents elicited by voltage steps and steady voltages in myocytes isolated from the rat basilar artery. J Physiol 469:535–548
25. Quayle JM et al (1993) Single calcium channels in resistance-sized cerebral arteries from rats. Am J Physiol 264:H470–H478
26. Ohya Y et al (1993) Voltage-dependent Ca2+ channels in resistance arteries from spontaneously hypertensive rats. Circ Res 73: 1090–1099
27. McHugh D, Beech DJ (1996) Modulation of Ca^{2+} channel activity by ATP metabolism and internal Mg^{2+} in guinea-pig basilar artery smooth muscle cells. J Physiol 492(Pt 2): 359–376
28. Yokoshiki H et al (1997) Regulation of Ca^{2+} channel currents by intracellular ATP in smooth muscle cells of rat mesenteric artery. Am J Physiol 272:H814–H819
29. Petkov GV et al (2001) Characterization of voltage-gated calcium currents in freshly isolated smooth muscle cells from rat tail main artery. Acta Physiol Scand 173:257–265
30. Matchkov VV et al (2004) A cyclic GMP-dependent calcium-activated chloride current in smooth-muscle cells from rat mesenteric resistance arteries. J Gen Physiol 123:121–134
31. Nikitina E et al (2007) Voltage-dependent calcium channels of dog basilar artery. J Physiol 580:523–541
32. Zhang J et al (2007) Role of Cav1.2 L-type Ca2+ channels in vascular tone: effects of nifedipine and Mg2+. Am J Physiol Heart Circ Physiol 292:H415–H425
33. Criddle DN et al (1994) Levcromakalim-induced modulation of membrane potassium currents, intracellular calcium and mechanical activity in rat mesenteric artery. Naunyn Schmiedebergs Arch Pharmacol 349: 422–430
34. Jackson WF et al (1997) Enzymatic isolation and characterization of single vascular smooth muscle cells from cremasteric arterioles. Microcirculation 4:35–50
35. Park JK et al (2007) Regulation of membrane excitability by intracellular pH (pHi) changers through Ca2+-activated K+ current (BK channel) in single smooth muscle cells from rabbit basilar artery. Pflugers Arch 454:307–319
36. Wu BN et al (2007) Hyposmotic challenge inhibits inward rectifying K+ channels in cerebral arterial smooth muscle cells. Am J Physiol Heart Circ Physiol 292:H1085–H1094
37. Morita H et al (2007) Membrane stretch-induced activation of a TRPM4-like nonselective cation channel in cerebral artery myocytes. J Pharmacol Sci 103:417–426
38. Welsh DG et al (2000) Swelling-activated cation channels mediate depolarization of rat cerebrovascular smooth muscle by hyposmolarity and intravascular pressure. J Physiol 527(Pt 1):139–148

Chapter 16

In Vitro Analysis of Hypertensive Signal Transduction: Kinase Activation, Kinase Manipulation, and Physiologic Outputs

Katherine J. Elliott and Satoru Eguchi

Abstract

Studying signal transduction in hypertension model systems in vitro will include several steps: (1) develop the cell culture model and induce hypertensive changes, (2) observe kinase activation, (3) manipulate signal transduction pathways, and (4) observe physiologic outputs. This chapter will provide the reader with overviews of the techniques our lab uses to inhibit signaling pathways with inhibitory RNAs and the outputs we use to monitor the effects.

Key words Tyrosine kinase, MAP kinase, Signal transduction, EGFR, ERK, Explant primary cell culture, miRNA, Adenovirus, VSMC, Angiotensin II

1 Introduction

This chapter will provide the reader with instructions on how to culture rat vascular smooth muscle cells (VSMC) and how to stimulate them with angiotensin II (Ang II) to induce a cellular hypertrophic phenotype similar to that observed in hypertension. Primary cell cultures, derived from dissection of living tissue and maintained in culture for a limited number of passages, provide a great tool to simplify the study of complex biologic disease processes such as hypertension and associated organ damage. The explant methods allow VSMC to migrate from the rat aorta onto a cell culture dish forming a monolayer of adherent cells, which will continue to proliferate for up to 12 passages [1, 2]. These cells can be stimulated by various agonists and manipulated genetically by adenovirus infection and downstream signal transduction pathways studied. This is a relatively easy-to-use and inexpensive model for the study of hypertensive signal transduction pathways.

This chapter will focus on epidermal growth factor receptor (EGFR) as an example of a tyrosine kinase and ERK as an example

Rhian M. Touyz and Ernesto L. Schiffrin (eds.), *Hypertension: Methods and Protocols*, Methods in Molecular Biology, vol. 1527, DOI 10.1007/978-1-4939-6625-7_16,

of MAP kinase (MAPK) and detail protocols to observe hypertensive signal transduction. The EGFR tyrosine kinases initiate signal transduction cascades that start with an autophosphorylation event, leading to activation of MAP kinases [3]. In vitro systems of cell culture lend themselves nicely to performing Western blot analysis to determine kinase activation by looking for the phosphorylation events by using phosphorylation-selective antibodies.

There are many ways to manipulate signaling events in cell culture, but we will focus here on inhibiting the kinase activity of EGFR or ERK through inhibitory RNA technologies using an adenoviral gene delivery system [4]. Primary cell cultures tend to be difficult to transfect; consequently, we have turned to infection with adenovirus to ensure close to 100% efficiency of gene transfer. Adenovirus can be constructed that will express siRNA-embedded micro inhibitory RNA (miR) and effectively block expression of endogenous kinases [5].

Finally, signal transduction events are best studies when physiologic outputs are monitored. The most critical change that occurs in VSMC with regard to hypertension is hypertrophy [6, 7]. We will discuss methodologies to monitor changes that occur in VSMC after stimulation.

2 Materials

2.1 Explant Method for VSMC Primary Cell Culture

This technique was adapted from Ross [2, 8].

1. 12-week-old male Sprague Dawley rat
2. Surgical scissors and tweezers.
3. VSMC growth medium: Dulbecco's modification of Eagle's medium (DMEM), 10% (v/v) fetal bovine serum, 1% (v/v) penicillin–streptomycin solution.
4. Trypsin.
5. HBSS.
6. CO_2 incubator.

2.2 Creating and miR-Expressing Adenovirus

1. BLOCK-iT™ Pol II miR RNAi Expression Vector Kit, Invitrogen.
2. Competent DH5α *E. coli.*
3. LB media and LB agar plates.
4. 1000× stock of spectinomycin (50 mg/ml in H_2O), kanamycin (50 mg/ml in H_2O), ampicillin (100 mg/ml in H_2O).
5. Commercial plasmid purification kit.
6. EagI and PacI restriction enzymes.
7. Phenol–chloroform–isoamylalcohol (25:24:1).

8. Chloroform.
9. TE: 10 mM Tris pH 8.0, 1 mM EDTA.
10. Gateway BP Clonase II, Invitrogen.
11. Gateway LR Clonase II, Invitrogen.
12. HEK 293 cells.
13. HEK 293 growth medium: DMEM, 1% (v/v) penicillin–streptomycin solution, 10% (v/v) fetal bovine serum, 2 mM L-glutamine.
14. Lipofectamine or other standard transfection reagents.
15. Fluorescent microscope.

2.3 Adenoviral Infection of VSMC

1. Serum-free medium: DMEM, 1% (v/v) penicillin–streptomycin solution.
2. FuGENE 6.

2.4 VSMC Stimulation with Angiotensin II

1. Serum-free medium: DMEM, 1% (v/v) penicillin–streptomycin solution.
2. Angiotensin II.

2.5 Western Blot

1. 1× SDS loading buffer: 0.05 M Tris–HCl pH 6.8, 2% (w/v) SDS, 6% (v/v) β-mercaptoethanol, 1% (w/v) bromophenol blue.
2. Sonicator.
3. 7.5 or 10% SDS PAGE gel, either preformed or make your own.
4. Nitrocellulose membrane.
5. Overnight transfer buffer: 4.5 g Tris–Base, 21.6 g glycine, 1200 ml H_2O, 330 ml methanol.
6. 10× TBS: 60.57 g Tris–Base, pH 7.5, 116.88 g NaCl, H_2O up to 1000 ml.
7. TBS-Tween: 100 ml 10× TBS, 1 ml Tween 20, 900 ml dH_2O.
8. Nonfat dry milk.
9. Primary antibody.
10. HRP-conjugated secondary antibody, usually anti-mouse or anti-rabbit.
11. ECL reagents.
12. X-ray film.
13. Autoradiography cassette and developer.

2.6 VSMC Hypertrophy

1. 0.5% SDS.
2. BCA protein assay kit.

3. Plate reader or spectrophotometer.
4. Trypsin.
5. HBSS.
6. PBS.
7. Coulter counter.
8. MTS assay kit.
9. Plate reader.

3 Methods

3.1 Explant Method for VSMC Primary Cell Culture

1. Excise the thoracic aorta of a male Sprague Dawley rat (200–250 g) directly below the left subclavian artery and above the diaphragm. Rapidly immerse in VSMC growth medium. Carefully remove connective tissue and adherent fat.
2. Longitudinally, cut open isolated aorta, and remove the endothelium by gently rubbing the intimal surface with a dull scissor (*see* **Note 1**).
3. Cut denuded aorta into approximately 3-mm square sections. Place the intimal side down into 6-well culture dish.
4. Gently add enough VSMC growth medium to minimally cover the tissue, about 100–200 μl, without disturbing the orientation of the explant and without causing the explant to float. Culture at 37 °C in 5% CO_2 incubator. Avoid handling the plate for 48 h after explant so as not to dislodge the tissue (*see* **Note 2**).
5. Beginning on day 2, monitor the plate for cell growth and add additional medium as necessary to avoid drying of tissue and migrating cells.
6. Allow VSMCs to grow out from the explant for 7–14 days (Fig. 1).
7. Once cells have established a monolayer culture surrounding the tissue, remove tissue and harvest cells by trypsin. Transfer collected cells to a 100-mm flask.
8. The cells obtained by this method should express the “hill and valley” growth characteristics of cultured VSMC. The expression of myosin light chain and smooth muscle α-actin can be confirmed by immunocytochemistry.
9. Cells should be maintained by passaging once a week with trypsin and seeding in 75-cm² flasks at approximately 0.5–1.0×10^6 cells. Cells should not be passaged more than 12 times and should never be frozen for storage (*see* **Note 3**).

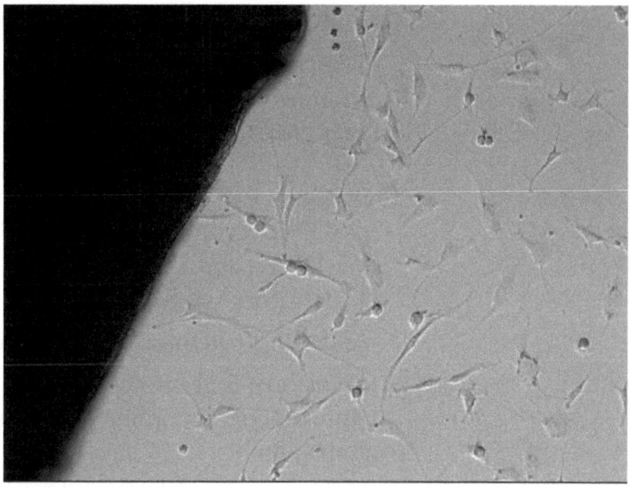

Fig. 1 VSMC explant culture, 14 days post explant

3.2 Creating an miR-Expressing Adenovirus

3.2.1 Cloning miR Sequence into pcDNA6.2-GW/EmGFP-miR

1. Input the sequence of target gene to be silenced (*see* **Note 4**) into Invitrogen's RNAi designer tool. The site will design "top" and "bottom" oligos that contain the correct inverted orientation of the miRNA sequence as well as the correct base overhangs for cloning (*see* **Note 5**).
2. Anneal oligos by mixing 50 μM oligos in 20 μL 1× annealing buffer. Boil for 4 min and then allow 10 min for the sample to cool at room temperature. Dilute annealed oligos 1:100 and then 1:50 in 1× annealing buffer.
3. Ligate annealed oligos into linearized pcDNA6.2-GW/EmGFP-miR with T4 DNA Ligase at room temperature for 60 min.
4. Transform 5 μL of the ligation product into high-competency *E. coli* DH5α. Plate transformants on LB agar plates with spectinomycin.
5. Use a commercial plasmid purification kit to isolate recombinant plasmid from 3 to 5 independent clones. Sequence across the miR sequence to confirm insertion.
6. This vector can be used in transient transfection assays to test the ability to knock down expression of the target gene.

3.2.2 Cloning GFP-miR Cassette into pDONR 221

1. Linearize 2 μg recombinant pcDNA6.2-GW/EmGFP-miR with EagI. Perform a phenol–chloroform–isoamylalcohol (PCI) extraction and chloroform extraction of the linearized vector, followed by ethanol precipitation. Resuspend in TE.
2. Perform BP recombination reaction with 150 ng linearized recombinant pcDNA6.2-GW/EmGFP-miR and 150 ng pDONR 221 with 2 μl Clonase II in final volume of 10 μl for 1 h at room temperature.

3. Add 1 μl Proteinase K and incubate for 10 min at 37 °C.
4. Transform 5 μl into competent DH5α *E. coli*. Plate a range of volumes (e.g., 5, 20, and 75 %) of the transformation onto LB agar plates with kanamycin.

3.2.3 Cloning GFP-miR Sequence into pAd/CMV/V5-DEST

1. Perform LR recombination reaction with 150 ng GFP-miR pDONR recombinant vector, 300 ng linearized pAd/CMV/V5-DEST, and 2 μl LR Clonase II in a final volume of 10 μl for 1 h at room temperature.
2. Add 1 μl Proteinase K and incubate for 10 min at 37 °C.
3. Transform 5 μl into competent DH5α *E. coli*. Plate a range of volumes of the transformation onto LB agar plates with ampicillin.
4. Use a commercial plasmid purification kit to isolate recombinant plasmid from 3 to 5 independent clones.
5. Assess for correct recombinants by sequencing or restriction enzyme analysis (*see* **Note 6**).

3.2.4 Packaging Adenovirus

1. Seed 5×10^5 HEK cells in a 60-mm culture plate 1 day before transfection.
2. Digest 3 μg GFP-miR pDEST with Pac1. Perform a PCI extraction and chloroform extraction of the DNA followed by ethanol precipitation. Resuspend the DNA in 5 μl TE.
3. Transfect HEK cells with 5 μl linearized GFP-miR pDEST using standard lipofectamine transfection methods (*see* **Note 7**).
4. 2 days post-transfection, transfer cells and media into 10-cm plate with additional 4 ml HEK growth media.
5. Allow infection to proceed until 80 % CPE is observed, usually 7–13 days post-transfection (*see* **Note 8**).
6. Collect adenovirus solution #1. Lyse cells by three consecutive freeze (−80 °C)–thaw (37 °C) cycles. Spin lysate for 30 min at $650 \times g$. Store the supernatant at −80 °C. Adenovirus solution #1 will be used to produce a high-titer stock of adenovirus.

3.2.5 Producing a High-Titer Stock of Adenovirus

1. Seed 3×10^6 HEK cells on a 10-cm plate 1 day before infecting to produce high-titer stock. Cells should be 80 % confluent upon infection.
2. Infect with 100 μl of adenovirus solution #1. Allow infection to proceed until 80–90 % of cells show CPE, usually 2–3 days.
3. Harvest adenovirus solution #2 in the same manner as adenovirus solution #1.

3.2.6 Rapid Adenoviral Titer

1. Seed 2.5×10^5 HEK cells per well of a 24-well culture dish (seven wells for one adenovirus) (*see* **Note 9**).

2. Using serum-free medium as diluent, prepare tenfold dilutions of your adenovirus solution (10^{-2}, 10^{-3}, 10^{-4}, 10^{-5}, 10^{-6}, 10^{-7}).
3. Add 50 μl of viral dilution to the well.
4. Incubate cells in CO_2 incubator for 48 h.
5. Count a minimum of three fields of GFP-positive cells using a microscope with a 20× objective.
6. Calculate infectious units (IFU)/ml for each well as follows:

$$\frac{\text{Mean number of positive cells} \times 239}{0.05 \times \text{dilution factor}}$$

3.3 Adenoviral Infection of VSMC

1. Seed 2×10^5 VSMC per well on 6-well culture plate (*see* **Note 10** and Table 1).
2. When cells become >80% confluent, wash twice with serum-free medium. Incubate with 2 ml infection medium for 1–3 days.
3. To prepare adenovirus infection solution, first calculate the appropriate multiplicity of infection (MOI) for the adenovirus stock solution (Table 1). In an Eppendorf tube, prepare the infection solution in a final volume of 100 μl per well, and mix adenovirus with serum-free medium and 3% FuGENE 6 (*see* **Note 11**).
4. Before infection, wash cells once with serum-free medium.
5. Add adenovirus infection solution to wells (100 μl/well) and incubate in CO_2 incubator for 90 min. Swirl the plate every 15 min making sure the infection solution covers the entire bottom to prevent cells from drying out.
6. Add 1 ml of serum-free medium to wells and continue to incubate for 48–72 h for maximal expression of transgene (*see* **Note 12**).

3.4 VSMC Stimulation with Angiotensin II (Ang II)

1. Serum starve 80–90% confluent VSMC for 24–72 h by removing growth medium, wash cells 1× with serum-free medium, and incubate with 1 ml serum-free medium or use adenovirus-infected cell (Fig. 2).

Table 1
Guidelines for seeding and adenoviral infection of VSMC in different sized culture wells

Plate size	Seeding density	Day of confluence	Approximate cell number at confluence	Infection volume, μl
6 well	2×10^5	3	5×10^5	100
12 well	1×10^5	2	2×10^5	50
24 well	5×10^4	2	1×10^5	40
96 well	3×10^3	2	2×10^4	40

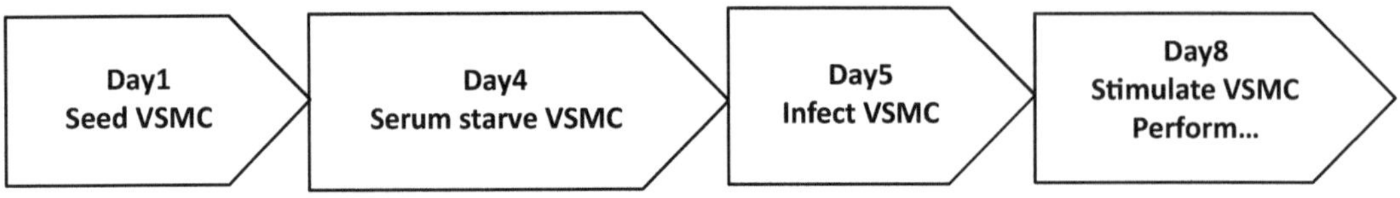

Fig. 2 Generalized flowchart of experimental design

2. On the day of stimulation, replace serum-free medium and let cells rest for 1 h in incubator.
3. Add Ang II at a final concentration of 100 nM. Stimulation time can be from 1–2 min to 24 h, depending on the signaling you wish to study (*see* **Note 13**).

3.5 Western Blot

3.5.1 Prepare Samples of Adenovirus-Infected and/or Adenovirus-Stimulated VSMC

1. Stop Ang II stimulation by aspirating media and immediately add 120 μl 1× SDS loading buffer to the well.
2. Scrape cells from the well with rubber scraper. Transfer to the Eppendorf tube.
3. Spin lysate for 3 min at 12,000 rpm.
4. Mild sonication for 10 s. Lysate can be stored at −20 °C for up to several months with negligible degradation of sample.

3.5.2 Run Western Blot

1. Run the sample on 7.5% or 10% SDS PAGE with stacking gel at 50 V until sample through stacking gel. Increase voltage to 100 V.
2. Transfer the protein to a nitrocellulose membrane by overnight transfer at 30 V in 4 °C using overnight transfer buffer.
3. Wash the membrane three times for 10 min in TBS-Tween, with slight rocking.
4. Block membrane with 5% (w/v) nonfat dry milk in TBS-Tween for 1 h at room temperature, with slight rocking.
5. Incubate blot with primary antibody in TBS-Tween overnight at 4 °C, with slight rocking.
6. Wash the membrane three times for 10 min in TBS-Tween, with slight rocking.
7. Incubate blot with secondary antibody (HRP-conjugated anti-mouse or anti-rabbit) in TBS-Tween for 1 h at room temperature, with slight rocking.
8. Wash the membrane three times for 10 min in TBS-Tween, with slight rocking.
9. Add ECL reagents, incubate at room temperature for 1 min, and expose to X-ray film (Fig. 3).

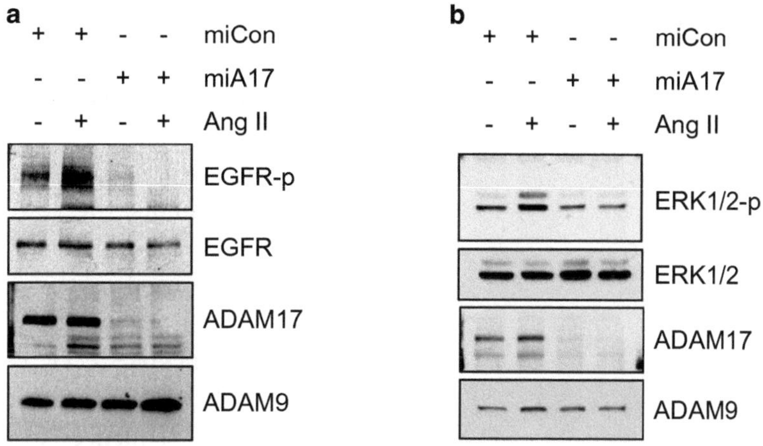

Fig. 3 Western blot of VSMC lysates. Cells were stimulated with 100 nM Ang II for 2 min (**a**) or 10 min (**b**). Cell lysates were subjected to immunoblot analysis as indicated [4]

3.6 VSMC Hypertrophy [6]

3.6.1 Cellular Protein Measurement

1. Seed VSMC in 24-well plates with $n=6$ for each sample. Stimulate cells with agonist and/or infect with adenovirus as needed for experiment.
2. Wash cells with PBS.
3. Lyse cells in 150 μl of 0.5 % SDS. Let it stand for 5 min.
4. Measure protein amount with the standard BCA protein assay kit.

3.6.2 Cell Volume/Coulter Counter Assay

1. Seed VSMC in 6-well plates with $n=3$ for each sample. Stimulate cells with agonist and/or infect with adenovirus as needed for experiment.
2. Wash cells twice with HBSS.
3. Remove cells from the plate with 250 μl of trypsin. Add 750 μl PBS to each well. Pipette up and down to disrupt cell clumps and transfer cell suspension to 1.5 ml tube.
4. Centrifuge tube at $250\times g$ for 3 min. Carefully remove supernatant.
5. Resuspend cells in 100 μl PBS.
6. Follow directions for Coulter counter setup.

3.6.3 MTS Cell Proliferation Assay

1. Seed VSMC in 96-well plate with $n=6$. Stimulate cells with agonist and/or infect with adenovirus as needed for experiment.
2. Use the standard MTS assay kit to read samples on plate reader.

4 Notes

1. From this point, procedure should be performed inside a tissue culture hood.
2. It is important that the tissue remains fixed with the intimal side facing the plate so that the VSMC can attach and migrate onto the floor of the culture well.
3. Seeding density may need to be adjusted according to how quickly the cells are growing.
4. The target sequence can be 5′UTR, coding sequence or 3′UTR of the gene to be silenced.
5. Pick 2–3 of the top sequences to test for silencing. These sequences must be checked to ensure they do not contain the restriction enzyme sites of Eag1 or Pac1, which will be used in later cloning steps.
6. Undigested samples of correct recombinants will run well above the standard DNA ladder, and a Pac1 digest will release the 2.0 kb fragment. Often, incorrect recombinants are either too small or have no Pac1 fragment and can be weeded out without sequencing.
7. Tube A: 10 μl lipofectamine with 90 μl Opti-MEM media. Tube B: 5 μg linearized vector in final 100 μl Opti-MEM media. Combine Tube A and Tube B at room temperature for 20 min, add 600 μl Opti-MEM media, and place all 800 μl of mixture onto prewashed cells for 3 h. Add 800 μl HEK growth media.
8. HEK growth media can be added if necessary.
9. Cells can be seeded and infected on the same day.
10. VSMC can be seeded onto 6-well plates at 2×10^5 cells per well. They should be nearing confluence in 3–4 days time. Some experiments may require using different size culture plates. An estimate of seeding density and other parameters is provided in Table 1.
11. FuGENE 6 should not be added directly to the plastic tube, and add to the tube already containing medium.
12. If adenoviral solution appears to be toxic to cells, wash cells 1× with serum-free medium after initial 90 min infection, and then add 1 ml serum-free medium for incubation.
13. Angiotensin II is prepared in DMSO and stored in small aliquots at −20 °C. Store 5 μl of 1 mM (10,000×) stock solution in small tube. Dilute 1:10 with water (1000×) solution.

References

1. Geisterfer AA, Peach MJ, Owens GK (1988) Angiotensin ii induces hypertrophy, not hyperplasia, of cultured rat aortic smooth muscle cells. Circ Res 62:749–756
2. Eguchi S, Hirata Y, Imai T, Kanno K, Marumo F (1994) Phenotypic change of endothelin receptor subtype in cultured rat vascular smooth muscle cells. Endocrinology 134: 222–228
3. Shirai H, Autieri M, Eguchi S (2007) Small gtp-binding proteins and mitogen-activated protein kinases as promising therapeutic targets of vascular remodeling. Curr Opin Nephrol Hypertens 16:111–115
4. Elliott KJ, Bourne AM, Takayanagi T, Takaguri A, Kobayashi T, Eguchi K, Eguchi S (2013) ADAM17 silencing by adenovirus encoding miRNA-embedded siRNA revealed essential signla transduction by angiotensin II in vascular smooth muscle cells. J Mol Cell Cardiol 62:1–7
5. Kuhn C, Frank D, Will R, Jaschinski C, Frauen R, Katus HA, Frey N (2009) Dyrk1a is a novel negative regulator of cardiomyocyte hypertrophy. J Biol Chem 284:17320–17327
6. Ohtsu H, Higuchi S, Shirai H, Eguchi K, Suzuki H, Hinoki A, Brailoiu E, Eckhart AD, Frank GD, Eguchi S (2008) Central role of GQ in the hypertrophic signal transduction of angiotensin II in vascular smooth muscle cells. Endocrinology 149:3569–3575
7. Ohtsu H, Dempsey PJ, Frank GD, Brailoiu E, Higuchi S, Suzuki H, Nakashima H, Eguchi K, Eguchi S (2006) Adam17 mediates epidermal growth factor receptor transactivation and vascular smooth muscle cell hypertrophy induced by angiotensin ii. Arterioscler Thromb Vasc Biol 26:e133–e137
8. Ross R (1971) The smooth muscle cell. II. Growth of smooth muscle in culture and formation of elastic fibers. J Cell Biology 50:172–186

Chapter 17

In Vitro and In Vivo Approaches to Assess Rho Kinase Activity

Vincent Sauzeau and Gervaise Loirand

Abstract

Increased arterial tone and the resulting rise in peripheral vascular resistance are major determinants of the elevated arterial pressure in hypertension. The RhoA/Rho kinase signaling pathways are now recognized as a major regulator of vascular smooth muscle contraction and arterial tone. Here we describe methods to directly and indirectly assess Rho kinase activity in vitro and in cells and tissues.

Key words Rho kinase, Myosin light-chain phosphatase, In vitro kinase assay, Immunoblot

1 Introduction

Arterial hypertension is a major risk factor of myocardial infarction and stroke that affects 25% of the adult population in industrialized societies. Increased arterial tone and the resulting rise in peripheral vascular resistance are major determinants of the elevated arterial pressure in hypertension [1]. Since the discovery of the essential role of RhoA/Rho kinase (ROCK) signaling in the regulation of vascular tone [2] and the antihypertensive effect of ROCK inhibitors [1, 3], much evidence has accumulated to implicate ROCK activation as a common component for the pathogenesis of hypertension. Accordingly, ROCK inhibitors are now considered as promising future therapies against cardiovascular diseases [4].

Vascular tone is regulated by arterial wall smooth muscle cell contraction that depends on the myosin light-chain phosphorylation [2]. Activation of the RhoA/ROCK pathway leads to increased myosin light-chain phosphorylation through inhibition of the myosin light-chain phosphatase activity by phosphorylation of its regulatory subunit MYPT-1 at inhibitory sites T696 and T850 [5]. T850 is considered to be a ROCK-specific phosphorylation site, whereas T696 can be phosphorylated by other kinases [5]. There are two isoforms of ROCK, ROCK 1 and ROCK2, that are both expressed in many tissues, including in vascular smooth muscle

Rhian M. Touyz and Ernesto L. Schiffrin (eds.), *Hypertension: Methods and Protocols*, Methods in Molecular Biology, vol. 1527, DOI 10.1007/978-1-4939-6625-7_17, © Springer Science+Business Media LLC 2017

cells. Nevertheless, although both ROCK1 and ROCK2 regulate myosin light-chain phosphatase and myosin light-chain phosphorylation, the control of vascular smooth muscle cell contractility essentially depends on ROCK2 [6].

All these data point out the need to assess ROCK activity both in vitro and in cells or tissues, and this chapter describes suitable methods for such ROCK assays. These methods are dedicated to ROCK2, but similar assays can be performed for ROCK1 with the corresponding specific tools. In vitro kinase assay with recombinant ROCK2 allows to directly measure the enzymatic activity and to screen putative ROCK inhibitors, while the same assay with ROCK2 immunoprecipitated from vascular cells and tissues from patients or animal models gives access to the kinase activity in different physiological or pathological situations. This assay consists in measuring, by scintillation counting, the ROCK-mediated incorporation of ^{32}P into a substrate peptide. The measurement of the level of phosphorylation of MYPT-1 by immunoblotting is an alternative but indirect method to assess ROCK in vascular smooth muscle cells and tissues with the advantage to be cheaper, easier, and safer to set up because of the absence of radioactivity.

2 Materials

The water used to prepare all solutions must be deionized and free of trace organic contaminants (ultrapure water). Solutions could be prepared previously and stored at 4 °C. For kinase assay, buffers should be used the same day it is prepared.

2.1 Rho Kinase Activity Assay

1. Kinase buffer: Tris 20 mM, β-glycerophosphate 25 mM, EGTA 1 mM, orthovanadate 0.1 mM, DTT 1 mM. Mix these chemical compounds and adjust pH to 7.5.
2. ROCK2 solution: ROCK2 from Merck Millipore (cat. number 14-338). Prepare a ROCK2 solution at 4 mU of specific enzyme activity/μL of kinase buffer (*see* **Note 1**).
3. $Mg^{2+}Cl_2$/ATP cocktail (Merck Millipore, cat. number 20-113): 20 mM MOPS, pH 7.2, 25 mM β-glycerophosphate, 5 mM EGTA, 1 mM Na_3VO_4, 1 mM dithiothreitol, 75 mM $MgCl_2$, and 500 μM ATP.
4. Long S6 kinase substrate peptide: Prepare a 1.1 mM S6 solution. Dilute 1 mg of S6 peptide (Merck Millipore, cat. number 12-420) in 250 μL of water.
5. [$\gamma^{32}P$] ATP solution: 1 mCi of [$\gamma^{32}P$] ATP (Perkin Elmer, cat. number NEG-502A).
6. Phosphoric acid solution 0.75 %.
7. 24-well/ P81 paper: Cut pieces of P81 paper (Whatman, cat. number 3698915) to cover each well of 24-well plate.

2.2 Immuno-precipitaion of ROCK2

1. Protein G Sepharose beads CL-4B (Pharmacia, cat. number 17-0618-01).
2. Lysis buffer: 10 mM Tris–HCl (pH 8.0), 1 % Triton X-100, 150 mM NaCl, 1 % aprotinin, 250 μM PMSF, 1 mM NaF, and 100 μM sodium orthovanadate.
3. Phosphate buffer solution (PBS).

2.3 Immunoblotting

1. Tris-buffered saline (TBS): 150 mM NaCl, 100 mM Tris–HCl, pH 7.4.
2. TBS-Tween solution: TBS containing 0.05 % Tween-20.
3. Blocking solution: 5 % milk in TBS.

3 Methods

3.1 In Vitro ROCK Assay

3.1.1 Purified Active ROCK Assay Protocol

1. Mix 978 μL of kinase buffer, 497 μL of $Mg^{2+}Cl_2$/ATP cocktail, 72 μL of long S6 kinase substrate peptide, and 50 μL of [γ^{32}P] ATP solution.
2. In a 96-well plate, add 15 μL of the mix, 5 μL of ROCK2 solution (20 mU), and 5 μL of putative ROCK inhibitor to be tested dissolved in the kinase buffer per well. Each molecule should be assayed at a minimum of two dilutions 5×10^{-7} and 5×10^{-5} M. Each dilution should be tested in duplicate (*see* **Note 2**). Each experiment must contain a minimum of two blanks (15 μL of the mix and 10 μL of kinase buffer), two positive controls (15 μL of the mix, 5 μL of ROCK2 solution, and 5 μL of kinase buffer), and two wells with a reference inhibitor at 10 μM (15 μL of the mix, 5 μL of ROCK2 solution, and 5 μL of 50 μM fasudil (Sigma, cat. number H139) or Y27632 (Sigma, cat. number Y0503)) solution in kinase buffer (*see* **Note 3**).
3. Heat the plate at 30 °C for 30 min.
4. Transfer 20 μL of each well in 24-well/ P81 paper and incubate 8 min at room temperature.
5. Add 1 mL of phosphoric acid solution for 6 min at room temperature and empty the wells. Repeat two times this step (*see* **Note 4**).
6. Dry and place P81 paper in a plastic tube. ROCK activity is measured by the radioactive label counting of [γ^{32}P] ATP in a scintillation counter.

3.1.2 Immuno-precipitated ROCK Assay Protocol

1. *Cell culture*: For each condition to be analyzed, a 10 cm culture dish with vascular smooth muscle cells at 80 % confluency is necessary (*see* **Note 5**). Wash the dish with ice-cold PBS, aspirate, and add 1 mL of ice-cold lysis buffer onto the dish (*see* **Note 6**). Incubate 5 min and scrape cells off the surface with a

cell scraper or a rubber policeman. Dissociate the mixture by pipetting up and down and transfer to a 2 mL tube.

3.1.3 Tissue Samples

Frozen tissues are dropped into five volumes of lysis buffer (5 mL/g of tissue). Homogenize the sample on ice using a Polytron-type homogenizer.

1. Centrifuge lysates at 1500 × *g* for 10 min at 4 °C.
2. Collect the supernatant and determine protein concentration of the supernatant.
3. Collect 1000 µg of total protein of the supernatant and bring the total volume to 1 mL using lysis buffer.
4. Add 2 µL of ROCK2 antibody (Santa Cruz, cat. number sc1851) and incubate 12 h at 4 °C.
5. Add 20 µL of Protein G Sepharose and incubate at 4 °C for 30 min.
6. Centrifuge tubes for 30 s at 1000 × *g*. Aspirate the supernatant and wash the beads with 1 mL of kinase buffer. Vortex and collect the beads again by centrifugation. Repeat this step three times. After the last centrifugation, resuspend the beads in 20 µL of kinase buffer.
7. In wells of a 96-well plate, incubate 20 µL of beads with 30 µL of the mix described in Subheading 3.1.1 (**step 1**).
8. Heat the plate at 30 °C for 30 min.
9. Transfer 40 µL of each well in 24-well/ P81 paper and incubate 8 min at room temperature.
10. Add 1 mL of phosphoric acid solution for 6 min at room temperature and empty the wells. Repeat two times this step (*see* **Note 3**).
11. Dry and place P81 paper in a plastic tube. ROCK activity is measured by the radioactive label counting of [γ^{32}P] ATP in a scintillation counter.

3.2 Evaluation of ROCK Activity by Western Blot Analysis

1. Total cellular lysates are obtained from primary vascular smooth muscle cells or vascular tissues as described in Subheading 3.1.2 (**steps 1–3**).
2. Dilute 30 µg of protein lysates in concentrated Laemmli buffer to finally obtain 25–50 µL of protein samples in 1× Laemmli buffer. Denature the proteins by heating the sample to 95 °C for 10 min.
3. Load protein samples in each lane of 7% SDS-polyacrylamide gel. Migrate at 30 mA till the dye front reaches the bottom of the gel.
4. Proceed to protein transfer on nitrocellulose membrane using semidry transfer method (*see* **Note 7**).

5. Block the membrane with the blocking solution for 30 min.
6. Incubate the membrane with pMYPT-1 antibody [rabbit antiphospho-specific T850-MYPT-1 antibody (Merck Millipore, Cat. Number 04-773) and/or goat antiphospho-specific T696-MYPT-1 antibody (Santa Cruz, cat. number sc-17556)] and rabbit anti-MYPT-1 polyclonal antibody, for 12 h at 4 °C. The final concentration of the antibodies is 1/1000 in blocking solution.
7. Wash three times with TBS-Tween solution (5 min each time) at room temperature.
8. Incubate the membrane with the appropriate secondary antibody conjugated to horseradish peroxidase for 1 h at room temperature. Dilute the secondary antibody in blocking solution.
9. Wash as in **step 7** and detect the immuno-complex using a chemiluminescent method (Pierce Biotechnology, cat. number 32132) (*see* **Note 8**).
10. After quantification of the immunoreactive bands, ROCK activity is expressed as the ratio of pMYPT-1:MYPT-1 in each sample.

4 Notes

1. To prevent decrease activity of ROCK2, avoid freeze and thaw. Prepare aliquots of ROCK2 enzyme and stock them at −70 °C.
2. Triplicate is strongly recommended for statistic analysis.
3. Positive and negative controls are crucial for the interpretation of the experiment. Quadriplate is recommended.
4. Avoid splash during washes to prevent radioactive contamination.
5. Culture of vascular endothelial cells or leukocyte suspension can be used in the same way.
6. Keep always the plate on ice to stop all enzymatic activities.
7. The efficiency of transfer can be evaluated by Ponceau stain.
8. Low or no signal could mean that the induction of the phosphorylation is not sufficient. Run a positive control with your samples to confirm the validity of the immunoblotting.

Acknowledgment

This work was supported by the Institut National de la Santé et de la Recherche Médicale (INSERM) and grants from the Agence National de la Recherche (ANR-09-JCJC-0115-01 and ANR-08-GENO-040-01) and the Fondation pour la Recherche Médicale (DEQ20090515416).

References

1. Loirand G, Pacaud P (2010) The role of Rho protein signaling in hypertension. Nat Rev Cardiol 7:637–647
2. Somlyo AP, Somlyo AV (2003) Ca2+ sensitivity of smooth muscle and nonmuscle myosin II: modulated by G proteins, kinases, and myosin phosphatase. Physiol Rev 83:1325–1358
3. Uehata M, Ishizaki T, Satoh H, Ono T, Kawahara T, Morishita T, Tamakawa H, Yamagami K, Inui J, Maekawa M, Narumiya S (1997) Calcium sensitization of smooth muscle mediated by a Rho-associated protein kinase in hypertension. Nature 389:990–994
4. Satoh K, Fukumoto Y, Shimokawa H (2011) Rho-kinase: important new therapeutic target in cardiovascular diseases. Am J Physiol Heart Circ Physiol 301:H287–296
5. Hirano K, Hirano M, Kanaide H (2004) Regulation of myosin phosphorylation and myofilament Ca2+ sensitivity in vascular smooth muscle. J Smooth Muscle Res 40:219–236
6. Wang Y, Zheng XR, Riddick N, Bryden M, Baur W, Zhang X, Surks HK (2009) ROCK isoform regulation of myosin phosphatase and contractility in vascular smooth muscle cells. Circ Res 104:531–540

Chapter 18

NADPH Oxidases and Measurement of Reactive Oxygen Species

Angelica Amanso, Alicia N. Lyle, and Kathy K. Griendling

Abstract

The NADPH oxidase (Nox) family of enzymes is expressed in many tissues that are involved in hypertension, including blood vessels, kidney, and brain. In these tissues, the products of NADPH oxidase activity, superoxide and ultimately hydrogen peroxide, act as intracellular and extracellular messengers during compartmentalized cellular signaling. The correct measurement of Nox activity and its products is crucial to enable studies of how these signaling pathways affect the molecular mechanisms underlying hypertension. Here, we describe methods for detection and measurement of hydrogen peroxide and superoxide derived from NADPH oxidases in biological samples such as cells and tissues.

Key words NADPH oxidases, Hydrogen peroxide, Reactive oxygen species measurement

1 Introduction

The Nox protein family is a major source of reactive oxygen species (ROS) in vascular cells, the kidney, and the brain [1]. The first member of this family to be described was gp91phox or Nox2, which generates large amounts of ROS in phagocytic cells, serving an important role in innate immunity [2]. Over the years, several additional members of the Nox family have been described (Nox1–Nox5, Duox1, and Duox2). The expression, subcellular localization, type of ROS produced, and mode of activation differ between the subtypes (for details, *see* reviews 1 and 3). Nox-derived ROS have physiological and pathophysiological roles in the cardiovascular system. In physiological conditions, Nox enzymes play important roles during development, in reparative processes, and in the regulation of vascular tone and oxygen sensing. In addition, Nox enzymes regulate cell growth, migration, inflammation, apoptosis, fibrosis, and proliferation, all of which contribute to the biology of cardiovascular pathologies and affect vascular relaxation, vascular and cardiac hypertrophy, salt retention, and central regulation of blood pressure [4, 5].

Rhian M. Touyz and Ernesto L. Schiffrin (eds.), *Hypertension: Methods and Protocols*, Methods in Molecular Biology, vol. 1527, DOI 10.1007/978-1-4939-6625-7_18, © Springer Science+Business Media LLC 2017

In hypertension, ROS derived from Nox enzymes induce vascular dysfunction, in part via the well-described inactivation of the vasodilator nitric oxide (NO) by superoxide [4, 6]. Vascular tone is directly correlated with local production and activity of NO by endothelial cells. Such regulation is modulated by alterations in local stimuli such as shear stress, as well as the presence of local vasodilators [7]. In response to these stimuli, increases and redistribution of blood flow occur in specific vascular networks. The presence of superoxide in this environment is an important buffer to NO action, because superoxide can rapidly interact with NO to form peroxynitrite [8]. Consequently, the bioavailability of NO is reduced and other reactive species are generated. Peroxynitrite has been shown to have a series of deleterious actions such as inhibition of superoxide dismutases, inactivation of prostacyclin synthase, and uncoupling of endothelial nitric oxide synthase (eNOS) [9]. Thus, Nox1 and Nox2, which produce superoxide, have potentially important roles for direct regulation of blood pressure [10–12].

In addition to reacting with NO to generate peroxynitrite, when produced in excess or at more acidic pH, superoxide can also spontaneously dismutate to hydrogen peroxide (H_2O_2; $Kd = 8 \times 10^4\ M^{-1}\ s^{-1}$) or dismutate to H_2O_2 via a reaction catalyzed by the superoxide dismutase enzymes (SOD; $Kd = 2 \times 10^9\ M^{-1}\ s^{-1}$). It has been shown in the literature that there are diverse roles for SOD isoforms in hypertension. The use of SOD mimetics or membrane-permeable SOD in animal models improves hypertension, markers of oxidative stress, media/lumen ratio, as well as endothelium-dependent relaxation by mechanisms related to the regulation of vascular remodeling and tone [13].

Of importance, H_2O_2 can induce and activate eNOS and can also promote vasodilation via activation of calcium-activated K+ channels to cause hyperpolarization [14]. Endothelial-specific overexpression of Nox4, which primarily produces H_2O_2, actually induces mild hypotension, suggesting that Nox4 may be beneficial for vascular function [15]. Other studies demonstrated that in rabbit mesenteric arteries precontracted with norepinephrine, H_2O_2 induces endothelium-independent relaxation [16]. It is thus clear that ROS critically regulate vascular tone, but that their effects may be dependent upon the type of ROS, the nature of the stimulus, and the vascular bed [17–19].

Measurement of ROS derived from Nox enzymes requires careful consideration of sample concentration in temporally and spatially reliable conditions. Such quantification can be a difficult challenge considering the well-controlled enzyme activation, low level production, stimulus-associated production, and compartmentalization [20, 21]. Although Nox enzyme activity is usually assessed by measuring its products ($O_2^{\cdot -}$ and H_2O_2), verification of Nox as the source requires the use of siRNA or Nox-specific inhibitors, such as apocynin and gp91-dstat. In this chapter, we describe general experimental procedures for H_2O_2 detection in tissue and cell culture using the Amplex® Red assay (horseradish peroxidase-based fluorometric assay), as well assessment of $O_2^{\cdot-}$ production by dihydroethidium (DHE)-HPLC quantitative analysis of the production of the oxidation product 2-hydroxyethidium.

2 Materials

Prepare all solutions using ultrapure water (prepared by purifying deionized water to attain a sensitivity of 18 MΩ•cm at 25 °C) and analytical grade reagents. Prepare and store all reagents at room temperature (unless indicated otherwise).

(A) Amplex Red Hydrogen Peroxide Kit [A22188, Molecular Probes-Invitrogen, USA]

Hydrogen peroxide reacts with Amplex Red reagent (N-acetyl-3,7-dihydroxyphenoxazine) at a stoichiometry of 1:1 in a reaction catalyzed by horseradish peroxidase (HRP) to generate the highly fluorescent and colored oxidation product resorufin. Specifically, HRP catalyzes the decomposition of H_2O_2 to the hydroxyl radical, which is reduced to water upon irreversible chemical oxidation of Amplex Red (colorless and nonfluorescent) to resorufin (colored and fluorescent). When resorufin is excited at 530 ± 12.5 nm, it strongly emits light at 590 ± 17.5 nm. Of importance, the excitation and emission of resorufin are sensitive to pH, where an ideal pH for this assay is pH 7.4 (pH range 7.0–8.0). When Amplex Red is performed at a pKa of ~6.0, the absorbance maximum shifts to 480 nM, and the amount of H_2O_2 detected is lower than what is present [22].

2.1 Amplex Red Kit Stock Solutions Preparation

2.1.1 10 mM Amplex Red Reagent Stock Solution

1. Prepare in the dark and keep covered with aluminum foil, as Amplex Red can undergo photooxidation to resorufin when exposed to light [23].
2. Allow Amplex Red reagent and DMSO (absolute) to warm to room temperature.
3. Just prior to use, dissolve the contents of the vial of Amplex Red reagent in 60 μl of DMSO. Use on the same day as prepared—*do not* store unused Amplex Red stock, as background may increase.

2.1.2 10 U/ml Horseradish Peroxidase (HRP) Stock

1. Dissolve the contents of the vial of HRP in 1.0 ml of 1× reaction buffer (supplied with kit as 5×). Add 400 μl of 5× reaction buffer to 1.6 ml of ultrapure H_2O to make 1×.
2. After the assay, any unused HRP stock solution should be divided into single-use aliquots of 100 μl and stored frozen at −20 °C.

2.1.3 H_2O_2 Standards

1. Prepare 20 mM H_2O_2 working solution by adding 22.7 μl of 3% H_2O_2 stock to 977 μl of 1× reaction buffer.
2. Dilute 20 mM H_2O_2 working solution further to 100 μM by adding 5 μl of 20 mM H_2O_2 to 995 μl of 1× reaction buffer.
3. Prepare the standard curve according to the chart below (Table 1):

2.2 Krebs HEPES Buffer

We recommend *Krebs HEPES buffer* (KHB) for performance of determination of intracellular and extracellular H_2O_2. Prepare fresh the day before or the day of assay. The composition of the buffer is 20 mM Na-HEPES, 99 mM NaCl, 4.69 mM KCl, 1 mM KH_2PO_4, 1.2 mM $MgSO_4$, 2.5 mM $CaCl_2$, 25 mM $NaHCO_3$, 5.6 mM glucose. For 1 L of KHB solution, combine:

1. Na-HEPES 5.206 g.
2. NaCl 5.786 g.
3. KCl 0.35 g.
4. KH_2PO_4 0.142 g.
5. $MgSO_4 \times 7H_2O$ 0.296 g.
6. $CaCl_2 \times 2H_2O$ 0.368 g.
7. $NaHCO_3$ 2.1 g.
8. D(+)Glucose 1.009 g.

Add the ingredients to 900 ml of ultrapure water, mix, and pH to 7.4. Once the pH has been reached, add additional water to reach 1 L.

(B) DHE [D11347, Molecular Probes-Invitrogen, USA]

Dihydroethidium (DHE) freely permeates cell membranes and is used extensively to monitor superoxide production. The reaction of DHE with $O_2^{\cdot-}$ yields 2-hydroxyethidium, which has a

Table 1
Preparation of standard curve for Amplex Red assay

H_2O_2 (μM final)	100 μM H_2O_2 (μl)	μl of 1× reaction buffer
0	0	200
2	4	196
4	8	192
6	12	188
8	16	184
10	20	180
50	100	100

molecular weight 16 U greater than DHE and is specific for $O_2^{\cdot-}$, and ethidium, which is not a $O_2^{\cdot-}$-specific product and most likely reflects the redox status of the cell [20, 21]. The superoxide-specific 2-hydroxyethidium can be readily separated from the parent DHE compound and the nonspecific ethidium by performing high-performance liquid chromatography (HPLC) using a C-18 reverse-phase column (Nucleosil 250, 4.5 mm; Sigma-Aldrich). Because each product elutes at a different time (DHE ~8.0 min, 2-hydroxyethidium ~14.5 min, and ethidium ~16.2 min), one can quantify each independent compound by calculating the area under each curve. To quantify, both ethidium and 2-hydroxyethidium are excited at a wavelength of 480 nm and emission is read at 580 nm, which detects both products. The area of the 2-hydroxyethidium peak can then be used to estimate the intracellular $O_2^{\cdot-}$ production.

2.3 Prepare DHE Stock Solution

1. Reconstitute DHE using only anhydrous DMSO. Stock solutions should be prepared immediately before use and used preferably for one batch of experiments.
2. Make a 10 mM stock solution by adding 315 μl of DMSO (absolute) to the 1 mg (pre-weighed vial) of DHE and then immediately cover the vial in aluminum foil to avoid exposure to light.
3. Vortex for 30 s to 1 min to ensure homogenous resuspension of DHE. Keep on ice until incubation with cells. Thaw at room temperature as DMSO freezes on ice.

(C) Cell and tissue preparation

Prepare standard lysis buffers to extract protein from cells (Subheading 3.1) and tissue (Subheading 3.2).

2.4 Triton Lysis Buffer (Stock): Cells

The composition is 25 mM HEPES pH 7.4, 100 mM NaCl, 1 mM EDTA, 10% (v/v) glycerol, and 1% (v/v) Triton X-100 [24]. For 250 ml:

1. HEPES 1.49 g.
2. NaCl 1.46 g.
3. EDTA 0.093 g.
4. 10% (v/v) glycerol 25 ml.
5. 1% (v/v) Triton X-100 0.25 ml.

Dissolve all of the solid compounds in a total volume of 200 ml of ultrapure water. Then add glycerol and Triton X-100 to the solution. Adjust pH to 7.4 and increase to a final volume of 250 ml with ultrapure water. This lysis buffer can be made ahead of time, aliquoted and stored at −20 °C. Just prior to use, thaw the stock Triton lysis buffer and add the ingredients below to make complete Triton lysis buffer:

1. 1 mM PMSF (phenylmethylsulfonyl fluoride). Prepare 100 mM stock solution by dissolving 0.0871 g PMSF in 5 ml of absolute ethanol. Aliquot and store at −20 °C.
2. 1 mM sodium orthovanadate. Prepare a 100 mM stock solution by dissolving 0.092 g sodium orthovanadate in 5 ml of ultrapure water. Adjust the pH to 10.0. At pH 10.0 the solution will be yellow. Boil the solution until it turns colorless (approximately 10 min). Cool solution to room temperature. Readjust the pH to 10.0 and repeat boil step until the solution remains colorless and the pH stabilizes at 10.0. Aliquot and store at −20 °C.
3. 10 ng/ml leupeptin. Prepare a 0.5 mg/ml stock solution dissolving 25 mg in 50 ml of ultrapure water. Aliquot and store at −20 °C.
4. 1 ng/ml aprotinin. Prepare a 0.5 mg/ml stock solution by dissolving 25 mg in 50 ml of ultrapure water. Aliquot and store at −20 °C.

2.5 Hunter's Lysis Buffer (Stock): Tissue

The composition is 25 mM HEPES pH 7.4, 150 mM NaCl, 1 mM EGTA, 10 mM of sodium pyrophosphate, 10 mM sodium fluorate, 10% glycerol, 1% Triton X-100, 1% Na deoxycholate, and 0.1% SDS. For 250 ml:

1. HEPES 1.49 g.
2. NaCl 2.19 g.
3. $MgCl_2$ 0.036 g.
4. EGTA 0.0951 g.
5. Na-pyrophosphate 1.12 g.
6. NaF 0.1 g.
7. 10% glycerol 25 ml.
8. 1% Triton X-100 2.5 ml.
9. 1% Na deoxycholate 2.5 g.
10. 0.1% SDS 0.5 g.

Add ingredients in the order indicated to 150 ml of ultrapure water. Add Na deoxycholate in small amounts over a period of ~1 h. This will help prevent Na deoxycholate from coming out of solution. Adjust pH to 7.4 and then bring to a final volume of 250 ml. This buffer can be made ahead of time and stored at −20 °C. Just prior to use, thaw the Hunter's buffer stock and add the ingredients below to make complete Hunter's buffer:

1. 1 mM PMSF (phenylmethylsulfonyl fluoride).
2. 1 mM sodium orthovanadate.
3. 10 ng/ml leupeptin.

4. 1 ng/ml aprotinin.

Prepare these solutions as indicated above for Triton lysis buffer.

2.6 Preparation of Membrane Fractions from Cells and Tissues

Membrane fraction preparation is required for NADPH oxidase activity measurement. Without isolation of the membrane fraction, the $O_2^{\cdot-}$ measured will be considered total $O_2^{\cdot-}$ instead of NADPH oxidase-dependent $O_2^{\cdot-}$. It is important to remember that cells have multiple sources of ROS that include NO synthases, mitochondria, and xanthine oxidase, some of which are contained in these membrane fractions.

Place the cell culture dish on ice, wash twice with ice-cold 1× phosphate-buffered saline (PBS-50 mM phosphate treated for 2 h with 5 g/100 ml Chelex-100 and filtered), and scrape cells from the dish. Centrifuge at 400×*g* (10 min) and resuspend the cell pellet in 1 ml of PBS containing the protease inhibitors aprotinin (10 μg/ml), leupeptin (0.5 μg/ml), pepstatin (0.7 μg/ml), and PMSF (0.5 mM) (pH 7.4). Sonicate the cell suspension (power 3 W, using a Microson 2425 from Misonix, Inc.) for 10 s on ice. Centrifuge at 28,000×*g* for 15 min at 4 °C. Resuspend the pellet in 150 μl of lysis buffer and measure the protein concentration using the Bradford assay (Subheading 3.5) [25].

3 Methods

3.1 Detection of H_2O_2 in Cell Culture with Amplex Red

This method can be used for whole-cell H_2O_2 detection. Alternatively, to measure NADPH oxidase-dependent H_2O_2 production, treat the cells with siRNA against the specific Nox isoform expressed in the cell line of interest. A negative control siRNA should be used when using siRNA to knockdown the gene of interest, as well as a transfection control. To find the best conditions to silence the Nox subunits, optimization of these conditions should be carried out for the Nox isoform of interest in the specific cell type used. Cells should be quiesced in serum-free media for at least 24 h and then stimulated with the growth factor or cytokine of interest. Alternatively, NADPH oxidase-dependent H_2O_2 production can be inferred by pretreating cells or tissues with a specific NADPH oxidase inhibitor, such as apocynin or gp91-dstat, as discussed earlier.

1. *In the dark*: Prepare a working solution of 100 μM Amplex Red reagent and 0.2 U/ml HRP by mixing the following:
   19.7 ml of Krebs HEPES buffer
   100 μl of 10 mM Amplex Red reagent stock solution
   200 μl of 10 U/ml HRP stock solution
2. *In the dark*: Aspirate existing media from cultured cell monolayer and add 1 ml of the working solution per 60 mm dish.

3. *In the dark*: Incubate cells in working solution at 37 °C in 5% CO_2. Roll the working solution across the cells once every 30 min for a predetermined optimal time point for the experimental purposes. In general, a time course between 1 and 8 h is recommended. Keep the remaining Amplex Red working solution (not added to cells) at 37 °C in the dark to use as a blank.
4. Include positive and negative controls: glucose oxidase (GOX) and catalase [7] enzymes, respectively. As a general rule, final solutions of GOX and CAT are 2 and 200 U/ml, respectively [26].
5. Transfer 100 μl of solution from each 60 mm dish and 100 μl of room temperature working solution to a 96-well black wall, optical bottom plate (Nunc).
6. Measure the fluorescence using a fluorescence microplate reader equipped for excitation in the range of 530 nm and emission detection at 590 nm. Subtract out the background (reaction buffer incubated without cells) from each sample reading.
7. Normalize readings to protein concentration following steps outlined in Subheading 3.5.

3.2 Detection of H_2O_2 in Tissues with Amplex Red

1. Prepare a working solution of 100 μM Amplex Red reagent and 0.2 U/ml HRP by mixing the following:
   19.7 ml of Krebs HEPES buffer
   100 μl of 10 mM Amplex Red reagent stock solution
   200 μl of 10 U/ml HRP stock solution
2. Incubate 1–3 mm of aorta or 10–100 μg of tissue from one mouse in 500–1000 μl of working solution at 37 °C in 5% CO_2 (in 24-well cell culture plates with enough volume to cover tissue). Incubate for 40 min to 2 h.
3. Take a 200 μl aliquot from the well containing the tissue sample and transfer it to the 96-well black wall, optical bottom plate (Nunc). Measure the fluorescence using a fluorescence microplate reader equipped for excitation in the range of 530 nm and emission detection at 590 nm. Subtract out the background (reaction buffer without tissue) from each sample reading.
4. Normalize readings to protein following steps outlined in Subheading 3.4 and 3.5.

3.3 Preparation of Lysate from Cell Culture for Protein Measurement

1. Place the cell culture dish on ice and wash the cells with ice-cold 1× PBS.
2. Aspirate PBS, then add ice-cold triton lysis buffer (1 ml per 10^7 cells/100 mm dish; 0.5 ml per 5×10^6 cells/60 mm dish).
3. Scrape adherent cells off the dish using a plastic cell scraper and then gently transfer the cell suspension into a microcentrifuge tube.
4. Sonicate at 6 W for 10 s per sample.

5. Pellet triton-insoluble fraction by centrifugation at 4 °C. Centrifugation force and time may vary by cell type; a guideline is 20 min at 10,000 × *g*.
6. Gently remove the tubes from the centrifuge and place on ice. Transfer the supernatant to a fresh, pre-chilled microcentrifuge tube on ice, and discard the triton-insoluble pellet.

3.4 Preparation of Lysate from Tissues for Protein Measurement

1. Dissect the tissue of interest, preferably on ice, with clean tools, as quickly as possible to prevent tissue degradation by proteases.
2. Place the tissue in round-bottom microcentrifuge tubes and immerse in liquid nitrogen to "snap freeze." Store samples at −80 °C for extraction of protein at a later date or keep on ice for immediate homogenization.
3. For a 10 mg piece of tissue, add ~300 μl lysis buffer rapidly to the tube, homogenize with an electric homogenizer, rinse the blade with another 300 μl Hunter's lysis buffer, and then homogenize again. Volumes of lysis buffer must be determined in relation to the amount of tissue present.
4. Centrifuge for 20 min at 10,000 × *g* at 4 °C in a microcentrifuge. Gently remove the tubes from the centrifuge and place on ice. Transfer the supernatant and place in a fresh, pre-chilled microcentrifuge tube on ice. Discard the pellet.

3.5 Protein Measurement by Bradford Assay

1. Dilute Bradford reagent 1:5. This dilution is stable at room temperature for 5–7 days.
2. Prepare BSA stock (1 mg/ml in ultrapure H_2O).
3. Prepare BSA standards and dilute the samples according to Table 1.

Bradford assay	BSA (1 mg/ml)	H_2O	Lysis buffer (1:10)	Sample dilute	(Dye 1:5 dilution)
BSA dilutions (μg /ml)					
Standard #1 0	0	100	100	10	190
Standard #2 2.50	10	90	100	10	190
Standard #3 3.75	15	85	100	10	190
Standard #4 5.00	20	80	100	10	190
Standard #5 7.50	30	70	100	10	190
Standard #6 10.00	40	60	100	10	190
Standard #7 15.00	60	40	100	10	190
Standard #8 20.00	80	20	100	10	190
	μl Protein suspension				
Samples	5	95		10	190

4. Add the standards and diluted samples to a 96-well plate in triplicate. Add the appropriate amount of dye (*see* Table 1) to the standard and sample wells and read the absorbance in a microplate reader at 595 nm. Once the Bradford reagent is added, the reaction is stable for up to 1 h at room temperature.
5. To calculate final protein concentration in µg/ml, multiply by the final dilution factor (× 400 if using Table 1 below).

3.6 Detection of Superoxide in Cell Culture with DHE

Assessment of whole-cell superoxide production

1. Rinse dishes with Krebs HEPES buffer (KHB) twice with 5 ml per 100 mm dish.
2. Add 2.5 ml fresh KHB per 100 mm dish and place dishes at 37 °C, 5 % CO_2.
3. *In the dark*: Add 2.5 µl of 10 mM DHE stock to the 2.5 ml of KHB already in the dish and mix well. Place dish at 37 °C, 5 % CO_2, and incubate for 30 min.
4. *In the dark*: Aspirate the DHE-KHB solution and add 100 µl of fresh KHB to each 100 mm dish.
5. *In the dark*: Harvest cells by scraping in the presence of the 100 µl of fresh KHB. Transfer the cells to an amber 1.5 ml microcentrifuge tube and add 300 µl of HPLC-grade methanol and vortex. Store the sample at −20 °C until the sample can be transferred to −80 °C.
6. Samples can be processed the same day or the next day. Vortex each sample and then homogenize with a glass homogenizer for 1 min or approximately 100 dounces at ~1000 rpm (or a power of 2 on a Wheaton Overhead Stirrer, cat# 903475).
7. Transfer 50 µl of homogenized sample to a separate microcentrifuge tube for protein measurement.
8. Pull the remaining sample volume into a 1 cc syringe and filter through a Nalgene PTFE 0.2 µm filter into a fresh amber 1.5 ml microcentrifuge tube. Store sample at −20 °C until ready to run the sample on HPLC.

Assessment of NADPH oxidase activity with DHE

9. Incubate 20 µg of membrane fraction isolated in KHB with DHE (50 µM) and NADPH (100 µM) in a final volume of 120 µl at 37 °C in the dark for 30 min. Stop the reaction by placing the samples on ice. Inject 100 µl into the HPLC system.

3.7 Detection of Superoxide in Tissues with DHE

(Aorta is used here as an example.)

1. Inject mice with heparin (100 units, 5 min) prior to euthanasia by CO_2.
2. Perfuse aortas with ice-cold KHB. Rapidly dissect out aortas without stretching and remove visible fat tissue under a dissecting microscope.

3. Cut each aorta into 10–12 2 mm rings in cold KHB.
4. *In dark*: Incubate three 2-mm rings in 1 ml of KHB containing 50 μM DHE solution for 30 min at 37 °C, 5% CO_2.
5. Transfer aortic rings to a new microcentrifuge tube and homogenize in 300 μl of methanol. Remove 50 μl of homogenate for protein measurements and filter the rest through a 0.22 μm syringe filter into a fresh amber tube. Store samples at −80 °C until analysis by HPLC.

3.8 Analysis of DHE Products by HPLC

1. For separation of ethidium, 2-hydroxyethidium, and dihydroethidium, the HPLC system should be equipped with a C-18 reverse-phase column (Nucleosil 250-4.5 mm, Sigma-Aldrich, St. Louis, MO, USA), in addition to both UV and fluorescence detectors. Fluorescence detection at 580 nm (emission) and 480 nm (excitation) is used to quantify ethidium and 2-hydroxyethidium, which are both excited at a wavelength of 480 nm and emit at 580 nm. The area of the 2-hydroxyethidium peak, which elutes at ~14.5 min, can then be used to estimate the intracellular $O_2^{\cdot-}$ production. UV absorption at 355 nm is used for detection of the parent DHE compound. The mobile phase used for separation on the column is composed of a gradient containing 60% acetonitrile and 0.1% trifluoroacetic acid. Dihydroethidium, ethidium, and hydroxyethidium are separated by a linear increase in acetonitrile concentration from 37% to 47% of mobile phase in 23 min at a flow rate of 0.5 ml/min.
2. Superoxide production is calculated from the amount of 2-hydroxyethidium generated, which is normalized to the protein concentration in the sample. Protein concentration is measured by Bradford assay (protocol in Subheading 3.5). PEG-SOD (100 U/ml) can be added to some samples 1 h prior to addition of DHE to determine the amount of signal that can be attributed to $O_2^{\cdot-}$.
3. The 2-hydroxyethidium HPLC peak corresponds to the amount of $O_2^{\cdot-}$ formed in the sample during the incubation and is expressed per milligram of protein.

4 Notes

4.1 Amplex Red Assay

1. The Amplex Red assay is highly specific and sensitive, with a limit of detection of ~5 pmol of H_2O_2 [29].
2. Resorufin is a very stable product that allows detection both in oxidative and reductive conditions. Another advantage is that HRP is active over a wide pH range; however, resorufin excitation and emission are sensitive to pH, and the reaction should be carried out in a pH range of 7.0–8.0 [29].

3. The signal is consistently abolished by addition of exogenous catalase 200 U/ml (negative control), and signal increases with the addition of glucose oxidase 2 U/ml (positive control) [21].
4. Addition of glucose in the media is not necessary for the glucose oxidase positive control. Standard low glucose media has sufficient glucose to support activity of the enzyme [26].
5. The stoichiometry of Amplex Red and H_2O_2 is 1:1, and, therefore, the assay results are linear over the range of values encountered in tissues and cells [29].
6. Amplex Red at high concentrations (50 μmol/L) can be auto-oxidized and produce $O_2^{\cdot -}$ and H_2O_2. Therefore, low concentrations of Amplex Red (10 μmol/L) are recommended [21].
7. Avoid exposing the Amplex Red assay to light. The reagent can easily be photooxidized to resorufin, thus artificially increasing the signal [29].
8. Single measurements of fluorescence are preferable to continuous measurements to minimize exposure to light from the fluorescent spectrometer or plate reader; therefore, time course experiments should be performed on individual samples. Continuous measurements invalidate the assay once Amplex Red is photooxidized [23].
9. It is recommended to perform the assay in 96-well black wall plates with an optical bottom, so all the samples are exposed to the same amount of light.
10. The lysis buffer (with inhibitors) should be ice-cold prior to homogenization.
11. Protein measurement can be performed using the Bradford assay, Lowry assay, or BCA assay. Bovine serum albumin (BSA) is a frequently used protein standard.
12. H_2O_2 release is calculated using H_2O_2 standards and expressed as picomoles per milligram of protein.
13. Confocal microscopy should be avoided for the Amplex Red assay. The laser light source is very powerful and will induce photooxidation [23].

4.2 DHE Assay

1. Reconstituted DHE solution should appear pink; a more intense color such as purple may be indicative of auto-oxidation of the dye.
2. DHE is a light-sensitive dye. For this reason, all of the procedures should be performed in dim light. DHE can react with oxygen in solution. It is recommended that DHE be prepared as a stock solution in argon-purged buffers using dark tubes [21].
3. A small background signal is expected from DHE stock solution.

4. One possible alternative if HPLC is not available is to measure NADPH oxidase by fluorometry. In the dark, incubate 10 μg protein from membrane fraction with KHB-DHE (10 μM) in the presence of NADPH (50 μM) and calf thymus DNA (1.25 μg/ml) in a final volume of 120 μl for 30 min at 37 °C. Total fluorescence is followed in a microplate reader using an acridine filter (excitation 490 nm and emission 570 nm). The acridine filter is more sensitive for 2-hydroxietidium [20].
5. The fluorometric assay described above has been used specifically for vascular smooth muscle cells [20]. For other cell types and conditions, validation by HPLC will be required to ensure that experimental conditions do not interfere with the ethidium product.
6. The presence of controls is extremely important in these protocols. It is highly recommended to incubate the same membrane fraction or cell preparation with superoxide scavengers, such as SOD (300–500 U/ml), as well as a specific NADPH oxidase inhibitor, such as apocynin (100 μM) or gp91-dstat (50 μM) [27] if determining NADPH oxidase activity is the goal.
7. As an alternative to this protocol, electron spin resonance (ESR) is an excellent approach to measure NADPH oxidase activity since it is able to detect radicals. Due to a lack of specificity for a broad range of fluorescent dyes, ESR is the gold standard for specific detection of superoxide [21]. This protocol was not included here because ESR machines are not widely available and require specific training.
8. Even with the use of membrane fractions, some results can be misinterpreted because other enzymes can be present in this fraction and produce superoxide. For example, in endothelial cells, NO synthase can generate $O_2^{\cdot-}$ in the absence of cofactors or substrate, shown previously in laminar shear stress conditions [20, 28]. For this reason, the use of siRNA specific for NADPH oxidases subunits is fundamental to accurately measuring NADPH oxidase activity.

References

1. Lassegue B, Griendling KK (2010) NADPH oxidases: functions and pathologies in the vasculature. Arterioscler Thromb Vasc Biol 30(4):653–661
2. Suh YA et al (1999) Cell transformation by the superoxide-generating oxidase Mox1. Nature 401(6748):79–82
3. Datla SR, Griendling KK (2010) Reactive oxygen species, NADPH oxidases, and hypertension. Hypertension 56(3):325–330
4. Amanso AM, Griendling KK (2012) Differential roles of NADPH oxidases in vascular physiology and pathophysiology. Front Biosci (Schol Ed) 4:1044–1064
5. Lassegue B, San Martin A, Griendling KK (2012) Biochemistry, physiology, and pathophysiology of NADPH oxidases in the cardiovascular system. Circ Res 110(10):1364–1390
6. Al Ghouleh I et al (2011) Oxidases and peroxidases in cardiovascular and lung disease: new concepts in reactive oxygen species signaling. Free Radic Biol Med 51(7):1271–1288
7. Nguyen Dinh Cat A, Touyz RM (2011) Cell signaling of angiotensin II on vascular tone:

novel mechanisms. Curr Hypertens Rep 13(2):122–128
8. Halliwell B, Zhao K, Whiteman M (1999) Nitric oxide and peroxynitrite. The ugly, the uglier and the not so good: a personal view of recent controversies. Free Radic Res 31(6):651–669
9. Price DT, Vita JA, Keaney JF Jr (2000) Redox control of vascular nitric oxide bioavailability. Antioxid Redox Signal 2(4):919–935
10. Grote K et al (2006) Critical role for p47phox in renin-angiotensin system activation and blood pressure regulation. Cardiovasc Res 71(3):596–605
11. Dikalova AE et al (2010) Upregulation of Nox1 in vascular smooth muscle leads to impaired endothelium-dependent relaxation via eNOS uncoupling. Am J Physiol Heart Circ Physiol 299(3):H673–H679
12. Wang HD et al (1998) Superoxide anion from the adventitia of the rat thoracic aorta inactivates nitric oxide. Circ Res 82(7):810–818
13. Fukai T, Ushio-Fukai M (2011) Superoxide dismutases: role in redox signaling, vascular function, and diseases. Antioxid Redox Signal 15(6):1583–1606
14. Ohashi J et al (2012) Mechanisms for enhanced endothelium-derived hyperpolarizing factor-mediated responses in microvessels in mice. Circ J 76(7):1768–1779
15. Schroder K et al (2012) Nox4 is a protective reactive oxygen species generating vascular NADPH oxidase. Circ Res 110(9): 1217–1225
16. Fujimoto S et al (2001) Mechanisms of hydrogen peroxide-induced relaxation in rabbit mesenteric small artery. Eur J Pharmacol 412(3):291–300
17. Lucchesi PA, Belmadani S, Matrougui K (2005) Hydrogen peroxide acts as both vasodilator and vasoconstrictor in the control of perfused mouse mesenteric resistance arteries. J Hypertens 23(3):571–579
18. Zhang DX et al (2012) H2O2-induced dilation in human coronary arterioles: role of protein kinase G dimerization and large-conductance Ca2+-activated K+ channel activation. Circ Res 110(3):471–480
19. Suvorava T et al (2005) Endogenous vascular hydrogen peroxide regulates arteriolar tension in vivo. Circulation 112(16):2487–2495
20. Laurindo FR, Fernandes DC, Santos CX (2008) Assessment of superoxide production and NADPH oxidase activity by HPLC analysis of dihydroethidium oxidation products. Methods Enzymol 441:237–260
21. Dikalov S, Griendling KK, Harrison DG (2007) Measurement of reactive oxygen species in cardiovascular studies. Hypertension 49(4):717–727
22. Rhee SG et al (2010) Methods for detection and measurement of hydrogen peroxide inside and outside of cells. Mol Cells 29(6):539–549
23. Zhao B, Summers FA, Mason RP (2012) Photooxidation of Amplex red to resorufin: implications of exposing the Amplex red assay to light. Free Radic Biol Med 53(5):1080–1087
24. Williams HC et al (2012) Role of coronin 1B in PDGF-induced migration of vascular smooth muscle cells. Circ Res 111(1):56–65
25. Dikalov SI et al (2008) Distinct roles of Nox1 and Nox4 in basal and angiotensin II-stimulated superoxide and hydrogen peroxide production. Free Radic Biol Med 45(9):1340–1351
26. Mueller S, Millonig G, Waite GN (2009) The GOX/CAT system: a novel enzymatic method to independently control hydrogen peroxide and hypoxia in cell culture. Adv Med Sci 54(2):121–135
27. Gupte RS et al (2009) Synergistic activation of glucose-6-phosphate dehydrogenase and NAD(P)H oxidase by Src kinase elevates superoxide in type 2 diabetic, Zucker fa/fa, rat liver. Free Radic Biol Med 47(3):219–228
28. Vasquez-Vivar J et al (1998) Superoxide generation by endothelial nitric oxide synthase: the influence of cofactors. Proc Natl Acad Sci U S A 95(16):9220–9225
29. Zhou M, Diwu Z, Panchuk-Voloshina N, Haugland RP. (1997) A stable nonfluorescent derivative of resorufin for the fluorometric determination of trace hydrogen peroxide: applications in detecting the activity of phagocyte NADPH oxidase and other oxidases.Anal Biochem. 253(2):162–168.

Chapter 19

Measurement of Superoxide Production and NADPH Oxidase Activity by HPLC Analysis of Dihydroethidium Oxidation

Denise C. Fernandes, Renata C. Gonçalves, and Francisco R.M. Laurindo

Abstract

The fluorogenic probe dihydroethidium (DHE) is widely used for detecting intracellular superoxide. DHE oxidation by superoxide generates specifically the compound 2-hydroxyethidium (2-E^+OH), so that 2-E^+OH detection confers specificity to superoxide assessment among many other reactive oxygen species. However, DHE oxidation in biological systems leads to formation of other fluorescent products, particularly ethidium, usually formed at higher quantities than 2-E^+OH. Since both 2-E^+OH and ethidium are fluorescent, their identification and quantification is possible only after their physical separation by HPLC. Here we describe the detailed procedures for superoxide measurement in cells (adhered or not) and fresh tissues fragments, followed by acetonitrile extraction and simultaneous fluorescent detection of 2-E^+OH and ethidium and absorbance detection of remaining unreacted DHE. In addition we report the use of DHE/HPLC for measuring NADPH oxidase activity in enriched-membrane fraction isolated from cells or tissues. These methods can improve accuracy and precision of quantitative superoxide measurements in biological samples.

Key words Dihydroethidium, Hydroethidine, Superoxide, Reactive species, NADPH oxidase, Oxidants, 2-hydroxyethidium, Ethidium, Fluorescence, HPLC

1 Introduction

Dihydroethidium (DHE, also named hydroethidine or HE) is a membrane-permeable nonfluorescent probe that is oxidized to different fluorescent products, among which the two most well studied are: 2-hydroxyethidium (2-E^+OH) and ethidium (E^+). The first is formed solely in the presence of superoxide anion, so that 2-E^+OH detection is a marker of superoxide formation and its identification confers specificity to superoxide assessment among many other reactive oxygen species (ROS) [1, 2]. Ethidium, the other fluorescent DHE-derived oxidation product, is formed in the presence of 1-electron oxidants or enzymatically, so E^+ identification will inform about total oxidant generation and is not specific for identifying

Rhian M. Touyz and Ernesto L. Schiffrin (eds.), *Hypertension: Methods and Protocols*, Methods in Molecular Biology, vol. 1527, DOI 10.1007/978-1-4939-6625-7_19, © Springer Science+Business Media LLC 2017

one particular ROS. Since both compounds (2-E^+OH and E^+) are fluorescent, their identification (and quantification) is possible only after their physical separation by liquid chromatography (HPLC). This implies that analysis by microscopy of total DHE-derived fluorescence in cells and tissues will not identify superoxide radical formation, although it will allow inferring about in situ oxidant formation [3, 4]. Discussion about the chemical basis, methodological advances and potential applications of these techniques has been provided in a number of previous article and reviews [5–10]. Here, we will concentrate in discussing details of the practical approach to detect superoxide in cells and tissues.

In this protocol, biological samples (cell or tissues) are incubated with DHE probe for 20–30 min. Within this incubation time, uncharged DHE will cross membranes, spread within cells and become oxidized by different intracellular oxidants (Fig. 1). DHE-derived products will be retained inside cells because they are charged and intercalate into DNA. Samples then are washed to remove extracellular DHE (that did not enter the cell/tissue) and DHE-derived oxidants are extracted from samples with organic solvent, acetonitrile. This solvent is the most efficient for detach DHE-derived compounds from DNA in vitro [3] and in tissues gives the best DHE-derived compounds recovery compared to chloroform or methanol (unpublished data). The obtained acetonitrile extract that contains DHE and its oxidation products is then dried and the powder can be stored frozen until HPLC analysis.

Chromatographic analysis of 2-E^+OH and other DHE oxidizing products from samples is preceded by optimization of 2-E^+OH/ethidium separation conditions, followed by development of standard curve calibrations with pure standards. Fluorescent products 2-E^+OH/ethidium are followed with a fluorescence detector, while DHE is followed using an absorbance detector (Fig. 2). Protocol optimization for peak separation will depend on the type of column, HPLC system, mobile phase and gradient conditions. Here, we describe our HPLC set-up conditions, as a starting material for each particular laboratory optimization, as well as calculations for obtaining the final result of 2-E^+OH in nmol/mg protein. It is important to note that quantification of 2-E^+OH by HPLC is a semi-quantitation of intracellular superoxide formation, since one or two molecules of superoxide are necessary for 2-E^+OH formation (Fig. 1).

Besides the quantification of 2-E^+OH by HPLC, it is also important to follow DHE consumption during analysis as an indicative of oxidant generation [4, 5]. Samples should retain some unreacted DHE (thus DHE should also be used in excess), indicating that DHE effectively trapped formed superoxide and was able to outcompete other superoxide targets, such as superoxide dismutase.

Dihydroethidium covalently joined with hexyl triphenylphosphonium cation, named Mito-DHE or Mito-SOX, targets to mitochondria [11]. Since this probe shows the same chemical characteristics and reactions described to DHE, the identification

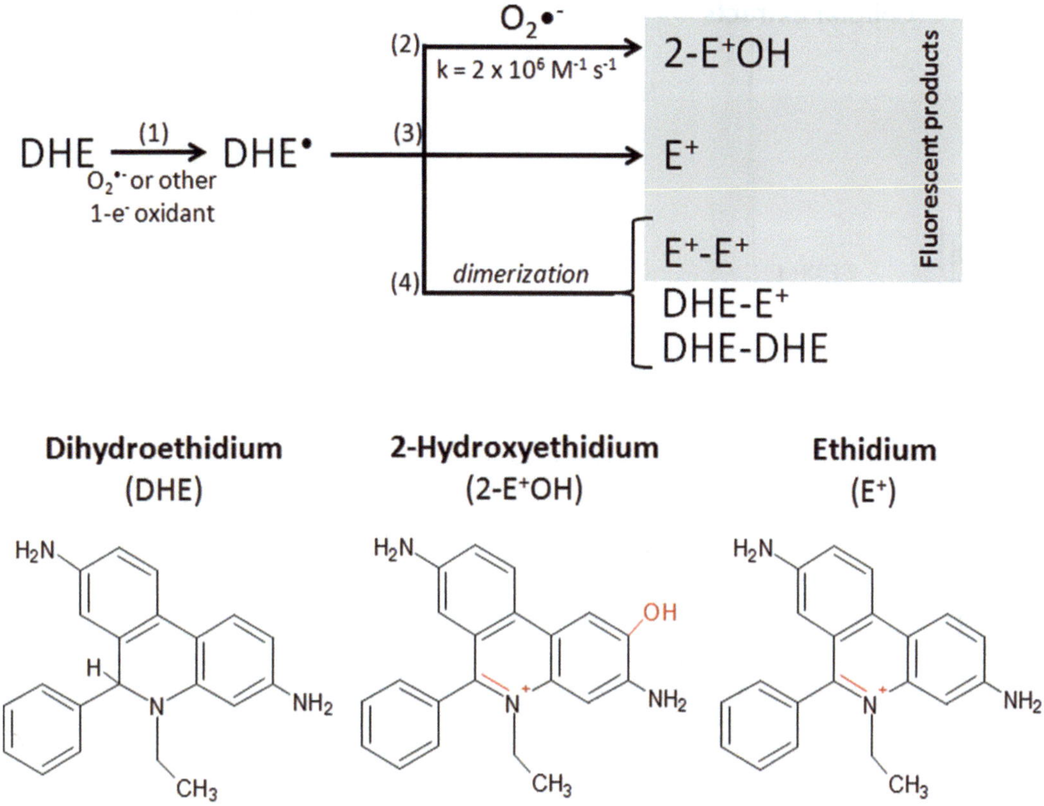

Fig. 1 DHE-derived oxidation products. The first step (*pathway 1*) of DHE oxidation is the formation of DHE radical ($DHE^{\cdot}$) by some 1-electron oxidant (hydroxyl radical or superoxide, for example). DHE radical will form specifically 2-E^+OH only by reacting with superoxide anion radical (*pathway 2*). DHE can also form other fluorescent products, independently of superoxide anion. Ethidium can be formed enzymatically, by 1-electron oxidants (*pathway 3*) or even directly from hydride transfer without DHE radical intermediate formation (pathway not shown). DHE radicals can also dimerise (DHE-DHE) and generate other dimers (DHE-E^+, E^+-E^+) by sequential oxidation steps (*pathway 4*). From these DHE-derived products, the most fluorescent (higher intensity signal, free in solution, λexc 490 nm, λem 570 nm) is 2-E^+OH, followed by E^+ and E^+-E^+ (intensity proportion is approximately 10:1:0.025, refs)

of mitochondrial superoxide production also requires chromatographic separation of Mito-2-E^+OH. DHE (or Mito-DHE) analysis by HPLC in cells and tissues can also be performed with other detectors, such as electrochemical or MS/MS [7]. These protocols were described step-by-step in Zielonka et al. [5], and allows the identification and quantification not only of the marker of superoxide production, 2-E^+OH, but also give insights about other oxidants formed during sample incubation with DHE that generate DHE dimers. Recently, DHE oxidation analyses by HPLC parallel with analysis of other fluorescent probes have been described for high-throughput real-time analysis in biological samples [8].

Finally, superoxide detection by HPLC can be used for measuring NADPH oxidase activity, a multi-subunit enzyme that specifically produces superoxide anion for defense or signaling and

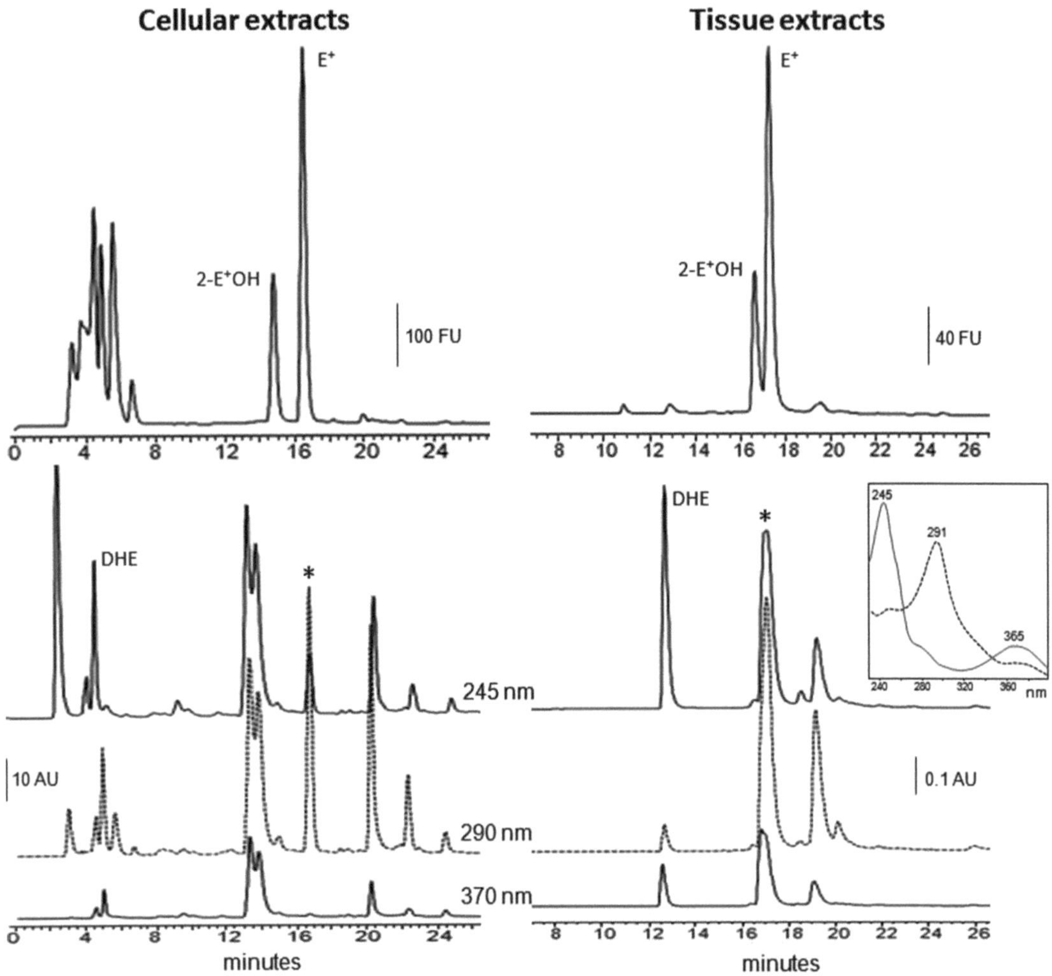

Fig. 2 Typical HPLC chromatogram of cellular (**a**) and tissue extracts (**b**). *Upper* are shown chromatograms for fluorescence detection (λexc 480 nm, λem 580 nm) for two different columns, Phenomenex (for cellular extracts) and Waters (for tissue extracts), following conditions described in Table 1. At *bottom* there are three chromatograms obtained in three different wavelengths with absorbance detector (245, 290 and 370 nm). Usually the first chromatogram (245 nm) is used for DHE peak area quantification, because at this wavelength is the highest DHE absorptivity compared to 370 nm (*see insert box* with absorbance DHE spectrum). At 290 nm is possible to detect a peak with time retention ~17 min (*asterisk*) that probably is the ethidium dimer (E^+-E^+; Zielonka dimers). Note that, although 2-E^+OH has the higher intensity signal when free in solution (legend of Fig. 1), in biological samples ethidium levels usually are higher than 2-E^+OH levels and show larger peaks and, thus, quantity after peak area conversion to concentration in biological extracts

whose main subunits (Nox and p22) are localized at membranes [12]. For this particular protocol, enriched-membrane fraction isolated from cells/tissues by sequential centrifugation is incubated with NADPH in the presence of DHE (the oxygen that will be reduced to superoxide anion by NADPH oxidase electron transfer is dissolved into solution, ~210 μM concentration at 37 °C and pH 7.4 [13]). Detection of 2-E^+OH will reflect superoxide formation by NADPH oxidase complex [3, 4].

2 Materials

Prepare all solutions with ultrapure and deionized water. Use analytical grade reagents. In many solutions diethylenetriamine pentaacetic acid (DTPA) is added for diminishing the concentration of transition metals ions that may interfere in oxidants production during incubation and/or extraction procedures. We also recommend (although it is not obligatory) treating solutions with Chelex-100 resin for 24 h to reinforce the removal of traces of metal ions. Be careful when preparing DHE or 2-E$^+$OH solutions, because these compounds are photosensitive, thus always avoid exposure to direct light during handling of DHE or 2-E$^+$OH.

2.1 DHE Incubation and Acetonitrile Extraction in Cells or Tissues

1. DHE stock solution: 10 mM. Add 1 mL of deoxygenated DMSO in 3 mg of DHE. Concentration should be confirmed at pH 7.4 at 265 nm ($\varepsilon = 1.8 \times 10^4$ $M^{-1} \cdot cm^{-1}$) or at 345 nm ($\varepsilon = 9.75 \times 10^3$ $M^{-1} \cdot cm^{-1}$) [14], especially if the solution was stored for more than 15 days. Store at −20 °C.
2. Acetonitrile (analytical or HPLC grade).
3. PBS: 7.78 mM Na_2HPO_4, 2.2 mM KH_2PO_4, 140 mM NaCl, and 2.73 mM KCl. Add in 900 mL of water 2.21 g of Na_2HPO_4, 3.2 g of KH_2PO_4, 16.2 g NaCl, and 0.405 g of KCl. Adjust pH to 7.4 and complete to 1 L with water. To sterilize the solution, filter into a vacuum filtering system with a 0.2-μm-filter or autoclave. Store at 4 °C.
4. PBS/DTPA: same as PBS described above, with the addition of 100 μM DTPA. Add 35.7 mg of DTPA, then adjust the pH and follow the PBS procedure.
5. Hanks/DTPA: $CaCl_2$ 1.3 mM, $MgSO_4$ 0.8 mM, KCl 5.4 mM, KH_2PO_4 0.4 mM, $NaHCO_3$ 4.3 mM, NaCl 137 mM, Na_2HPO_4 0.3 mM, DTPA 0.1 mM, glucose 5.6 mM, pH 7.4 Add in 900 mL of water 147 mg of $CaCl_2 \cdot 2H_2O$, 200 mg $MgSO_4 \cdot 7H_2O$, 400 mg KCl, 60 mg KH_2PO_4, 360 mg $NaHCO_3$, 8 g NaCl, 91 mg $Na_2HPO_4 \cdot 7H_2O$, 35.7 mg DTPA, adjust the pH to 7.4, add 1 g of glucose and make up to 1 L with water. To sterilize the solution, filter into a vacuum filtering system with a 0.2-μm-filter. Store at 4 °C.
6. Lysis buffer A: Tris-base 20 mM pH 8.0, NaCl 137 mM, NP-40 1%, Triton 2%, glycerol 10%. Add in 40 mL of water 121 mg of Tris-base and 0.4 g of NaCl. Adjust the pH for 8.0 and add 0.5 mL of NP-40, 1 mL of Triton and 5.0 mL of glycerol. Make up to 50 mL with water. Store at 4 °C. For daily use, in 8.8 mL of lysis buffer A add 100 μL of aprotinin 10 μg/mL, 100 μL of leupeptin 10 μg/mL, and 1 mL of PMSF 1 mM and maintain the solution at 4 °C.

7. Aprotinin stock solution: 1 mg/mL. Add 1 mL of Hepes buffer 20 mM pH 7.5 in 1 mg of aprotinin. Store at −20 °C in aliquots.
8. Hepes buffer 20 mM: Add 40 mL of water in 238 mg of Hepes. Adjust the pH at 7.5 and make up to 50 mL with water.
9. Leupeptin stock solution: 1 mg/mL. Add 1 mL of Hepes buffer 20 mM pH 7.5 in 1 mg of leupeptin. Store at −20 °C in aliquots.
10. Phenylmethylsulfonyl fluoride stock solution: 100 mM. Add 1 mL of analytical grade ethanol in 174 mg of PMSF. Store at −20 °C in aliquots.
11. Vacuum concentrator.
12. Mortar and pestle (for tissues).
13. Liquid nitrogen (for tissues).

2.2 Chromatographic Solutions

1. Mobile phase A (cellular extracts): In a 1 L flask add 800 mL of water, 100 mL of acetonitrile and 1 mL of trifluoroacetic acid. Make up to 1 L with water. Filter the solution into a vacuum filtering system with a 0.2-μm-filter. Store the mobile phase at 4 °C.
2. Mobile phase A (tissue extracts): In a 1 L flask add 900 mL of water, 50 mL of acetonitrile and 1 mL of trifluoroacetic acid. Make up to 1 L with water. Filter the solution into a vacuum filtering system with a 0.2-μm-filter. Store the mobile phase at 4 °C.
3. Mobile phase B (cellular extracts): In a 1 L flask add 500 mL of water, 400 mL of acetonitrile and 1 mL of trifluoroacetic acid. Make up to 1 L with water. Filter the solution into a vacuum filtering system with a 0.2-μm-filter. Store the mobile phase at 4 °C.
4. Mobile phase B (tissues extracts): Filter HPLC grade acetonitrile into a vacuum filtering system with a 0.2-μm-filter.
5. 2-Hydroxyethidium stock solution: Dissolve 33 mg of xanthine in NaOH 1 M. Prepare DHE 1 mM: add 10 μL of DHE 10 mM stock solution in 90 μL of HCl 1 mM (*see* **Note 1**). In 40 μL of PBS/DTPA add 5 μL of xanthine solution, 2.5 μL of xanthine oxidase 1 U/mL, and 2.5 μL of DHE 1 mM. Incubate at 37 °C for 30 min in the dark. Calculate the final concentration of 2-EOH by measuring the absorbance of this solution at 470 nm ($\varepsilon = 9.4 \times 10^3$ $M^{-1} \cdot cm^{-1}$) [14]. The concentration of 2-EOH stock solution is generally around 30 μM. Store at −20 °C (*see* **Note 2**).
6. Ethidium stock solution: 50 μM. Dilute 2 μL of commercially obtained ethidium bromide (10 mg/mL) in 998 μL of PBS/DTPA. Ethidium concentration is determined at pH 7.4 at 480 nm ($\varepsilon = 5.8 \times 10^3$ $M^{-1} \cdot cm^{-1}$) [14].

7. 2-Hydroxyethidium standard curve solutions: Dilute the 2-EOH stock solution (~30 μM) in mobile phase A in different concentrations (generally between 10 μM and 0.5 nM). The lowest concentration is the one that allows a reliable peak area measurement.
8. Dihydroethidium standard curve solutions: Dilute the DHE stock solution (10 mM) in mobile phase A in different concentrations (50 μM to 10 nM).
9. Ethidium standard curve solutions: Dilute the ethidium bromide stock solution (50 μM) in mobile phase A in different concentrations (generally between 5 μM and 0.5 nM).

2.3 HPLC Components and Calibration

1. HPLC device: For 2-E^{+}OH analysis in samples a HPLC system equipped with an absorption and fluorescence detectors, and a C_{18} column for proceeding with compound separation is necessary. In Table 1 are described our instrumental setup for DHE and its derived products analysis, that may be altered depending on particular characteristics of column/HPLC device. Tissue extracts probably have great content of lipids and thus after repeated sample injections into HPLC will likely increase column pressure. In turn to diminish this problem, we recommend cleaning HPLC system with pure acetonitrile after five to six tissue injections and use more robust columns, such as Waters. Phenomenex C_{18} column generates better 2-E^{+}OH/E^{+} separation than Waters C_{18} column, but its half-life is strongly reduced with tissue sample injections. In addition, addition of pre-columns (C_{18} microcolumns) into HPLC line is indispensable to increase column half-life and to avoid contaminant peaks (compounds from previous injections that were retained into the column).
2. HPLC calibration: After chromatographic conditions were established for optimal 2-E^{+}OH/E^{+} separation in your HPLC device, inject pure standards (DHE, 2-E^{+}OH and E^{+}) to generate the calibration curves necessary for further quantitation of DHE and DHE-derived products in sample extracts.

2.4 Enriched-Membrane Fraction (for NADPH Oxidase Activity Measurement)

1. DHE 1 mM: add 10 μL of DHE stock solution (10 mM) in 90 μL of PBS/DTPA.
2. NADPH 2 mM: add 1 mL of phosphate buffer 10 mM pH 8 in 1.67 mg of NADPH. Store at −20 °C for 2 weeks. Protect from light.
3. Lysis buffer B: Tris–HCl 50 mM pH 7.4 containing DTPA 0.1 mM, ethylene glycol-bis(2-aminoethyl-ether)-N,N,N′,N′-tetraacetic acid (EGTA) 0.1 mM, 0.1% β-mercaptoethanol, aprotinin 10 μg/mL, leupeptin 10 μg/mL and phenylmethylsulfonyl fluoride 1 mM. Add in 150 mL of water 30.3 g of Tris-base, 7.9 mg of DTPA and 7.6 mg of EGTA. Adjust the pH for 7.4. Make up to 200 mL with water. Store at 4 °C. For daily use, in 8.8 mL of lysis buffer B add 10 μL

Table 1
Instrumental set up for DHE and its derived products analysis for cellular and tissue extracts

<table>
<tr><th></th><th>Cellular extracts</th><th>Tissue extracts</th></tr>
<tr><td>Column</td><td>Phenomenex Synergil C_{18}, 150 × 4.6 mm, 4 μm, 80 A</td><td>Waters Nova-Pak C_{18}, 150 × 3.9 mm, 4 μm, 100 A</td></tr>
<tr><td>Mobile phase A</td><td>90 % H_2O 10 % CH_3CN 0.1 % TFA</td><td>95 % H_2O 5 % CH_3CN 0.1 % TFA</td></tr>
<tr><td>Mobile phase B</td><td>60 % H_2O 40 % CH_3CN 0.1 % TFA</td><td>100 % CH_3CN</td></tr>
<tr><td>Flow rate</td><td>0.6 mL/min</td><td>0.4 mL/min</td></tr>
<tr><td>Volume for sample resuspension</td><td>80 μL</td><td>80 μL</td></tr>
<tr><td>Injection volume</td><td>60 μL</td><td>60 μL</td></tr>
<tr><td>Gradient</td><td><table>
<tr><th>Time (min)</th><th>A (%)</th><th>B (%)</th></tr>
<tr><td>0</td><td>60</td><td>40</td></tr>
<tr><td>5</td><td>60</td><td>40</td></tr>
<tr><td>25</td><td>0</td><td>100</td></tr>
<tr><td>35</td><td>0</td><td>100</td></tr>
<tr><td>40</td><td>60</td><td>40</td></tr>
<tr><td>43</td><td>60</td><td>40</td></tr>
</table></td><td><table>
<tr><th>Time (min)</th><th>A (%)</th><th>B (%)</th></tr>
<tr><td>0</td><td>100</td><td>0</td></tr>
<tr><td>10</td><td>60</td><td>40</td></tr>
<tr><td>20</td><td>20</td><td>80</td></tr>
<tr><td>25</td><td>20</td><td>80</td></tr>
<tr><td>30</td><td>100</td><td>0</td></tr>
<tr><td>35</td><td>100</td><td>0</td></tr>
</table></td></tr>
<tr><td>Photodiode array detector</td><td>245, 370 nm</td><td></td></tr>
<tr><td>Fluorescence detector</td><td>λexcitation: 480 nm; λemission: 580 nm</td><td></td></tr>
<tr><td>Retention time</td><td>DHE 5.0 min
2-E^+OH 15.2 min
E^+ 16.8 min</td><td>DHE 12.7 min
2-E^+OH 16.2 min
E^+ 17.2 min</td></tr>
</table>

β-mercaptoethanol, 100 μL of aprotinin 10 μg/mL, 100 μL of leupeptin 10 μg/mL, and 1 mL of PMSF 1 mM and maintain the solution at 4 °C.

4. Trichloroacetic acid 10%: dilute 1 mL TCA 100% in 9 mL water. For obtaining a TCA 100% stock solution, dissolve 500 g TCA (as shipped) into 350 mL water. Store at room temperature.
5. Ultracentrifuge.

3 Methods

3.1 Adherent Cells

Dihydroethidine is a light-sensitive probe, thus procedures that involve DHE must be performed in a place protected from direct lighting (for example, into a laminar flow hood with its lights turned off). Carry all steps at room temperature, unless otherwise specified. Cells can be cultured in different dishes (p100 or p-6 well). Run a control with superoxide dismutase is strongly recommended (*see* **Note 3**). Procedures will be described for p-6 well and in parenthesis/italic information for p100 is also added.

1. After specific treatment of confluent cells (85–90%), remove the medium and add to each well 0.5 mL (*3 mL*) of Hanks/DTPA and add 2.5 μL (*15 μL*) of DHE stock solution and incubate for 30 min, in cell culture incubator (37 °C) (*see* **Note 4**).
2. Identify two Eppendorf tubes for each sample and put them on a rack.
3. Remove the buffer containing DHE (*see* **Note 5**) and wash carefully the cells with 0.5 mL (*3 mL*) PBS/DTPA (*see* **Note 6**).
4. Add 0.5 mL (*1 mL*) of acetonitrile and scrape the cells (*see* **Note 7**).
5. Transfer the acetonitrile lysate into an identified tube and place it on ice.
6. Centrifuge the samples for 15 min at 18,000 × *g* at 4 °C.
7. Transfer the supernatant to the second identified tube. Keep pellets on ice with opened cap for remaining acetonitrile evaporation.
8. Dry the supernatants in a vacuum concentrator at room temperature (approximately 2 h for 0.5 mL of acetonitrile) (*see* **Note 8**). Store the pale pink dried pellet at −80 °C for further HPLC analysis (*see* **Note 9**).
9. Add 50 μL of lysis buffer to samples pellet maintained on ice (**step 8**), strongly vortex for 1 min, sonicate (3 times at 6 W for 10 s) and keep samples on ice for 30 min. Determine the protein concentration.

3.2 Non-adherent Cells

1. After specific treatment of cells ($\geq 5 \times 10^5$ cells), centrifuge cells at 1000 × *g* for 5 min.
2. Remove the medium by aspiration and add 0.5 mL of Hanks/DTPA and 2.5 μL of DHE 10 mM stock solution.
3. Incubate for 30 min at 37 °C.
4. Identify 2 Eppendorf tubes for each sample and put them on a rack.
5. Centrifuge the samples at 1000 × *g* for 5 min at 4 °C.

6. Remove the Hanks/DTPA and add 0.5 mL of PBS/DTPA; repeat **steps 5** and **6** for the second wash.
7. Add 0.5 mL of acetonitrile and vortex for 1 min.
8. Centrifuge the samples for 15 min at 18,000 × *g* at 4 °C. Follow the same steps described for adherent cells (**steps 7–9**).

3.3 Tissues

As recommended for cells, procedures involving manipulation of DHE or its derived products must be performed under protection from direct light. Carry each step at room temperature unless otherwise specified. All tissues should be carefully cleaned, because any remaining blood, clots, or thrombi will rapidly oxidize DHE to ethidium or nonfluorescent products. Perfuse tissues with saline before remove them from the animal. If necessary, clean the tissue with scalpel (always maintaining the tissue in iced PBS). We strongly suggest developing one initial experiment with few samples to optimize DHE concentration (50–150 μM), DHE time incubation (15–30 min) and tissue weight (minimal that allows reliable 2-E^{+}OH quantification by HPLC). One important experimental control is to add superoxide dismutase before DHE incubation (*see* **Note 3**).

1. Identify 2 Eppendorf tubes for each sample and put them on a rack.
2. Cut the cleaned tissue in fragments around 50–150 mg. For myocardium, we recommend 150 mg, for arteries such as iliac or aorta, we cut segments of 3 mm (about 30 mg) (*see* **Note 10**).
3. Weigh the tissue in an analytical weighing-machine.
4. Gently transfer the tissue into an identified tube (*see* **Note 11**).
5. Add 0.5 mL of PBS/DTPA and 2.5 μL of DHE stock solution (10 mM).
6. Incubate the tissue with DHE for 30 min at 37 °C (*see* **Note 12**).
7. Carefully wash the tissue in iced PBS twice in order to remove excess DHE that eventually did not permeate the tissue.
8. Pulverize the segment into a mortar with a pestle in the presence of liquid nitrogen (*see* **Note 13**). Transfer the powder with a spatula for a tube and add 0.5 mL of acetonitrile (*see* **Note 14**).
9. Sonicate samples 3 times for 10 s (6 W) with minimal intervals of 10 s. Maintain tubes all the time immersed into the ice.
10. Centrifuge the samples for 15 min at 18,000 × *g* at 4 °C.
11. Transfer the supernatant to the second identified tube. Keep pellets on ice with opened cap for remaining acetonitrile evaporation.

12. Dry the supernatants in a vacuum concentrator at room temperature (approximately 2 h for 0.5 mL of acetonitrile) (*see* **Note 8**). Store the pale pink dried pellet at −80 °C for further HPLC analysis (*see* **Note 9**).
13. Add 50 μL of lysis buffer to the sample pellet kept on ice (**step 11**), strongly vortex for 1 min, sonicate (3 times at 6 W for 10 s) and keep samples on ice for 30 min. Determine the protein concentration (*see* **Note 15**).

3.4 HPLC Analysis and Calculations

Avoid direct lighting during **steps 1** and **2**.

1. Add 60 μL of mobile phase A to dried sample, vortex and, if necessary, homogenize with a pipette (*see* **Note 16**).
2. Inject 60 μL of sample into HPLC device, that was previous set up with the conditions described in Table 1 (*see* **Note 17**).
3. Convert sample peak areas into concentration, using standard curve calibrations. Simultaneous detection of DHE, 2-E^+OH and E^+ allows the ideal situation of using DHE as an internal control during organic extraction of each sample. Thus, DHE-derived products are expressed as ratios of 2-E^+OH and E^+ generated per DHE consumed (initial DHE concentration minus remaining DHE) (2-E^+OH/DHE and E^+/DHE). Then, 2-E^+OH and E^+ ratios are normalized by protein concentration (*see* **Note 18**).

3.5 Membrane-Enriched Fraction (Measurement of NADPH Oxidase Activity)

Membrane-enriched fraction can be isolated from cells or tissues. Cells should be grown on p100 dishes for a sufficient quantity of isolated membrane fraction (in general ~10% of total protein content). For tissues, fragments usually ≥50 mg are appropriate, along one to get enough material, but sometimes running a pilot test is necessary to verify the purification yield. In this protocol, HPLC device is equilibrated under tissue extract conditions displayed in Table 1, due to lipid content in samples. It is indispensable to run a blank control (without protein) in parallel with samples that will be injected at each day work. This control indicates how much contaminant 2-E^+OH there is in DHE working solution (1 mM), and all samples defined to produce superoxide during NADPH incubation are detected as those show higher 2-E^+OH levels than daily blank control. Other important controls are the use of NADPH oxidase inhibitors in membrane-enriched fraction incubations before NADPH and DHE additions (*see* **Note 19**).

3.5.1 For Cells

1. After specific treatment, wash cells that were grown in p100 dishes with 3 mL of cold PBS twice.
2. Add 500 μL of lysis buffer B and scrape cells.
3. Sonicate samples 3 times for 10 s (6 W) with minimal intervals of 10 s. Maintain tubes all the time into the ice.

4. Centrifuge samples for 5 min at 1000 ×*g* at 4 °C.
5. Centrifuge the supernatants for 15 min at 18,000 ×*g* at 4 °C (*see* **Note 20**).
6. Centrifuge the supernatants for 15 min at 100,000 ×*g* at 4 °C.
7. Remove the supernatant and resuspend the transparent pellet with 100 μL of lysis buffer B (*see* **Note 21**).
8. Determine the protein concentration (*see* **Note 22**).
9. Pipette membrane fraction in PBS/DTPA. The volume of membrane fraction is that corresponds to 20 μg of protein. The volume of PBS/DTPA is 48 μL minus the volume of membrane fraction for 20 μg of protein (*see* **Note 23**).
10. Add 3 μL of DHE 1 mM and 9 μL of NADPH 2 mM.
11. Incubate at 37 °C in the dark for 30 min.
12. Add 60 μL of trichloroacetic acid 10%, vortex, and maintain samples on ice for 20 min.
13. Centrifuge samples for 10 min at 15,000 ×*g* at 4 °C.
14. Collect the supernatant and maintain tubes on ice until HPLC injection. Samples should be injected in the same day in HPLC (*see* **Notes 24** and **25**).

3.5.2 For Tissues

1. Add 1 mL of lysis buffer B in tissue.
2. Homogenize the tissue with a polytron, maintaining the tubes with samples into the ice.
3. Follow the same steps described for cells (**steps 3–14**) (*see* **Notes 26** and **27**).

3.5.3 Calculations

1. Convert sample 2-E^+OH peak areas into concentrations, using standard curve calibrations. Subtract 2-E^+OH concentration of each sample from 2-E^+OH concentration of blank control. This difference is the superoxide production obtained during incubation of membrane-enriched fraction with NADPH. There is no need to normalize for protein concentration because all incubations will have been performed with equal protein quantities.

4 Notes

1. It is also recommended for fresh DHE solutions to be kept in HCl 1 mM to minimize autooxidation [14].
2. In order to obtain pure 2-E^+OH compound, prepare c.a. 50 mL 2-E^+OH as described, inject sequentially into HPLC and collect the corresponding 2-E^+OH peak with care for not collecting ethidium compound. After dried, the reddish pellet obtained is re-suspended in DMSO and its concentration

calculated by absorbance. Another way is to prepared 2-$E^{+}OH$ by reacting DHE with Fremy's salt [14]. 2-hydroxyethidium can also be obtained commercially (Noxygen).

3. One important experimental control with cells or tissues is to add SOD conjugated to polyethylene-glycol (PEG-SOD; 25 U/mL) before DHE incubation. Peg-SOD should be incubated for 30–60 min; lower time incubation will result in interference of ROS produced during PEG penetration into cells that promotes disturbances in membrane fluidity [15], and higher time incubation may reflect moderate nonspecific decrease in 2-$E^{+}OH$ levels [4]. In addition, another relevant control is PEG-Catalase (200 U/mL) incubation, especially in samples with high heme protein content.
4. DHE incubation is performed in Hanks/DTPA buffer instead of cellular medium for decreasing extracellular superoxide targets, mainly bovine serum albumin that is in high concentration in fetal bovine serum.
5. Depending on the experiment, HPLC analysis of Hanks/DTPA containing DHE can be a powerful tool. Supernatants can be injected directly in HPLC, and 2-$E^{+}OH$ generation will inform about extracellular superoxide production; for example in neutrophils during oxidative burst.
6. Do not drop PBS/DTPA directly on the cells, otherwise cells can detach. Drop the buffer in the dish wall and gently mix the plate for washing. After washing, remove carefully all PBS/DTPA from each well by aspiration. Any remaining PBS/DTPA will significantly delay the acetonitrile evaporation step.
7. Since acetonitrile is a volatile organic solvent, we strongly recommend to add acetonitrile and scrape only two wells at a time.
8. Sample evaporation should also be performed in the dark. Depending on the vacuum equipment used for sample concentration, the transparent lid will allow light to reach samples during this procedure. In this case, wrap the lid of equipment with aluminum foil. Some vacuum concentration devices instead contain an internal lamp to increase temperature inside the vacuum concentrator and thus diminish the evaporation time. In this case, do not turn on vacuum concentration light and develop the evaporation at room temperature.
9. Dried samples can be stored at −80 °C at least for 3 months without decreasing 2-$E^{+}OH$ levels.
10. It is not recommended to first freeze tissues and then perform DHE incubation. For good results DHE incubation should occur in the same day that tissues were removed from animals. Tissue can be maintained into ice PBS for some hours (2–6 h). Our observation with iliac arteries from rabbits after 14 days from angioplasty [3] is that DHE oxidation analyses in frozen

vessels generally do not show results with statistical differences that are obtained with fresh ones. We have also performed some measurements in mouse aorta and myocardium, and DHE consumption in fact increased in frozen compared to fresh tissues (unpublished data). This increase may be due to less efficient organic extraction in frozen versus fresh tissues, and/or due to artifactual ROS production during tissue defrosting. Thus, if using frozen tissues is unavoidable, DHE initial concentration should be higher than 50 μM.

11. How tissue is manipulated since its removal and during all steps is critical for reactive oxygen species production. It is important to gently handle the tissue and to procedure in a similar manner among all experiments for ensuring reproducibility.
12. Incubation time may vary, depending on the tissue. If there is no measurable remaining DHE in HPLC analysis, it will be necessary diminish incubation time and/or increase DHE concentration.
13. Liquid nitrogen will freeze water present in the atmosphere, so it will be not very easy to "find" the tissue powder inside the white powder of solidified water. Carefully remove all white powder to the identified tube, even some frozen water come together.
14. Some tissues cannot be pulverized because are too small and/or soft. For those particular cases, washing can be performed by centrifugation (1000 × *g* for 2 min), followed by careful cleaning of buffer drops from each tube with a swab, and then acetonitrile addition directly to the tissue (without tissue pulverization). Follow the procedure from **step 9**.
15. For some tissues it is not possible to determine protein concentration in remaining pellet after acetonitrile extraction, thus HPLC results can be normalized by weight.
16. Defreeze only samples that will be analyzed during the working day, what depends on the chromatographic run time. After sample resuspension in the mobile phase, samples cannot be stored any longer.
17. Injection volume will depend on loop size from HPLC device. In this protocol volumes of sample resuspension and injection were based on a loop size of 50 μL, but these volumes can be changed depending on the loop size of your HPLC equipment.
18. The overall baseline values obtained under optimal conditions with 50 μM DHE at 80 % VSMC confluence were 180 ± 40 nmol 2-E^{+}OH/μmol DHE and 200 ± 50 nmol E/μmol DHE (ca. ~20 % of initial DHE concentration). In all protocols, data can also be normalized for the amount of protein or number of cells; results will be analogous, although variability tends to be higher. In particular cases that cell number may vary (e.g., with

an apoptotic reagent), it is necessary normalize data for the amount of protein or cell number.

19. For measuring NADPH oxidase activity some controls are necessary; it is important to compare incubation of same membrane fraction with or without superoxide scavengers, such as SOD (25 U/mL) or tiron (20 μM). In addition, it is recommended to validate the assay using compounds known to inhibit NADPH oxidase activity, such as the flavoprotein inhibitor diphenyleneiodonium chloride (DPI, 10–20 μM), despite its lack of specificity [16], or some of emerging NADPH oxidase inhibitors such as triazolopyrimidines or pyrazolopyridine derivatives (respectively VAS- or GK-family compounds) [16]. These controls confer specificity for NADPH oxidase measurement and avoid misinterpretation of other superoxide sources in membrane-enriched fractions, such as endothelial nitric oxide synthase [4].
20. While the first step of centrifugation will pellet whole cells that were not lysed during sonication procedure, the second centrifugation will pellet mitochondria and nuclei.
21. The volume of lysis buffer B for resuspending enriched-membrane fraction may vary. One hundred microliters is recommended for the pellet obtained from a cellular culture at 85–90 % confluence in a p100 dish. For lower cell confluence or cellular loss during treatment, this volume can be decreased. For enriched-membrane fraction from tissues, lysis buffer B volume will depend on purification yield.
22. If HPLC analysis will not be performed at the same day of membrane fraction isolation, we recommend freeze samples at −80 °C and determine protein concentration in the day that they will be incubated with DHE and injected into HPLC, because freezing samples also diminishes total protein content in samples.
23. Some membrane fraction samples remain turbid after defrosted, and maybe show some aggregates in suspension. For properly protein solubilisation we recommend to sonicate them once (3 s of 6 W) before determining protein concentration.
24. Samples that were incubated with NADPH cannot be frozen for further HPLC analysis. Instead, incubate with DHE only the number of samples that can be injected into HPLC in the same day. In addition, enriched-membrane fractions can be stored at −80 °C for 1–2 weeks, with a small daily decrease in NADPH oxidase activity.
25. When analysis of NADPH oxidase activity by HPLC from a specific cell/tissue shows only increase in 2-E^{+}OH peak (with ethidium peak area constant), it is possible develop this measurement with fluorescence detection (λexc 490; λem 590 nm)

in microplate spectrofluorometer. This adaptation decreases time and costs expenditures; however, this method will be inaccurate if ethidium levels change among samples. For more details *see* ref. [3].

26. If the mechanical homogenization was not enough to disrupt the tissue, the volume of pellet obtained in the first centrifugation (1000 × *g*) may be similar or even higher than the volume of supernatant. In this case, sonicate again samples and observe the pellet size; if it remains the same, increase buffer volume and sonicate the samples (probably there is too much tissue for 1 mL of buffer).
27. Some tissues, such as large blood vessels, cannot be homogenized with polytron because of their high content of elastic fibers. These tissues can instead be pulverized into a mortar with a pestle in the presence of liquid nitrogen and the powder transferred to a tube for lysis buffer B addition.

Acknowledgment

The authors are members of the CEPID Redoxoma (Fundação de Amparo à Pesquisa do Estado de São Paulo - FAPESP Grant 2013/07937-8). Work also supported by FAPESP Grant 2009/54764-6 and Fundação Zerbini. RCG was recipient of MD studentship (FAPESP 2013/03363-7).

References

1. Zhao H, Kalivendi S, Zhang H, Joseph J, Nithipatikom K, Vasquez-Vivar J, Kalyanaraman B (2003) Superoxide reacts with hydroethidine but forms a fluorescent product that is distinctly different from ethidium: potential implications in intracellular fluorescence detection of superoxide. Free Radic Biol Med 34:1359–1368
2. Zhao H, Joseph J, Fales HM, Sokoloski EA, Levine RL, Vasquez-Vivar J, Kalyanaraman B (2005) Detection and characterization of the product of hydroethidine and intracellular superoxide by HPLC and limitations of fluorescence. Proc Natl Acad Sci U S A 102:5727–5732
3. Fernandes DC, Wosniak J Jr, Pescatore LA, Bertoline MA, Liberman M, Laurindo FR, Santos CX (2007) Analysis of DHE-derived oxidation products by HPLC in the assessment of superoxide production and NADPH oxidase activity in vascular systems. Am J Physiol Cell Physiol 292:C413–C422
4. Laurindo FR, Fernandes DC, Santos CX (2008) Assessment of superoxide production and NADPH oxidase activity by HPLC analysis of dihydroethidium oxidation products. Methods Enzymol 441:237–260
5. Zielonka J, Hardy M, Kalyanaraman B (2009) HPLC study of oxidation products of hydroethidine in chemical and biological systems: ramifications in superoxide measurements. Free Radic Biol Med 46:329–338
6. Zielonka J, Vasquez-Vivar J, Kalyanaraman B (2008) Detection of 2-hydroxyethidium in cellular systems: a unique marker product of superoxide and hydroethidine. Nat Protoc 3:8–21
7. Zielonka J, Kalyanaraman B (2010) Hydroethidine- and MitoSOX-derived red fluorescence is not a reliable indicator of intracellular superoxide formation: another inconvenient truth. Free Radic Biol Med 48:983–1001
8. Zielonka J, Zielonka M, Sikora A, Adamus J, Joseph J, Hardy M, Ouari O, Dranka BP,

Kalyanaraman B (2012) Global profiling of reactive oxygen and nitrogen species in biological systems: high-throughput real-time analyses. J Biol Chem 287:2984–2995

9. Georgiou CD, Papapostolou I, Patsoukis N, Tsegenidis T, Sideris T (2005) An ultrasensitive fluorescent assay for the in vivo quantification of superoxide radical in organisms. Anal Biochem 347:144–151
10. Georgiou CD, Papapostolou I, Grintzalis K (2008) Superoxide radical detection in cells, tissues, organisms (animals, plants, insects, microorganisms) and soils. Nat Protoc 3:1679–1692
11. Robinson KM, Janes MS, Pehar M, Monette JS, Ross MF, Hagen TM, Murphy MP, Beckman JS (2006) Selective fluorescent imaging of superoxide in vivo using ethidium-based probes. Proc Natl Acad Sci U S A 103:15038–15043
12. Lassègue B, San Martín A, Griendling KK (2012) Biochemistry, physiology, and pathophysiology of NADPH oxidases in the cardiovascular system. Circ Res 110:1364–1390
13. Robinson J, Coope JM (1970) Method of determining oxygen concentrations in biological media, suitable for calibration of the oxygen electrode. Anal Biochem 33: 390–399
14. Zielonka J, Zhao H, Xu Y, Kalyanaraman B (2005) Mechanistic similarities between oxidation of hydroethidine by Fremy's salt and superoxide: stopped-flow optical and EPR studies. Free Radic Biol Med 39:853–863
15. Beckman JS, Minor RL Jr, White CW, Repine JE, Rosen GM, Freeman BA (1988) Superoxide dismutase and catalase conjugated to polyethylene glycol increases endothelial enzyme activity and oxidant resistance. J Biol Chem 263: 6884–6892. Laurindo FR, de Souza HP, Pedro Mde A, Janiszewski M (2002) Redox aspects of vascular response to injury. Methods Enzymol 352:432–454
16. Drummond GR, Selemidis S, Griendling KK, Sobey CG (2011) Combating oxidative stress in vascular disease: NADPH oxidases as therapeutic targets. Nat Rev Drug Discov 10: 453–471

Chapter 20

Assessment of Caveolae/Lipid Rafts in Isolated Cells

G.E. Callera, Thiago Bruder-Nascimento, and R.M. Touyz

Abstract

This chapter outlines protocols to evaluate protein localization, recruitment or phosphorylation levels in cholesterol/sphingolipids-enriched cell membrane domains and recommends experimental designs with pharmacological tolls to evaluate potential cell functions associated with these domains. We emphasize the need for the combination of several approaches towards understanding the protein components and cellular functions attributed to these distinct microdomains.

Key words Caveolae, Lipid rafts, Detergent-free method, Methyl-β-cyclodextrin, Statins

1 Introduction

Lipid rafts are key players in the integration of cellular responses. These dynamic ordered cholesterol/sphingolipids-enriched cell membrane domains are transient platforms and aggregate interacting signaling proteins [1, 2]. Two major kinds of free cholesterol, sphingomyelin, and glycosylphosphatidylinositol (GPI)-containing microdomains are now recognized to coexist within the plasma membrane [2, 3]. Lipid rafts are flattened structures, with GPI-anchored proteins that float freely in cell membranes and lack distinctive properties. Caveolae constitute a subset of lipid rafts with morphologically defined cell surface flask-shaped invagination that contain caveolin as a major structural protein [3–5].

Compartmentalization of signaling proteins is likely required to provide the appropriate molecular proximity necessary for rapid, efficient and specific regulation of downstream events. Lipid rafts as dynamic distinct structures can aggregate and include or exclude proteins creating a restricted and integrative microenvironment. Extracellular stimuli drive specific lipid–lipid, protein–lipid, and protein–protein oligomerizing interactions, giving rise to larger, more stable and functional raft domains, which initiate signal transduction from the cell surface [1, 3, 6–8]. The mechanisms whereby humoral or mechanical factors trigger the ordered assembly of

Rhian M. Touyz and Ernesto L. Schiffrin (eds.), *Hypertension: Methods and Protocols*, Methods in Molecular Biology, vol. 1527, DOI 10.1007/978-1-4939-6625-7_20, © Springer Science+Business Media LLC 2017

lipids and proteins are variable. Post translational modification of protein, caveolin interactions and lipid modifications modulate raft assembly and determine protein recruitment into lipid rafts and/or increase residency time in these microenvironments [1, 3, 7–9]

As it is now increasingly appreciated, cholesterol/sphingolipids-enriched domains are important for the activation of protein signaling pathways in disease-associated organ target damage [10–15]. Given the complexity of lipid rafts/caveolae, investigating protein trafficking and raft assembly as well as the biological responses attributed to these domains requires critical use of methodologies and interpretation of data in order to draw conclusions of these cellular processes.

Generally, methods used to investigate caveolae/lipid raft protein interaction exploit their biophysical, biochemical, and morphological properties. Cholesterol and sphingolipids have the tendency to associate with each other, thus segregating into more ordered state in the cell membrane. The structure of their hydrophobic moieties allows a tight lipid packing which resists to non-ionic detergent extraction. This detergent insoluble residue is enriched with cholesterol, sphingolipids, and raft-associated proteins. The low density of the lipid rafts allows for their separations from the remaining soluble membrane components by flotation in discontinuous sucrose gradient centrifugation. Proteins with strong interaction within these highly ordered domains retain their association with lipids and are recovered in the detergent resistant membrane fraction [1, 3, 16–18].

Criticisms have been directed to the use of detergent resistance as a defining factor for raft components [1, 3, 19]. Variations in raft-associated protein composition may occur depending on the method employed. Experimental conditions may interfere with partitioning dynamics of the signaling proteins toward lipid rafts. Detergent extraction disrupts lipid–protein weak interactions, so that most membrane proteins are solubilized. Thus, proteins that are only weakly associated with lipid raft membranes can be solubilized. Furthermore, lipid rafts are cytoskeletal-associated structures and detergents disrupt cytoskeletal–membrane interactions and compromise this assessment. The use of non-ionic detergents and sucrose gradient fractionation also has limitations regarding the contamination from non-raft plasma membranes or intracellular membranes. Protein content in detergent resistant membrane fraction may not reflect the components of native lipid rafts in cell membranes.

Depletion or sequestration of free cholesterol from the plasma membrane has been carried out with pharmacological tools to manipulate lipid raft association of proteins. Disruption of domains whose integrity depends on cholesterol is not a procedure specific for lipid rafts [1, 3, 18–20]. Many cellular functions can be perturbed by cholesterol depletion. The disruption of lipid rafts releases proteins promoting the activation of several signaling pathways, interferes with the lateral movement of proteins, and alters membrane polarization leading to intracellular calcium increase. For cell protocols with cholesterol modifying drugs, experimental controls are required to reassure the role of raft-associated proteins and cellular functions attributed to lipid rafts. Cholesterol reload may provide the restoration of the responses abrogated by the disruption of the domains. Methyl-β-cyclodextrin (MβCD) that extracts cholesterol from plasma membrane is employed to disrupt lipid rafts. The water-soluble MβCD is known to form inclusion complexes with cholesterol, thereby enhancing its solubility in aqueous solution. The hydrophobic cholesterol molecule is trapped inside the cyclodextrin rings and can be further removed. Inhibition of cholesterol biosynthetic pathway also interferes with lipid raft association of proteins. Statins inhibit 3-hydroxy-3-methylglutaryl-coenzyme A (HMG-CoA) reductase leading to reduction of membrane cholesterol. As a complementary experimental control, the replenishment of the HMG-CoA reductase product, mevalonate, must be performed.

As cholesterol modifying drugs remove cholesterol from lipid rafts and caveolae, these reagents cannot distinguish between signaling events occurring in these compartments. Taking into account the morphological aspects of lipid rafts, molecular approaches may be applied to knockdown caveolins, which are essential in forming the flask-shaped membrane invaginations [1, 3, 15]. Small interference (siRNA) provides an efficient method to knockdown caveolin-1 expression and downregulate caveolae-derived signaling. Cell lines derived from primary cultures isolated from caveloin-1 knockout mice are powerful tools to investigate contribution of this subset of lipid rafts to cell function in association with siRNA protocols. The limitation of using protein knockdown methods is the potential for compensatory effects.

Microscopy techniques for studying lipid rafts in live cells have been developed. The main downside is the requirement of highly specialized equipment besides the technical expertise. Some of them, similarly to the other methods used to define spatial raft-dependent processes and raft-associated proteins are prone to artifacts due to the use of fluorescent probes. These methods have been highlighted in recent reviews [19].

To minimize the pitfalls, the general consensus is the combination of several approaches towards understanding the protein components and cellular functions attributable to these distinct microdomains. To date, the use of biochemical, pharmacological and molecular approaches in association with fluorescence microscopy techniques, as well as the useful caveolin knockout models constitute the best approach to evaluate the functional and spatial importance of lipid rafts/caveolae in cell signaling.

Here we provide detailed protocols to evaluate protein localization recruitment or phosphorylation levels in cholesterol/

sphingolipids-enriched cell membrane domains and recommend experimental designs with pharmacological tolls to evaluate potential cell functions associated with these domains.

2 Materials

2.1 Reagents

1. Potassium phosphate monobasic (KH_2PO_4, Sigma, cat. no. P3786).
2. Sodium phosphate dibasic (Na_2HPO_4, EMD, cat. no. SX0720-5).
3. Sodium chloride (NaCl, EMD, cat. no. CASX0420-5).
4. Potassium chloride (KCl, EMD, cat. no. PX1405-1).
5. Sodium carbonate (Na_2CO_3, EMD, cat. no. SX0395-1).
6. Calcium chloride dihydrate ($CaCl_2{\cdot}2H_2O$, EMD, cat. no. CX0130-1).
7. Magnesium chloride hexahydrate ($MgCl_2{\cdot}6H_2O$, EMD, cat. no. MX0045-1).
8. Tris-base (VWR, cat. no. CA80503-542).
9. Sucrose (Sigma, cat. no. S9378).
10. Sodium hydroxide (NaOH, Sigma, cat. no. S5881).
11. 2-(*N*-morpholino)ethanesulfonic acid (MES, Calbiochem, cat. no. 4755893).
12. Trichloroacetic acid (TCA, VWR, cat. no. CATX1045-1).
13. OptiPrep™ (60% Iodixanol, Fresenius Kabi Norge AS, cat. no. 01-63-15-001-A).
14. Aprotinin (stock 1 mg/mL, Sigma, cat. no. A1153).
15. Pepstatin A (stock 1 mg/mL, Sigma, cat. no. P5318).
16. Leupeptin (stock 1 mg/mL, Sigma, cat. no. L2884).
17. Phenylmethylsulfonyl fluoride (PMSF, stock 1 mg/mL, Sigma, cat. no. P7626).
18. Sodium orthovanadate (Na_3VO_4, stock 1 mg/mL, Sigma, cat. no. 450243).
19. Dulbecco's Modified Eagle's medium (DMEN, Gibco, cat. no. 31600-083).
20. Fetal bovine serum (FBS, Wisent, cat. no. 080-150).
21. Methyl-β-cyclodextrin (MβCD, Sigma, cat. no. C4555).
22. Atorvastatin (EMD, cat. no. 189291).
23. Cholesterol-water soluble (Sigma, cat. no. C4951).
24. Mevalonic acid (Mevalonate, Sigma, cat. no. 79849).

2.2 Equipment

1. SW-41 Beckman rotor.
2. 14×89 mm Ultra-clear centrifuge tube (Beckman 344059) or 14×89 mm polycarbonate centrifuge tube (Beckman 331372).

2.3 Reagent Setup

1. *PBS (Phosphate-buffered saline)—1 L*
   Dissolve 8 g NaCl, 0.2 g KCl, 1.44 g Na_2HPO_4, and 0.24 g KH_2PO_4 in double-distilled water (ddH_2O) and bring to a final volume of 1 L. Adjust the pH to 7.4 using HCl.
2. *500 mM Na2CO3, pH 11*
   Dissolve 26.5 g Na_2CO_3 in ddH_2O and bring to a final volume of 500 mL. Adjust the pH to 11 using NaOH.
3. *Raft buffer-250 mM MES-buffered saline (10× MBS, pH 6.5)*
   Dissolve 24.4 g MES, and 39.5 g NaCl in ddH_2O and bring to a final volume of 500 mL. Adjust the pH to 6.5 using NaOH.
4. *85 % Sucrose*
   Add 10 mL 10× MBS to 85 mg sucrose and bring to a final volume of 100 mL with ddH_2O (~30 mL). Moderate heat is needed to dissolve the sucrose.
5. *30 % Sucrose*
   Combine 5 mL 10× MBS, 25 mL 500 mM Na_2CO_3, 17.6 mL 85 % sucrose, and 2.4 mL ddH_2O.
6. *5 % Sucrose*
   Combine 2 mL 10× MBS, 10 mL 500 mM Na_2CO_3, 1.2 mL 85 % sucrose, and 6.8 mL ddH_2O.
7. *TCA 20 %*
   Dissolve 10 g trichloroacetic acid in ddH_2O and bring to a final volume of 500 mL.
8. *Additives for Na_2CO_3*
   Prepare 20 mL of 500 mM Na_2CO_3 containing 2 μg/mL aprotinin, 2 μg/mL pepstatin, 2 μg/mL leupeptin, 1 mM PMSF, and 1 mM Na_3VO_4.
9. *Base buffer for the OptiPrep protocol (20 mM Tris–HCl, pH 7.8, and 250 mM sucrose)*
   Dissolve 0.6 g Tris base in ddH_2O and bring to a final volume of 100 mL and Adjust the pH to 7.8 using HCl. Dissolve 8.5 g sucrose in 20 mM Tris–HCl to a final volume of 100 mL.
10. *1 M $CaCl_2$ stock*
    Dissolve 1.47 g in ddH_2O and bring to a final volume of 10 mL.
11. *1 M $MgCl_2$ stock*
    Dissolve 2.03 g in ddH_2O and bring to a final volume of 10 mL.
12. *0.1 M PMSF stock*

Dissolve 0.17 g in ethanol and bring to a final volume of 10 mL. Store at −20 °C.

13. *0.1 M Na_3VO_4 stock*

Dissolve 0.18 g in ddH_2O and bring to a final volume of 10 mL. Store at −20 °C.

14. *Additives for OptiPrep*

Prepare 10 mL base buffer containing 2 μg/mL aprotinin, 2 μg/mL pepstatin, 2 μg/mL leupeptin, 1 mM PMSF and 1 mM Na_3VO_4, 1 mM $CaCl_2$, and 1 mM $MgCl_2$.

15. *0.1 M NaOH*

Dissolve 0.2 g NaOH in ddH_2O and bring to a final volume of 50 mL.

3 Methods

3.1 Non-detergent-Based Isolation of Raft Membranes Fractionation

Biochemical isolation of lipid raft membranes and their subsequent analysis is a useful and simple method to determine if signaling components are located, or had their content increased in raft microdomains. Two common techniques described here are used to evaluate protein localization or phosphorylation levels to rafts prior to, and after cell stimulation. These protocols were tested for rat vascular smooth muscle cells (VSMCs) in culture (Figs. 1 and 2).

3.1.1 Detergent-Free Membrane Analysis with Sodium Carbonate Buffer in pH 11

This procedure does not involve detergent extraction for the isolation of lipid rafts, and it is based on pH and sodium carbonate resistance [21, 22]. Cold sodium carbonate, at high alkaline pH, separates proteins that are firmly attached to membranes from those that are more peripherally associated. Rafts, due to their higher lipid/protein ratio, are isolated by centrifugation in a discontinuous sucrose gradient and fractions are harvested. This high pH method requires a cell disruption step.

Procedure:

1. Prepare VSMCs grown to sub-confluence (~95%) in 100 mm dishes (growth arrest for 24 h).

   Critical step: All solutions, materials, and handling must be at 0–4 °C.

2. After the stimulation protocol, wash the cells three times with ice-cold PBS.

3. Scrape cells with a rubber policeman, into 1 mL 500 mM Na_2CO_3, pH 11 (plus protease/phosphatase inhibitors; see reagents setup).

   Comment: Extraction with cold alkaline carbonate prepares an insoluble membrane fraction whose buoyant density permits its flotation in discontinuous sucrose gradients.

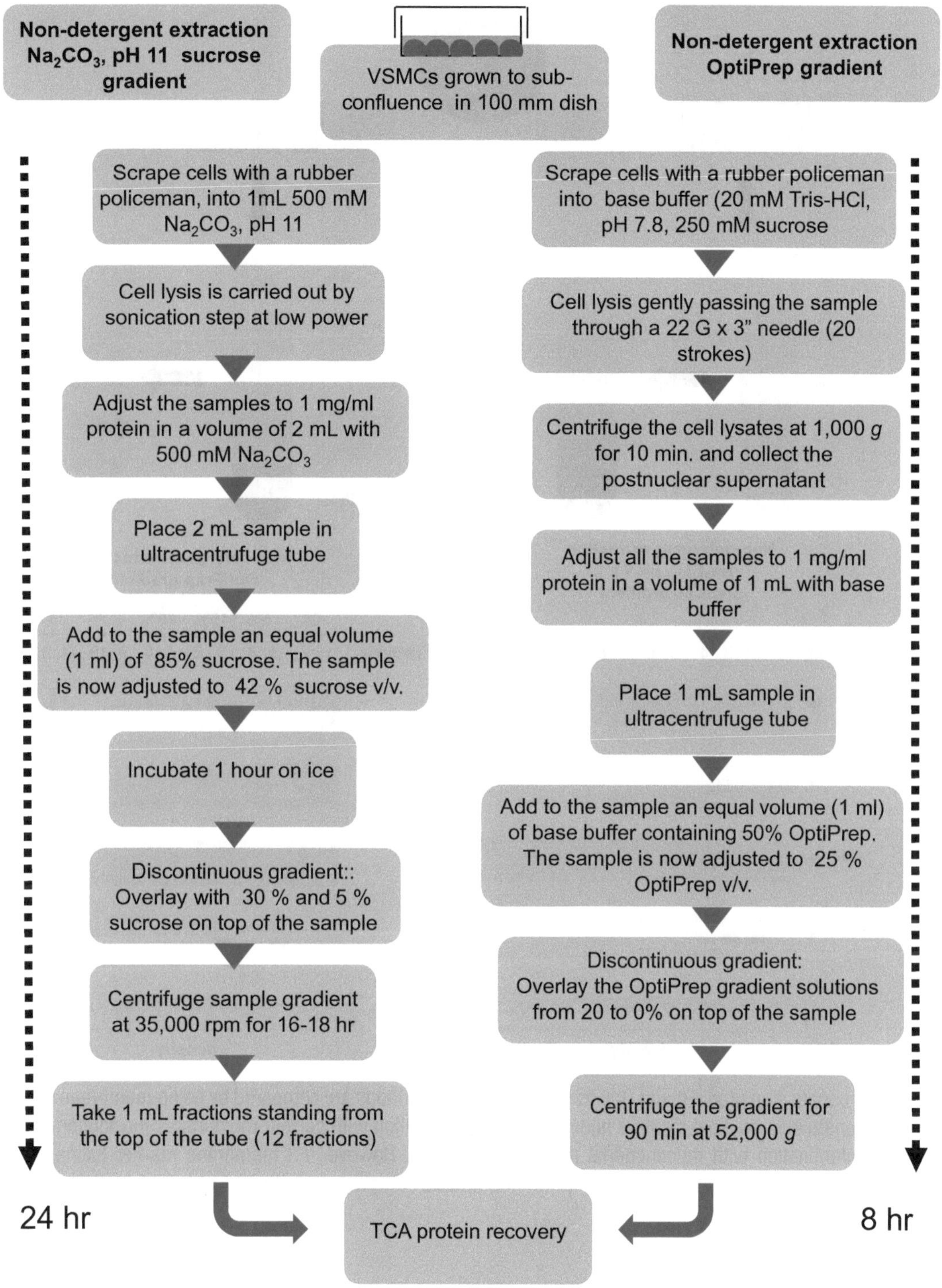

Fig. 1 Flow diagram showing the major steps in the methods for the preparation of detergent-free lipid rafts procedures. *Left*, Na_2CO_3 buffer in pH 11 and sucrose gradient; *right*, OptiPrep step gradient

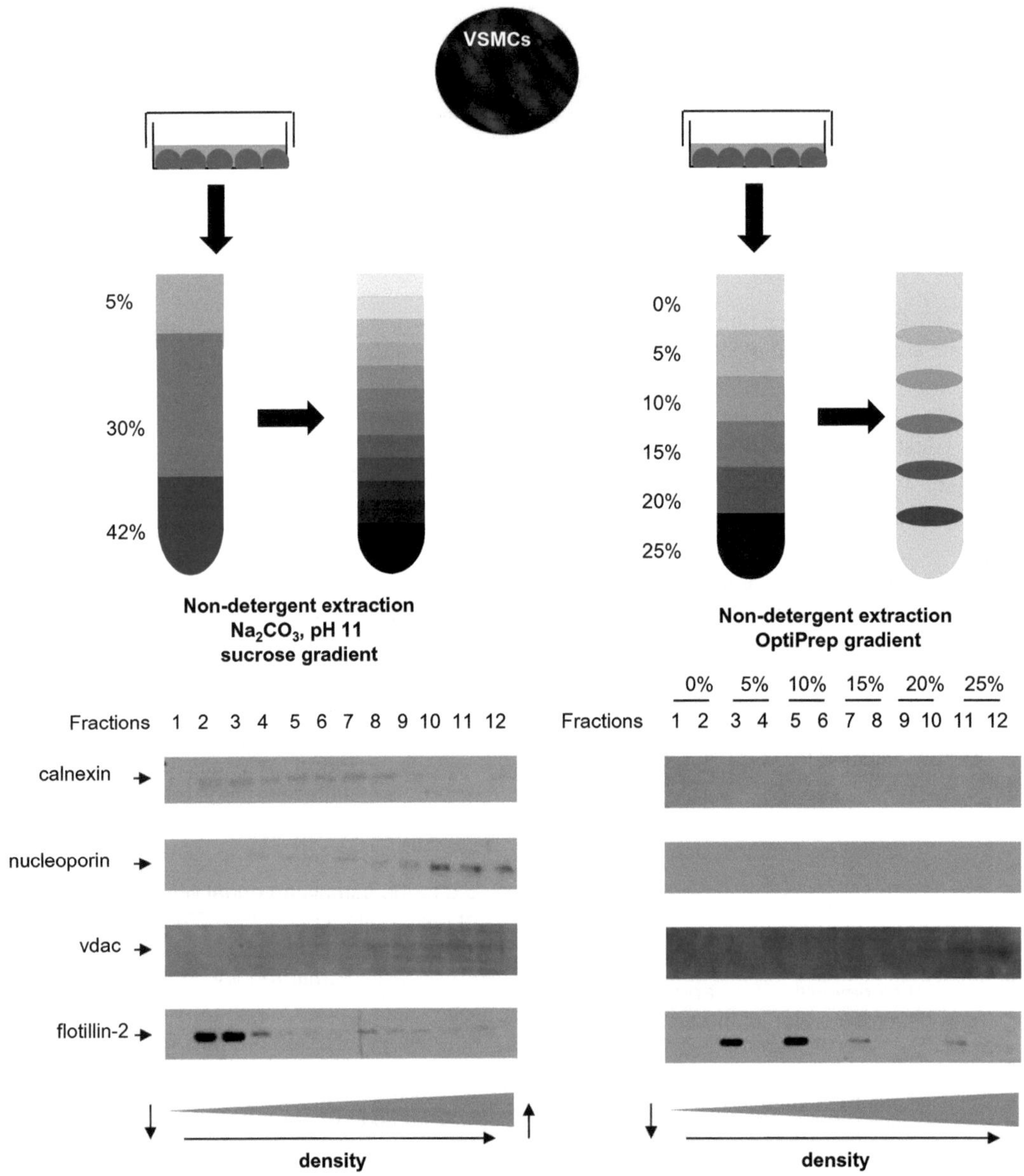

Fig. 2 Carbonate step gradient and OptiPrep detergent free methods are compared by using membrane markers. Carbonate step gradient displays undetectable contamination with nuclear membranes (nucleoporin) and slight contamination with mitochondrial membranes (VDAC). However, ER membrane marker (calnexin) is detected throughout the gradient. OptiPrep method offered raft preparation with lack of intracellular membranes contamination

4. Cell lysis is carried out by a sonication step at low power (three times, 10 s bursts)

   Comment: Such step is introduced to finely disrupt cellular membranes. It must be gentle to preserve the relationship between membrane, protein and cytoskeletal components.

Optional: gently pass the sample through a 22 G×3″ needle (20 strokes) plus dounce homogenizer (10 strokes).

5. Determine the total protein content of each individual sample lysate.
6. Adjust all the samples to 1 mg/mL protein in a volume of 2 mL with 500 mM Na_2CO_3 (plus protease/phosphatase inhibitors).
7. Place the 2 mL sample in a 14×89 mm Ultra-clear centrifuge tube (Beckman 344059).

   Comment: 14×89 mm polycarbonate centrifuge tube (Beckman 331372) can be employed.
8. Add 2 mL 85 % sucrose in raft buffer (MBS, 2-(*N*-morpholino) ethanesulfonic acid (MES)-buffered saline) to each sample and mix gently by pipetting up and down. The sample is now adjusted to ~42 % v/v sucrose.
9. Let stand for 1 h on ice.
10. A discontinuous gradient is formed above the sample in 42 % sucrose. Overlay with 6 mL of 30 % sucrose in MBS and overlay again with 2 mL of 5 % sucrose in MBS.

    Comment: The buoyant density of lipid rafts permits their flotation in and recovery from discontinuous sucrose gradients after centrifugation.
11. Centrifuge sample gradient at 100,000×*g* for 16–18 h in a SW-41 Beckman rotor at 4 °C.

    Critical step: During the centrifugation step, the brake must be turned off. It will take over 1 h for the full stop.

    Comment: The SW-41 6 allows the centrifugation of six samples at the time. This information should be considered to design the time course for cell stimulation.
12. Take 1 mL fractions starting from the top of the tube (total 12 fractions).

    Comment: There should be a light scattering band confined to the 5–35 % sucrose interface (around fractions 2 and 3) that contains raft associated proteins.
13. Divide each fraction to equal parts, resulting in two sets of 12 fractions.

    Break point: At this point, the sample sets can be processed or stored at −80 °C to be processed later.
14. Trichloroacetic acid (TCA) is used for further protein recovery. On ice, take 500 μL of each fraction and add 500 μL of TCA 20 % (v/v).

    Comment: The use of a 2 mL microcentrifuge tubes is recommended due to the bubbling following the TCA addition.
15. Incubate on ice for 1 h to allow protein precipitation.

16. Centrifuge for 10 min at 16,000 × *g*, 4 °C.
17. Discard the supernatant.
18. Spin down the remaining supernatant (30 s) in order to completely eliminate it.

    Comment: Residual TCA will affect the pH of the Laemmli buffer in the further step.
19. Resuspend the pellet in 42 μL of 0.1 M NaOH to neutralize the TCA.
20. Add 7 μL of 6× Laemmli sample buffer and boil 5 min.

    Comment: Use the total volume of each sample for sodium dodecyl sulfate polyacrylamide (SDS-PAGE) gel electrophoresis.

3.1.2 OptiPrep Step Gradient-Simplified Method for the Preparation of Detergent-Free Lipid Rafts

Another simplified method for the purification of detergent-free lipid rafts that requires shorter-density gradient centrifugation was described to provide a highly purified raft fraction [23]. OptiPrep is an iodixanol-based density gradient medium that can form a gradient from a solution of uniform density under the influence of the centrifugal field. Flotation on OptiPrep step gradient offers raft preparation with lack of intracellular membranes contamination. This method requires short ultracentrifugation and omits the sonication step.

Procedure:

1. Prepare VSMCs grown to sub-confluence (~95 %) in 100 mm dishes (growth arrest for 24 h).

    Critical step: All solutions, materials, and handling must be at 0–4 °C.
2. After the stimulation protocol, wash the cells three times with ice-cold PBS.
3. Scrape cells with a rubber policeman into base buffer (20 mM Tris–HCl, pH 7.8, 250 mM sucrose) to which has been added 1 mM $CaCl_2$ and 1 mM $MgCl_2$ and protease/phosphatase inhibitors (see reagents setup).
4. Pellet cells by centrifugation for 2 min at 250 × *g*.
5. Resuspend cells in 500 μL of base buffer (plus 1 mM $CaCl_2$, 1 mM $MgCl_2$ and protease/phosphatase inhibitors).
6. Cell lysis is carried out by gently passing the sample through a 22 G × 3″ needle (20 strokes).
7. Centrifuge the cell lysates at 1000 × *g* for 10 min.
8. Collect the resulting postnuclear supernatant and transfer to a separate microcentrifuge tube.
9. Determine the total protein content of each individual sample lysate.

10. Adjust all the samples to 1 mg/mL protein in a volume of 1 mL with base buffer (plus 1 mM $CaCl_2$, 1 mM $MgCl_2$, and protease/phosphatase inhibitors).
11. Place the 1 mL sample in a 14 × 89 mm Ultra-clear centrifuge tube (Beckman 344059).

    Comment: 14 × 89 mm polycarbonate centrifuge tube (Beckman 331372) may be employed.
12. Add to the sample an equal volume (1 mL) of base buffer containing 50% OptiPrep.
13. Prepare a 10 mL density gradient from solutions of base buffer and OptiPrep as follows: 0% (2 mL), 5% (2 mL), 10% (2 mL), 15% (2 mL), and 20% (2 mL).
14. Overlay the gradient solutions (from 20 to 0%) on top of the cell lysate, which is now 25% in OptiPrep.
15. Centrifuge the gradient for 90 min at 52,000 × *g* using an SW-41 rotor in a Beckman ultracentrifuge.

    Critical step: During the centrifugation step, the brake must be turned off.
16. Take 1 mL fractions starting from the top of the tube (total 12 fractions).

    Optional: Take 2 mL fractions starting from the top of the tube (total 6 fractions).

    Comment: Do not aliquot the fractions, this method allows for only one set of samples.

    Break point: At this point, the sample sets can be processed or stored at −80 °C to be processed later.
17. As for sodium carbonate extraction, recover the protein with TCA (following the **step 14**).

    Comment: For 2 mL fractions add 2 mL of 20% TCA. The use of a 5 mL microcentrifuge tubes is recommended due to the bubbling following the TCA addition.

4 Protocols for Cholesterol Modifying Drugs

Cell protocols with cholesterol modifying drugs are recommended, in association with cell fractionation, to evaluate the potential cell functions associated with caveolae/lipid rafts. The following protocols were tested in mouse and rat mesenteric VSMCs.

4.1 Cell Protocol for Cholesterol Depletion with MβCD and Cholesterol Reloading

Depletion of cholesterol from the VSMC plasma membrane can be carried out MβCD [24]. Cholesterol depletion and cholesterol reload are performed prior to cell stimulation in growth arrested cells (Fig. 3).

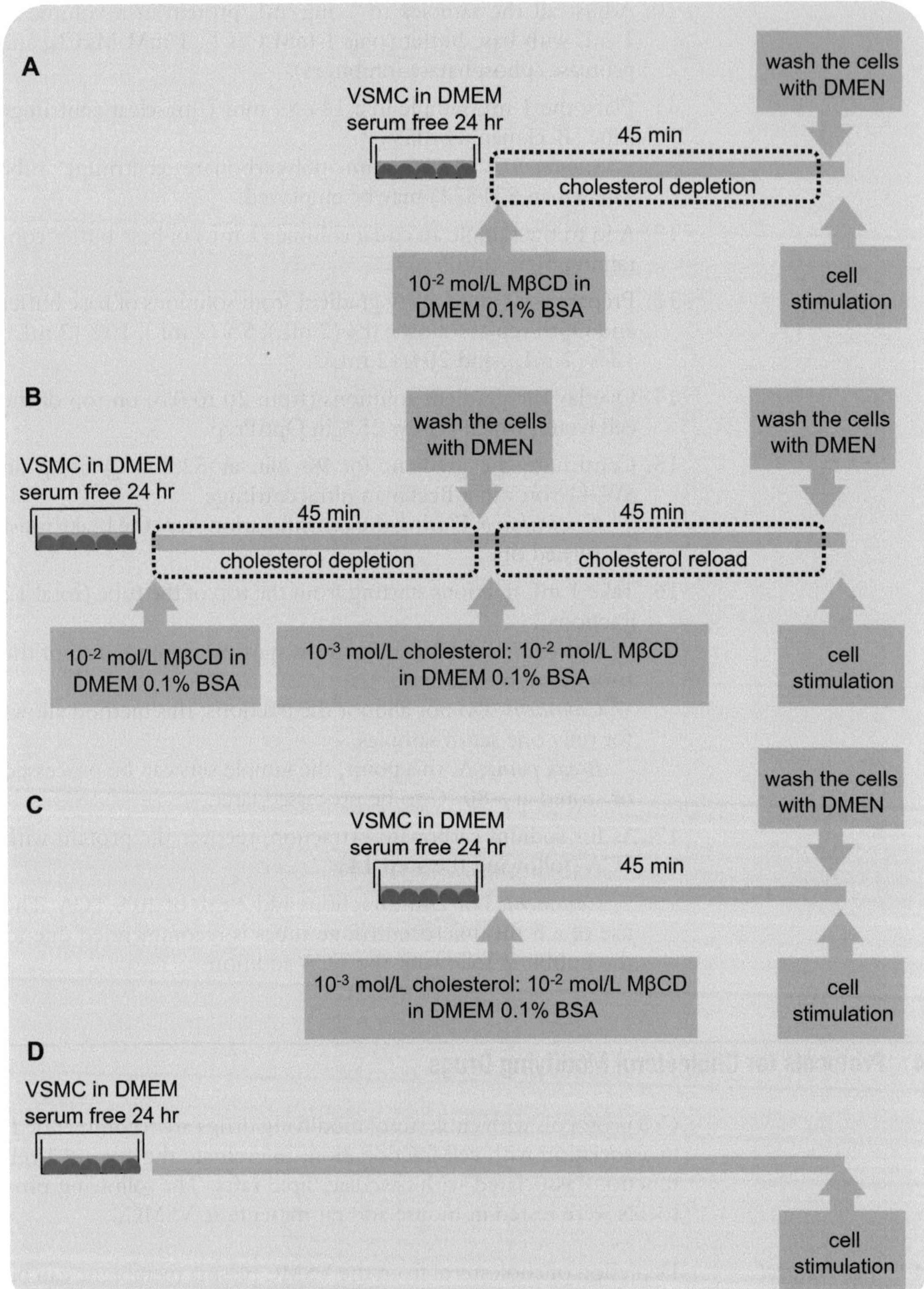

Fig. 3 Protocol for cholesterol depletion with methyl-β-cyclodextrin (MβCD) and cholesterol reloading. (**a**) Experimental group 1 for cholesterol depletion: cells are incubated with 10^{-2} mol/L MβCD in DMEM containing 0.1 % BSA for 45 min at 37 °C; after incubation period, MβCD is washed off. (**b**) Experimental group 2 for

Protocol:

1. Prepare VSMCs grown to sub-confluence (~95 %) in 100 mm dishes (growth arrest for 24 h) for four experimental groups.
   Comment: The choice of the dish size is based on the experimental procedure to be performed after cell stimulation.
   Experimental group 1: *Cholesterol depletion.*
2. Incubate the cells with 10^{-2} mol/L MβCD in DMEM containing 0.1 % BSA for 45 min at 37 °C.
   Comment: In this group, cholesterol is depleted with MβCD without further reload.
3. Wash the cells with DMEM serum free.
   Comment: In this step cholesterol associated with MβCD is removed.
   Experimental group 2: *Cholesterol depletion followed by cholesterol reload.*
4. Incubate the cells with 10^{-2} mol/L MβCD in DMEM containing 0.1 % BSA for 45 min at 37 °C.
5. Wash the cells with DMEM serum free.
   Comment: In this step cholesterol associated with MβCD is removed.
6. Cholesterol (water-soluble) is reloaded by incubating cholesterol-depleted cells with 10^{-3} mol/L cholesterol: 10^{-2} mol/L MβCD complex in DMEM-0.1 % BSA for 45 min at 37 °C.
   Comment: The complex prevents the overload of the plasma membrane with cholesterol.
7. Wash the cells with DMEM serum free.
   Comment: In this step MβCD and unincorporated cholesterol are removed.
   Experimental group 3: *Control for cholesterol reload.*
8. Incubate the cells with cholesterol: MβCD complex for 45 min at 37 °C, without previous cholesterol depletion.
9. Wash the cells with DMEM serum free.

   Critical step: MβCD potentially incorporates drugs utilized for cell stimulation depending on their chemical structure. For experimental groups 1, 2, and 3, cells must be washed to remove the MβCD and unincorporated cholesterol and immediately used for stimulation.

Fig. 3 (continued) cholesterol depletion followed by cholesterol reloading: cells are incubated with 10^{-2} mol/L MβCD in DMEM containing 0.1 % BSA for 45 min at 37 °C; after incubation period, MβCD is washed off; Cholesterol is reload to the cell by incubating cholesterol: 10^{-2} mol/L MβCD complex in DMEM-0.1 % BSA for 45 min at 37 °C; the complex and unincorporated cholesterol is washed off. (**c**) Experimental group 3 as a control for cholesterol reload: cells are incubated with cholesterol: MβCD complex for 45 min at 37 °C; the complex is washed off. (**d**) Experimental group 4 is the control without cholesterol manipulation

Experimental group 4: Control without cholesterol manipulation.

Comment: All experimental groups must be carried out at the same time.

4.2 Cell Protocol for Cholesterol Biosynthetic Pathway Inhibition with Statins

Statins interfere with cholesterol biosynthesis by inhibiting HMG-CoA reductase leading to reduction of membrane cholesterol. Cholesterol synthesis starts with one molecule of acetyl CoA and one molecule of acetoacetyl-CoA, which are hydrated to form HMG-CoA. HMG-CoA is then reduced to mevalonate by the enzyme HMG-CoA reductase. Mevalonate is then converted to farnesyl pyrophosphate and the subsequently squalene, the precursor for cholesterol. Statins, which inhibit HMG-CoA reductase, inhibit the production of cholesterol and can be used as a toll to study lipid rafts. The following protocol was developed by using atorvastatin to inhibit cholesterol synthesis 72 h prior to cell stimulation (Fig. 4).

Protocol:

1. Prepare VSMCs grown to sub-confluence (~70%) in 100 mm dishes for three experimental groups.

   Comment: The choice of the dish size is based on the experimental procedure to be performed after cell stimulation.

   Experimental group 1: Cholesterol synthesis inhibition with atorvastatin.
2. Cells are incubated with 10^{-7} mol/L atorvastatin in DMEM containing 10% FBS for 48 h, at 37 °C.
3. Cell medium is replaced with DMEM serum free and cells are incubated with 10^{-7} mol/L atorvastatin for an additional 24 h.

   Experimental group 2: Mevalonate supplementation.
4. Cells are incubated with 10^{-4} mol/L mevalonate in DMEM 10% FBS 1 h prior to atorvastatin treatment.
5. Cells are incubated with 10^{-7} mol/L atorvastatin which is added to DMEM containing 10% FBS supplemented with mevalonate for 48 h at 37 °C.
6. Cell medium is replaced with DMEM serum free and cells are incubated with 10^{-7} mol/L atorvastatin plus 10^{-4} mol/L mevalonate for an additional 24 h.

   Experimental group 3: Control without cholesterol synthesis inhibition.
7. For the control group, in absence of the pharmacological agents, DMEM 10% FBS is replaced with serum free media for 24 h.

   Comment: All experimental groups must be carried out at the same time.

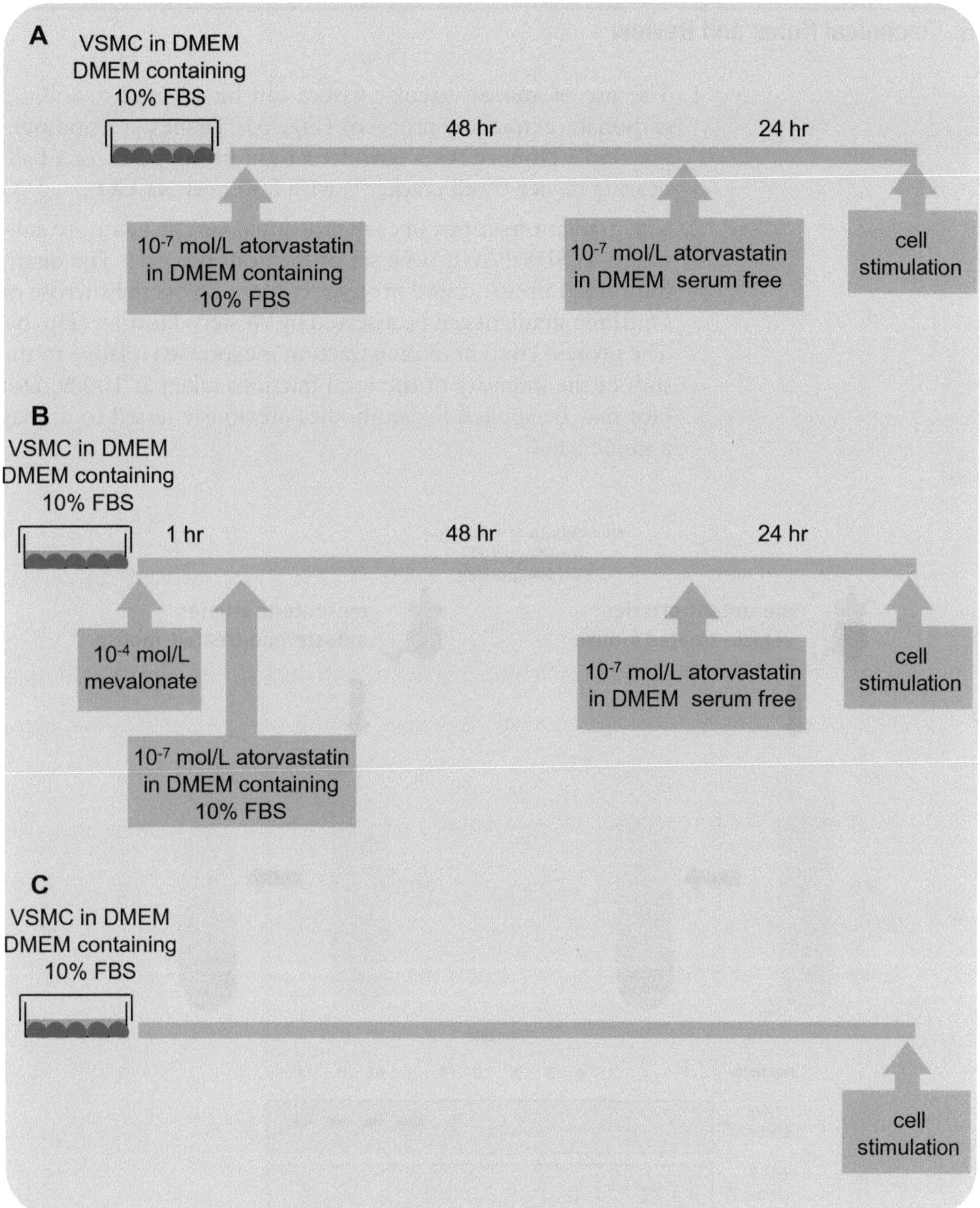

Fig. 4 Cell protocol for cholesterol biosynthetic pathway inhibition with atorvastatin. (**a**) Experimental group 1 for cholesterol synthesis inhibition with atorvastatin: cells are incubated with 10^{-7} mol/L atorvastatin in DMEM containing 10 % FBS for 48 h, at 37 °C; cell medium is replaced with DMEM serum free and cells are incubated with 10^{-7} mol/L atorvastatin for an additional 24 h. (**b**) Experimental group 2 for mevalonate supplementation: cells are incubated with 10^{-4} mol/L mevalonate in DMEM 10 % FBS 1 h prior to atorvastatin treatment; cells are incubated with 10^{-7} mol/L atorvastatin which is added to DMEM containing 10 % FBS supplemented with mevalonate for 48 h at 37 °C; cell medium is replaced with DMEM serum free and cells are incubated with 10^{-7} mol/L atorvastatin plus 10^{-4} mol/L mevalonate for an additional 24 h. (**c**) Experimental group 3 is the control without cholesterol synthesis inhibition

5 Technical Notes and Review

1. The use of animal vascular tissues can be adapted to sodium carbonate extraction protocol (Fig. 5). Tissues are homogenized in a Dounce tissue grinder a tight fitting pestle or a ball-bearing device ("cell cracker") with 500 mM Na_2CO_3.
2. The gradient fractions of each individual sample lysate are subjected to SDS-PAGE (one set of fractions per gel). The distribution of raft-associated proteins content across the sucrose or OptiPrep gradient can be assessed by Western blotting (Fig. 6). The protein content in each fraction is expressed relative to the sum of the intensity of the total fractions taken as 100 %. Dot blot may be applied for antibodies previously tested to display a single band.

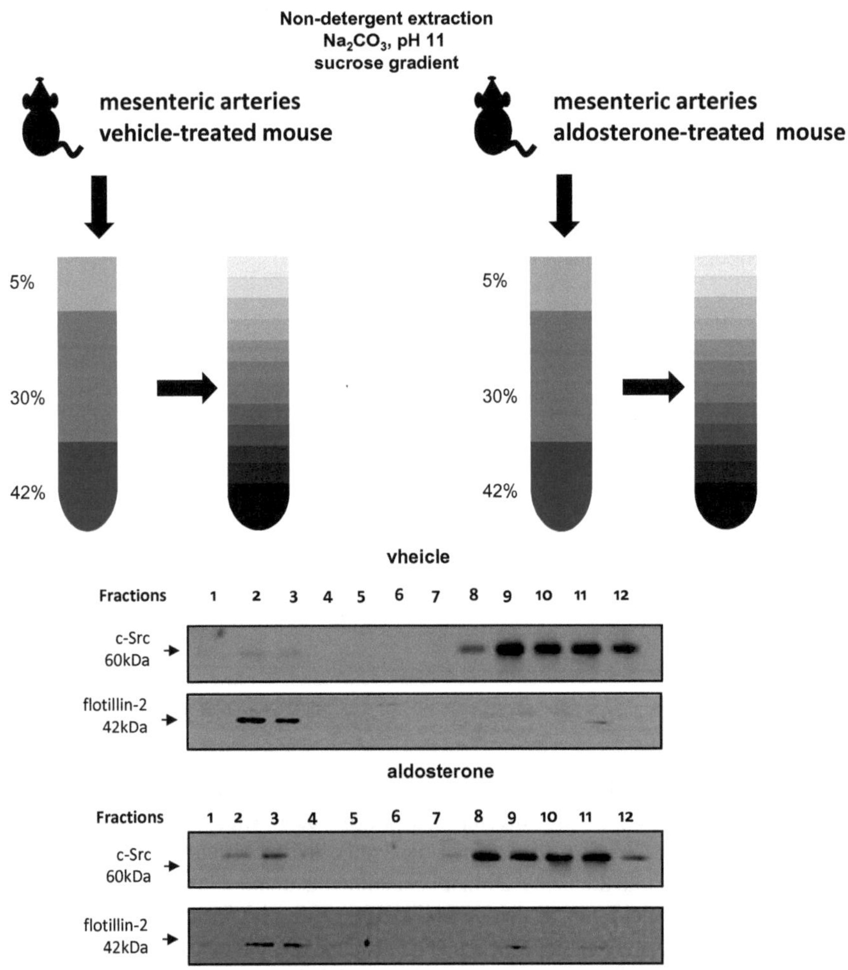

Fig. 5 Effect of in vivo aldosterone infusion on c-Src content in raft fractions from mesenteric arteries. Representative immunoblots of c-Src and flotillin-2 content of sucrose gradient fractions of mesenteric arteries from mice infused with aldosterone or vehicle

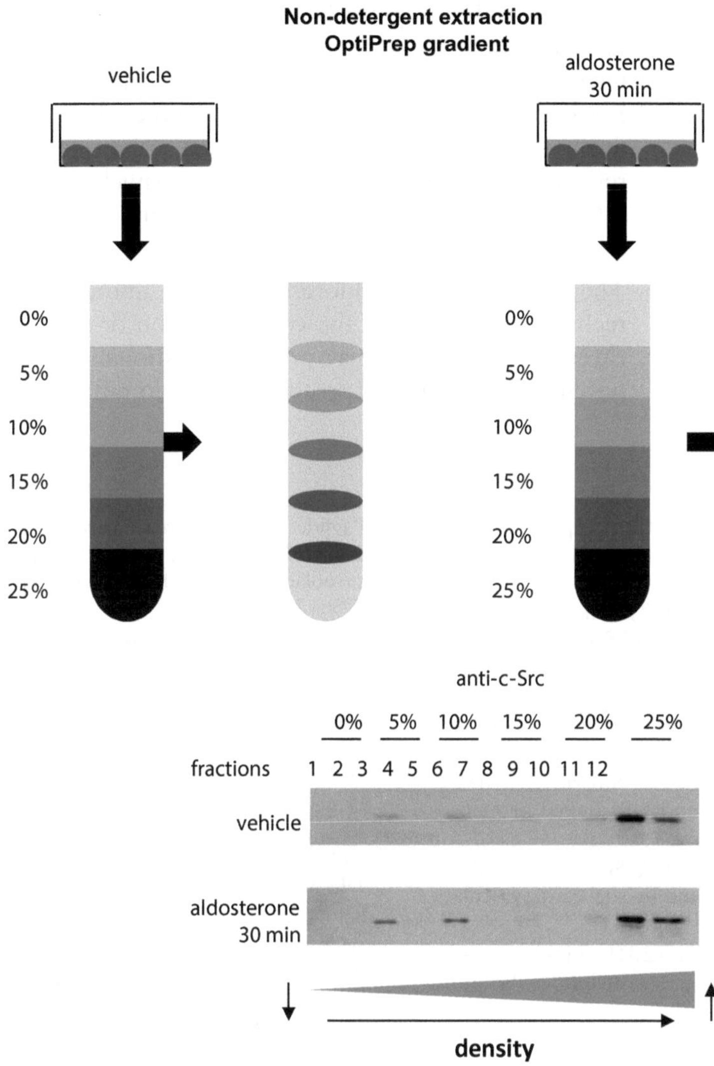

Fig. 6 Effect of aldosterone stimulation on c-Src content in the low density cholesterol-enriched fractions of VSMC membrane (OptiPrep method)

3. Monitoring the level of cholesterol present in sucrose fractions obtained from either method confirms that cholesterol-enriched membrane domains are present or absent within given fractions.
4. Due to the structural diversity of caveolae and lipid rafts, it is difficult to establish differential markers for these domains. However, raft-associated proteins are used as markers during biochemical fractionation procedures designed to identify the fractions containing these plasma membrane domains. Peripheral

proteins, such as annexin II or transmembrane proteins, such as flotillin-2 are used to identify raft fractions. Markers for intracellular membranes or the non-raft plasma membrane markers are however supposed to be excluded from the raft fractions: transferrin receptor (non-raft membranes), calnexin (endoplasmic reticulum membrane), nucleoporin (nuclear membrane), β-COP (Golgi marker), and voltage-dependent anion channels (VDAC, mitochondrial membrane).

5. The use of immunofluorescence and immunoprecipitation techniques to evaluate the co-localization or interaction with caveolin or flotilin-2 may provide additional support for the potential association of proteins with lipid rafts.

References

1. Simons K, Toomre D (2000) Lipid rafts and signal transduction. Nat Rev Mol Cell Biol 1:31–39
2. Simons K, Ikonen E (1997) Functional rafts in cell membranes. Nature 387:569–572
3. Allen JA, Halverson-Tamboli RA, Rasenick MM (2007) Lipid raft microdomains and neurotransmitter signalling. Nat Rev Neurosci 8:128–140
4. Reeves VL, Thomas CM, Smart EJ (2012) Lipid rafts, caveolae and GPI-linked proteins. Adv Exp Med Biol 729:3–13
5. Gratton JP, Bernatchez P, Sessa WC (2004) Caveolae and caveolins in the cardiovascular system. Circ Res 94:1408–1417
6. Lingwood D, Simons K (2010) Lipid rafts as a membrane-organizing principle. Science 327:46–50
7. Pike LJ (2003) Lipid rafts: bringing order to chaos. J Lipid Res 44:655–667
8. Thomas CM, Smart EJ (2008) Caveolae structure and function. J Cell Mol Med 12:796–809
9. Pike LJ (2009) The challenge of lipid rafts. J Lipid Res 50:S323–S328
10. Insel PA, Patel HH (2009) Membrane rafts and caveolae in cardiovascular signaling. Curr Opin Nephrol Hypertens 18:50–56
11. Chidlow JH Jr, Sessa WC (2010) Caveolae, caveolins, and cavins: complex control of cellular signalling and inflammation. Cardiovasc Res 86:219–225
12. Williams TM, Lisanti MP (2004) The Caveolin genes: from cell biology to medicine. Ann Med 36:584–595
13. Li XA, Everson WV, Smart EJ (2005) Caveolae, lipid rafts, and vascular disease. Trends Cardiovasc Med 15:92–96
14. Pavlides S, Gutierrez-Pajares JL, Danilo C, Lisanti MP, Frank PG (2012) Atherosclerosis, caveolae and caveolin-1. Adv Exp Med Biol 729:127–144
15. Callera GE, Montezano AC, Yogi A, Tostes RC, Touyz RM (2007) Vascular signaling through cholesterol-rich domains: implications in hypertension. Curr Opin Nephrol Hypertens 16:90–104
16. Smart EJ, Graf GA, McNiven MA, Sessa WC, Engelman JA, Scherer PE, Okamoto T, Lisanti MP (1999) Caveolins, liquid-ordered domains, and signal transduction. Mol Cell Biol 19:7289–7304
17. Schuck S, Honsho M, Ekroos K, Shevchenko A, Simons K (2003) Resistance of cell membranes to different detergents. Proc Natl Acad Sci U S A 100:5795–5800
18. Lucero HA, Robbins PW (2004) Lipid rafts-protein association and the regulation of protein activity. Arch Biochem Biophys 426:208–324
19. Simons K, Gerl MJ (2010) Revitalizing membrane rafts: new tools and insights. Nat Rev Mol Cell Biol 11:688–699
20. Patel HH, Insel PA (2009) Lipid rafts and caveolae and their role in compartmentation of redox signaling. Antioxid Redox Signal 11:1357–1372
21. Song KS, Li S, Okamoto T (1996) Co-purification and direct interaction of Ras with caveolin, an integral membrane protein of caveolae microdomains. J Biol Chem 271:9690–9697
22. Smart EJ, Ying YS, Mineo C, Anderson RG (1995) A detergent-free method for purifying caveolae membrane from tissue culture cells. Proc Natl Acad Sci U S A 92: 10104–10108

23. Macdonald JL, Pike LJ (2005) A simplified method for the preparation of detergent-free lipid rafts. J Lipid Res 46:1061–1067
24. Callera GE, Yogi A, Briones AM, Montezano AC, He Y, Tostes RC, Schiffrin EL, Touyz RM (2011) Vascular proinflammatory responses by aldosterone are mediated via c-Src trafficking to cholesterol-rich microdomains: role of PDGFR. Cardiovasc Res 91:720–731

Chapter 21

Isolation and Characterization of Circulating Microparticles by Flow Cytometry

Dylan Burger and Paul Oleynik

Abstract

Microparticles are small fragments (0.1–1.0 μm) of cellular membrane which are shed by cells under conditions of stress. As levels of circulating microparticles are elevated in disease, there has been significant interest in their assessment and quantification under pathological conditions. Here we describe a protocol for the isolation of microparticles from plasma samples and their characterization/quantification by flow cytometry. This assay has been employed for the assessment of microparticle levels in both human and animal plasma and may also be modified for the characterization of microparticles from culture media or from other biological samples (i.e., urine).

Key words Microparticle, Microvesicle, Ectosome, Biomarker, Flow cytometry, Membrane, Plasma

1 Introduction

Microparticles, also referred to as ectosomes or microvesicles, are submicron (0.1–1.0 μm) membrane fragments which are formed through exocytic blebbing of the plasma membrane under conditions of cell stress or injury [1, 2]. They are physically and functionally distinct from larger (>1 μm) apoptotic bodies which are formed exclusively during late-stage apoptosis [3] and from the smaller (40–100 nm) exosomes which are constitutively secreted [2–4]. Microparticles may be further characterized by the externalization of phosphatidylserine, and the presence of surface antigens from their cell of origin. Originally identified as "platelet dust" [5], microparticles (platelet, leukocyte, erythrocyte, or endothelial origin) may be found in plasma samples and are increased in multiple diseases including hypertension, diabetes, and chronic kidney disease [1]. Accordingly, microparticles have garnered significant attention as biomarkers of vascular and nonvascular pathologies. Such clinical utility is underscored by the observations that microparticle levels reflect vascular health/function and that increases in circulating microparticle populations predict future cardiovascular risk [6–8].

Rhian M. Touyz and Ernesto L. Schiffrin (eds.), *Hypertension: Methods and Protocols*, Methods in Molecular Biology, vol. 1527, DOI 10.1007/978-1-4939-6625-7_21, © Springer Science+Business Media LLC 2017

Despite the pervasiveness of microparticle research, a major impediment to the field has been the vast array of methodologies employed for both handling and quantification of circulating microparticles [9]. A number of methodologies have been utilized for the assessment/quantification of microparticles including immunoassays, flow cytometry, electron microscopy, atomic force microscopy, and dynamic light scattering [10]. Amongst the various approaches, flow cytometry is most widely employed for quantification due to its relative simplicity and the widespread availability of equipment. At present, no standardized approach exists for handling and quantification of microparticles although efforts to establish such a standard are underway [11].

Our laboratory has established and regularly employs a flow cytometry-based approach for the enumeration of endothelial and Annexin V-positive microparticles in plasma samples and culture media [12, 13]. This approach involves the separation of microparticles from other extracellular vesicles by differential centrifugation (outlined in Subheading 3.1), labeling of cell-specific surface antigens using fluorescently conjugated antibodies (Subheading 3.2), and finally enumeration and characterization by flow cytometry (Subheading 3.3).

2 Materials

2.1 Instruments

1. Low speed centrifuge: Beckman Coulter Allegra 6R equipped with GH-3.8A swing bucket rotor (Beckman Coulter).
2. High speed centrifuge: Sorvall RC6 Plus, equipped with F-20/micro rotor (Thermo Scientific).
3. MoFlo XDP High Speed Cell Sorter and Flow Cytometer equipped with appropriate lasers (i.e., 488 nm, 640 nm) and Summit software (Beckman Coulter).
4. Thermo Forma −86 °C ULT freezer (Thermo Scientific, *optional*).
5. IsoTemp 210 Water Bath (Fisher Scientific, *optional*).
6. LabQuake Tube Rotator (Thermo Scientific).

2.2 Reagents

1. Heparin-coated Vacutainer—13 × 100 mm (Becton Dickinson, *see* **Note 1**).
2. 21 G needle (Becton Dickinson, *see* **Note 2**).
3. 15 ml polypropylene tube (Becton Dickinson).
4. 1.5 ml microcentrifuge tubes (Fisher Scientific, *see* **Note 3**).
5. Annexin V Binding Buffer (*see* **Note 4**).
6. Fluorescent-conjugated Annexin V (*see* **Note 5**).
7. Fluorescent-conjugated antibodies (*see* Table 1, **Notes 5** and **6**).

Table 1
Surface markers/antigens used for the detection of circulating microparticles

Origin/phenotype of microparticles		Antigen/marker	Reference(s)
Nonspecific	Externalized phosphatidylserine	**Annexin V**	[12–15]
Nonspecific	Cell incorporating dyes	CFSE, calcein	[13, 16]
Platelets		CD41, CD42a	[17–19]
Erythrocytes		CD235a	[19, 20]
Leukocytes		**CD45**, CD11a	[15, 18, 20]
	Neutrophil	CD66b	[19, 21]
	Monocytes	CD14	[15, 19, 22, 23]
	T-cell lymphocytes	CD3	[19, 23]
	Helper T-cell lymphocyte	CD4	[20, 24]
	Cytotoxic T-cell lymphocyte	CD8	[24]
	B lymphocyte	CD19	[19, 23]
Endothelial cells		**CD144**, CD31, CD54, CD106, CD105, CD34, CD62E	[13, 15, 18, 19]
Multiple origins	Tissue factor	CD142	[15]

Antigens validated and employed by our laboratory are *bolded*

8. 5 ml polypropylene round bottom tubes—12 × 75 mm (Becton Dickinson).
9. 1 μm polystyrene microspheres for size calibration (Molecular Probes, *optional*—*see* **Note 7**).
10. Ethylenediaminetetraacetic acid (EDTA, Sigma-Aldrich, *optional*).

3 Methods

The assessment of microparticles first involves separation from other classes of extracellular vesicles. Microparticles are isolated from plasma, or other biological samples, by differential centrifugation, and resuspended in a labeling medium. Microparticles are then fluorescently labeled based on surface characteristics and assessed by flow cytometry. An initial low-speed centrifugation removes cells and large particles (including platelets) from suspension while microparticles remain suspended. It is critical that this spin be performed rapidly to prevent artificial platelet activation and subsequent formation of platelet-derived microparticles. This step is particularly critical should samples be frozen for future analysis. A subsequent high-speed centrifugation sediments microparticles, while exosomes and smaller vesicle populations remain in suspension. We utilize Beckman Coulter Allegra 6R and Sorvall RC6 centrifuges for low and high-speed centrifugation however any centrifuge capable of 1500 × *g* (low speed) and 20,000 × *g* (high speed) is sufficient. Once isolated, microparticles are labeled for externalized phosphatidylserine using Annexin V, and/or for cell-specific surface markers. Table 1 summarizes the most common markers used for the identification and quantification of circulating microparticles by flow cytometry.

3.1 Blood Collection and Processing for Analysis

3.1.1 Human Samples

1. Collect whole blood into a heparinized BD Vacutainer tube (13 × 100) by phlebotomy.
2. Immediately transfer the sample into a 15 ml polypropylene tube and centrifuge for 15 min (Allegra 6R) at room temperature and 1500 × *g* to a obtain platelet-poor plasma supernatant.
3. Transfer the microparticle-containing supernatant to a fresh 15 ml polypropylene tube being careful not to disturb the pellet. Discard the pellet which contains platelets, red blood cells, and large cell debris (i.e. apoptotic bodies).
4. Centrifuge the sample (Allegra 6R) a second time for 15 min at 4 °C and 1500 × *g* to obtain a platelet-free plasma supernatant. Discard the pellet.
5. Transfer a minimum of 200 μl aliquots of the microparticle-containing supernatant (platelet-free plasma) into 1.7 ml microcentrifuge tubes.
6. Snap freeze the platelet-free plasma in liquid nitrogen and store at −80 °C or continue with isolation of microparticles (*see* **Note 8**).

3.1.2 Mouse/Animal Samples

1. Collect blood by cardiac puncture into heparinized (17 U/ml) 1.7 ml microcentrifuge tubes.
2. Centrifuge the sample (RC6 Plus) for 15 min at room temperature and 1500 × *g*.
3. Transfer the microparticle-containing supernatant to a fresh microcentrifuge tube and discard the pellet.
4. Centrifuge the sample again (RC6 Plus) for 15 min at 4 °C and 1500 × *g*.
5. Transfer a minimum of 200 μl aliquots of the microparticle-containing supernatant (platelet-free plasma) to 1.7 ml microcentrifuge tubes.
6. Snap freeze the platelet-free plasma in liquid nitrogen and store at −80 °C or continue directly with the isolation of microparticles.

3.1.3 Preparation of Microparticles from Platelet-Free Plasma

1. Thaw (if frozen) samples rapidly in a 37 °C water bath. Remove samples from water bath immediately after thawing (*see* **Note 8**).
2. Centrifuge the samples (RC6 Plus) at 20,000 × *g* for 20 min at 4 °C to obtain microparticle-containing pellet, discard supernatant.
3. Resuspend microparticles in annexin V binding buffer by gentle rotation using a LabQuake tube rotator for at least 5 min at 4 °C.

3.2 Labeling of Microparticles

3.2.1 Labeling of Externalized Phosphatidylserine with Annexin V

1. Incubate microparticle-containing samples with fluorescence-conjugated annexin V (0.5 μg/ml) in annexin V binding buffer for 15 min at room temperature in the dark.
   (a) As Annexin V binds to phosphatidylserine in a Ca^{2+}-dependent manner, the appropriate negative control for determining autofluorescence is a population of microparticles incubated in Annexin V-binding buffer lacking $CaCl_2$. Alternatively microparticles incubated in Annexin V-binding buffer containing 25 mM EDTA which chelates Ca^{2+} may also be used.
2. Centrifuge the samples (RC6 plus) at 20,000 × *g* for 20 min at 4 °C, discard supernatant.
3. Resuspend samples in annexin V binding buffer (or Ca^{2+}-free buffer for negative controls) by gentle rotation using a LabQuake tube rotator for 5 min at 4 °C.

3.2.2 Labeling of Microparticles Using Antibodies for Surface Antigens

Note: this step may be performed in conjunction with annexin V surface labeling.

1. Incubate microparticle samples with the appropriate dilution of antibody for approximately 15 min in annexin V binding buffer (*see* **Note 6**).
   (a) The appropriate negative control for determining autofluorescence is a matched, fluorescence-conjugated isotype control incubated under the same conditions and at the same concentration as the chosen antibody.
2. Centrifuge the samples (RC6 Plus) at 20,000 × *g* for 20 min at 4 °C, discard supernatant.
3. Resuspend samples in 1× annexin V binding buffer by gentle rotation using a LabQuake tube rotator for 5 min at 4 °C.

3.3 Flow Cytometry

We utilize a MoFlo Legacy High Speed Cell Sorter (Beckman Coulter) equipped with Summit software version 4.3 for multicolor flow cytometry and analysis. However, several other cytometers (i.e., EPICS, LSRII, FC500) have also been employed successfully [10, 25].

1. Calibrate the cytometer using Flow-Check Fluorospheres (Beckman Coulter) for alignment of the 488 nm excitation laser and AlignFlow Plus flow cytometry alignment beads, 6 μm (Invitrogen) for alignment of the 640 nm excitation laser.
   (a) If using any other excitation lasers be sure to align them with an appropriate method before commencing any analysis.
2. Set side scatter (SSC) and desired fluorescence channels to logarithmic (Log) mode and forward scatter (FSC) to linear (Lin) mode.
3. Set the threshold level of event detection to just above the noise level in order to observe the smallest detectable particles.
4. Establish an upper size limit for identifying microparticles. This may be achieved by using a sample of standard 1 μm polystyrene microspheres plot SSC Log versus FSC Lin. Include all events with a FSC less than or equal to that of the 1 μm microspheres (Region 1 in Fig. 1a). As the lower limits of detection for cytometry is greater than 0.1 μm a lower size gate is unnecessary.
   (a) Note that the FSC generated by microspheres may not directly correlate with that generated by equivalently sized microparticles. Accordingly it is recommended that any FSC size gate be verified by sorting microparticles using the established gate and examining them by electron microscopy (Fig. 2, *see* also refs. 13, 26).
5. Exclude doublet events by including only singlets from a plot of FSC Lin versus Pulse Width (Region 2 in Fig. 1b).
6. Individual (i.e., single-labeled) populations may be plotted as SSC versus fluorescence (Fig. 1c), while double labeled populations should be plotted using double fluorescence plots (Fig. 1d). To be sure that only singlet microparticles of appropriate size (<1 μm) are analyzed for their fluorescence apply a gate of Region 1 + Region 2 onto each fluorescence plot.
7. Establish applicable detector voltages for each fluorescence signal by analyzing a representative unlabeled (autofluorescence) control while adjusting the voltage for each detector so that the autofluorescence signal lies in the first decade of signal detection.
8. Analyze isotype controls (for antibody-based microparticle labeling) or annexin V-samples labeled in Ca^{2+}-free buffer (for annexin V labeling) and draw positive regions to the right of the brightest isotype control signals.
9. Acquire labeled microparticle samples at a rate that does not exceed 10,000 events per second with the total acquired events typically being in the range of 1000–500,000. For analysis of

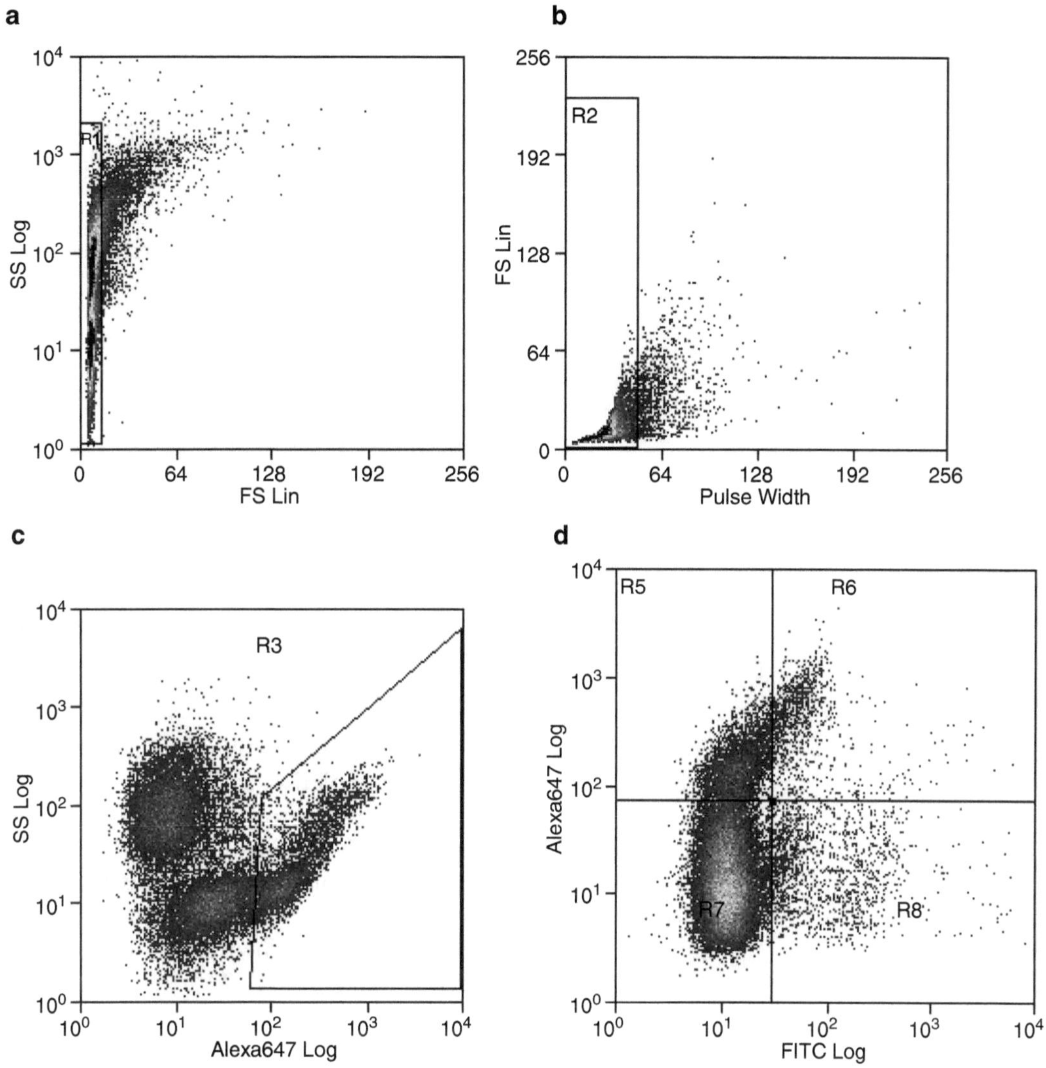

Fig. 1 Representative tracings of flow cytometric analysis of annexin V (Alexa 647) and CD144 (FITC)-labeled microparticles from mouse plasma samples. (**a**) SSC (log) versus FSC (lin) tracing with established size gate (R1). (**b**) FS (lin) versus pulse width to ensure non-doublet events (R2). (**c**) SS (log) versus Alexa 647 (log) for analyzing single-labeled Annexin V^{+ve} microparticles. (**d**) Alexa 647 (log) versus FITC (log) for analyzing Annexin V^{+ve}, $CD144^{+ve}$ endothelial microparticles

multiple-labeled MPs it is necessary to ensure that the fluorescence emission spectra of the fluorescence labels do not overlap. If they do overlap then compensation must be performed (*see* **Note 5**). For analysis of single-labeled MP populations this is not necessary.

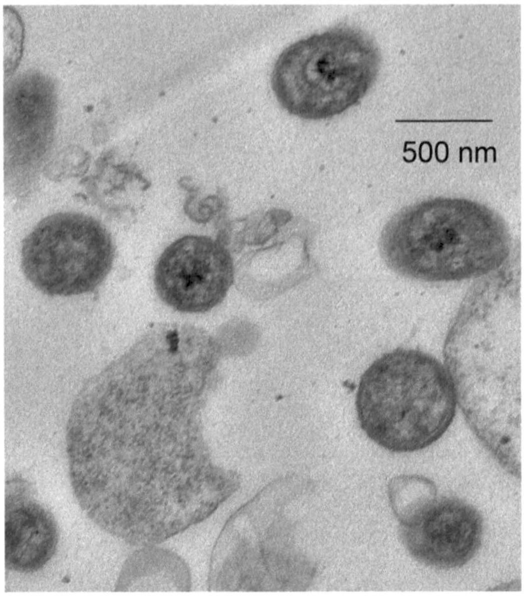

Fig. 2 Electron micrograph of sorted Annexin V positive microparticles using the gating strategy established in Fig. 1a/b

10. For quantification, run a standardized volume of labeled MPs (we typically use 200 μl) to completion and identify microparticles as those events which shift into a region of positivity. Calculate the number of positive events as a fraction of the volume analyzed (i.e., MPs/ml plasma). Alternatively, or for cytometers for which running a defined volume is not possible, fluorescent microbeads with a predefined concentration may be employed as a reference standard [17, 27].

4 Notes

1. We primarily use heparin (17 U/ml) as an anticoagulant. Alternatively sodium citrate (0.32%) has also successfully been employed.
2. It is important to ensure that a sufficiently large gauge needle be used so as to avoid artificial microparticle formation from platelets and erythrocytes in response to shear.
3. Certain brands of microcentrifuge tube may not be capable of handling higher speed centrifugation. Ensure that the centrifuge tubes chosen are rated for centrifugation at 20,000 × *g* or higher. We use Fisherbrand Premium microcentrifuge tubes which are rated up to 30,000 × *g*.

4. Annexin V binding buffer is often available as a component of commercially available annexin V labeling kits. Alternatively, such a buffer may be prepared as follows. For calcium-free annexin V binding buffer simply omit the addition of $CaCl_2$.

1× Annexin V Binding Buffer

Reagent	Final concentration (mM)	For 50 ml
HEPES (1 M, pH 7.4)	10	500 μl
NaCl	140	409 mg
$CaCl_2$	2.5	13.8 mg

5. The choice of fluorescent label(s) will depend on availability of conjugated antibodies as well as the fluorescence emission spectra, if using multiple labels. Avoid fluorescent labels with too similar of fluorescence emission spectra. For example, FITC or PE combined with APC or Alexa647 are good candidate pairs.
6. Antibodies should be titrated to ensure antibody labeling is done under saturating conditions. Similarly, the appropriate incubation time for antibody should be determined experimentally. In our experience, titrating antibody or setting compensation levels should be done with purified microparticle populations rather than the parent cells as the appropriate antibody dilutions can differ between microparticles and their parent cells.
7. When initially establishing a size gate it may be beneficial to analyze the FSC of a population of appropriately sized (~1 μm) microspheres. However, the scatter produced by a population of microspheres may not be equivalent to that produced by membrane microparticles. Accordingly it is recommended that any established size gate for microparticles be verified by subanalysis of sorted microparticles (i.e., electron microscopy or dynamic light scattering) to ensure that membrane vesicles of the desired size range (0.1–1.0 μm) are being identified.
8. Where possible, avoid freezing of microparticle-containing samples as long-term freezing has been reported to impact on microparticle levels, potentially through antigen degradation [28]. If freezing is required, rapid snap freezing of platelet-free plasma and storage at −80 °C is recommended. We have found that storage in this manner has little effect on measured microparticle levels for up to 1 year. When thawing microparticle samples, a rapid thaw at 37 °C is recommended, followed by placement at 4 °C. Avoid prolonged incubation at 37 °C which may also lead to antigen degradation.

Acknowledgments

D.B. is supported by a Kidney Research Scientist Core Education and National Training Program (KRESCENT) New Investigator Award.

References

1. Burger D et al (2013) Microparticles: biomarkers and beyond. Clin Sci 124(7):423–441
2. Boulanger CM (2010) Microparticles, vascular function and hypertension. Curr Opin Nephrol Hypertens 19(2):177–180
3. Gyorgy B et al (2011) Membrane vesicles, current state-of-the-art: emerging role of extracellular vesicles. Cell Mol Life Sci 68(16):2667–2688
4. Mathivanan S, Ji H, Simpson RJ (2010) Exosomes: extracellular organelles important in intercellular communication. J Proteomics 73(10):1907–1920
5. Wolf P (1967) The nature and significance of platelet products in human plasma. Br J Haematol 13(3):269–288
6. Sinning JM et al (2011) Circulating CD31+/Annexin V+ microparticles correlate with cardiovascular outcomes. Eur Heart J 32(16): 2034–2041
7. Amabile N et al (2005) Circulating endothelial microparticles are associated with vascular dysfunction in patients with end-stage renal failure. J Am Soc Nephrol 16(11):3381–3388
8. Amabile N et al (2012) Predictive value of circulating endothelial microparticles for cardiovascular mortality in end-stage renal failure: a pilot study. Nephrol Dial Transplant 27(5): 1873–1880
9. Jy W et al (2004) Measuring circulating cell-derived microparticles. J Thromb Haemost 2(10):1842–1843
10. Lacroix R et al (2010) Overcoming limitations of microparticle measurement by flow cytometry. Semin Thromb Hemost 36(8):807–818
11. Lacroix R et al (2012) Impact of pre-analytical parameters on the measurement of circulating microparticles: towards standardization of protocol. J Thromb Haemost 10(3):437–446
12. Burger D et al (2012) Microparticles induce cell cycle arrest through redox-sensitive processes in endothelial cells: implications in vascular senescence. J Am Heart Assoc 2012:e001842
13. Burger D et al (2011) Endothelial microparticle formation by angiotensin II is mediated via Ang II receptor type I/NADPH oxidase/Rho kinase pathways targeted to lipid rafts. Arterioscler Thromb Vasc Biol 31(8):1898–1907
14. Simak J, Holada K, Vostal JG (2002) Release of annexin V-binding membrane microparticles from cultured human umbilical vein endothelial cells after treatment with camptothecin. BMC Cell Biol 3:11
15. Flores-Nascimento MC et al (2009) Microparticles in deep venous thrombosis, antiphospholipid syndrome and Factor V Leiden. Platelets 20(6):367–375
16. Bernimoulin M et al (2009) Differential stimulation of monocytic cells results in distinct populations of microparticles. J Thromb Haemost 7(6):1019–1028
17. Robert S et al (2009) Standardization of platelet-derived microparticle counting using calibrated beads and a Cytomics FC500 routine flow cytometer: a first step towards multicenter studies? J Thromb Haemost 7(1):190–197
18. Chirinos JA et al (2005) Elevation of endothelial microparticles, platelets, and leukocyte activation in patients with venous thromboembolism. J Am Coll Cardiol 45(9):1467–1471
19. Guiducci S et al (2008) The relationship between plasma microparticles and disease manifestations in patients with systemic sclerosis. Arthritis Rheum 58(9):2845–2853
20. Rautou PE et al (2012) Abnormal plasma microparticles impair vasoconstrictor responses in patients with cirrhosis. Gastroenterology 143(1):166–176, e6
21. Gasser O et al (2003) Characterisation and properties of ectosomes released by human polymorphonuclear neutrophils. Exp Cell Res 285(2):243–257
22. Jayachandran M et al (2008) Characterization of blood borne microparticles as markers of premature coronary calcification in newly menopausal women. Am J Physiol Heart Circ Physiol 295(3):H931–H938
23. Baka Z et al (2010) Increased serum concentration of immune cell derived microparticles in polymyositis/dermatomyositis. Immunol Lett 128(2):124–130
24. Kornek M et al (2011) Human T cell microparticles circulate in blood of hepatitis patients and induce fibrolytic activation of hepatic stellate cells. Hepatology 53(1):230–242

25. Lacroix R et al (2010) Standardization of platelet-derived microparticle enumeration by flow cytometry with calibrated beads: results of the International Society on Thrombosis and Haemostasis SSC Collaborative workshop. J Thromb Haemost 8(11):2571–2574
26. Eyre J et al (2011) Monocyte- and endothelial-derived microparticles induce an inflammatory phenotype in human podocytes. Nephron Exp Nephrol 119(3):e58–e66
27. Pattanapanyasat K et al (2004) Flow cytometric quantitation of red blood cell vesicles in thalassemia. Cytometry B Clin Cytom 57B(1):23–31
28. Shah MD et al (2008) Flow cytometric measurement of microparticles: pitfalls and protocol modifications. Platelets 19(5):365–372

Chapter 22

Isolation of Mature Adipocytes from White Adipose Tissue and Gene Expression Studies by Real-Time Quantitative RT-PCR

Aurelie Nguyen Dinh Cat and Ana M. Briones

Abstract

The study of adipose tissue and more specifically of adipocytes is considered pivotal for dissecting molecular mechanisms responsible for alterations in several organs and systems, including adipose tissue, not only in obesity but also in other diseases (hypertension, heart failure). Adipose tissue is a complex tissue composed of adipocytes and the stromal vascular fraction which includes a heterogeneous population of preadipocytes, blood cells, endothelial cells, and macrophages. In the present chapter, methods are detailed to generate purified mature adipocytes from white adipose tissue by using enzymatic digestion. Such methods should help laboratories to study the specific roles of adipocytes in different pathologies and are easily adaptable to different animal models. Moreover, as gene activity is controlled at both transcriptional and posttranscriptional levels, it is very important to determine the levels of messenger ribonucleic acid (mRNA) of genes of interest. This process involves the isolation of total RNA and subsequent analysis of the mRNA of interest by real-time quantitative reverse transcription polymerase chain reaction (qRT-PCR). Given the unique nature of adipose tissue and adipocytes (i.e., containing high amounts of lipid), we have set up a special RNA isolation technique in both white adipose tissue and isolated mature adipocytes from mice. In summary, isolation and culture of adipocytes in vivo and gene expression studies will help to understand the mechanisms that control adipocyte function in physiological and pathological states and may lead to design interventions that might affect the adipocyte birth-death balance or phenotype.

Key words White adipose tissue, Mature adipocytes isolation, Total RNA, qRT-PCR

1 Introduction

Adipocytes are now recognized as metabolically active endocrine/paracrine/autocrine cells that synthesize, store and secrete a wide spectrum of hormones, regulatory cytokines and vasoactive factors that play crucial roles in regulating cell turnover and function, not only locally within the adipose tissue but also in adjacent blood vessels and other key metabolic organ systems [1–4].

To characterize adipocytes function under normal and pathophysiological conditions, a huge variety of culturing techniques, mostly based on enzymatic digestion, can be used [5–9]. However,

Rhian M. Touyz and Ernesto L. Schiffrin (eds.), *Hypertension*: Methods and Protocols, Methods in Molecular Biology, vol. 1527, DOI 10.1007/978-1-4939-6625-7_22, © Springer Science+Business Media LLC 2017

significant variability might exist between adipocyte isolation and cell culture methods depending on the adipose tissue depot or the species used. A number of clonal preadipocyte cell lines of rodent origin have been available for more than 20 years, and have provided extremely important information about the study of the mechanisms involved particularly in adipocyte differentiation [10, 11]. However, in a primary culture system, cells maintain the physiological characteristics of the donor animals and are a useful model for studying the biological functions of the tissues. We should always be aware of both the metabolic and physiologic differences between various cell types (cell lines vs. primary culture) used in experiments. Therefore, depending of the specific questions concerning adipocyte function it might be necessary to use specific cell culture models [11]. In fact, throughout the years the different experimental models of fat cells have provided priceless information about its role in hormone actions, metabolic processes and formation of new fat cells and this has been exhaustively reviewed recently [12]. In the present communication, we provide a simple method which with minor modifications will allow for the isolation of purified cultures of mature adipocytes from different fat tissues.

Long or short-term adaptations to hormonal, nutritional, and other diverse factors take place throughout the life of the adipocyte and can affect either cell survival or the production of adipocyte secretory proteins. The mechanisms underlying these metabolic alterations may involve pretranscriptional or posttranscriptional events that change the amount or the activity of the protein. Therefore, the study of gene expression patterns of these factors in adipocytes and/or white adipose tissue (WAT) under basal and pathological conditions has grown in significance during the past decade.

As its name implies, real-time quantitative RT-PCR involves two major steps: RT and real-time PCR. Similar to other mRNA detection methods, the success of qRT-PCR relies primarily on the quality (i.e., purity) of total RNA [13], without any contamination of genomic DNA. Here, because of the unique nature of white adipose tissue and adipocytes (i.e., extremely high lipid content), we describe an in-house developed protocol that makes use of conventional RNA extraction reagents and isolation protocols, which has given us consistently high purity and quantity total RNA.

For real-time PCR, we describe dye-based (i.e., SYBR Green I dye) PCR protocols. The major advantage of the dye-based method is the reduced cost, especially when running multiple assays for multiple mRNAs, because no probes are required. However, the main disadvantage is that it may generate false-positive signals because the dye binds to any double-stranded DNA (i.e., both the target and nonspecific sequences).

Absolute or relative quantitation can be used. The absolute quantitation assay is used to determine the absolute amount of the target mRNA by interpolating its quantity from a standard curve. However, the absolute quantities of the standards must first be known by independent means. In contrast, the relative quantitation will analyze changes in gene expression in a given sample relative to a reference sample (e.g., an untreated control sample). Given that it is often unnecessary to know the absolute amount of a target mRNA, relative quantitation assays are preferred and described here.

There are two calculation methods used for relative quantitation: standard curve and comparative C_T (threshold cycle number). Although these two methods give equivalent results, we have routinely used the standard curve method because it requires the least amount of optimization and validation. We run the target and reference (i.e., housekeeping gene) amplifications in separate wells using their respective standard curves for the following two reasons: (1) to use the comparative C_T method, a validation experiment must be performed to show that the efficiencies of the target and reference amplifications are more or less equal; (2) to amplify the target and reference genes in the same tube, limiting primer concentrations must be identified and shown not to affect C_T values. However, we need to construct a standard curve for every assay to use the standard curve method, and this can increase the potential adverse effect of any dilution errors.

2 Materials

2.1 Adipocytes Isolation

1. Krebs-Ringer bicarbonate HEPES buffer.

   Composition: 125 mM NaCl, 4.8 mM KCl, 0.5 mM NaH_2PO_4, 1.2 mM $MgSO_4$, 2.6 mM $CaCl_2$, 25 mM Hepes, 2 mM $NaHCO_3$, 5.5 mM glucose, 1% BSA. Weight 1.46 g NaCl, 0.07 g KCl, 0.012 g NaH_2PO_4, 0.058 g $MgSO_4$, 0.0764 g $CaCl_2$, 1.19 g Hepes (*see* **Note 1**) in a final volume of 200 mL ultrapure water. Add 0.0336 g $NaHCO_3$, 0.198 g glucose, and 2 g BSA.

2. DMEM/F12 medium.

   Dulbecco's modified Eagle's medium (DMEM)/Ham's F12 (F12) and antibiotics (100,000 units/L penicillin, 100 mg/L streptomycin). Both DMEM and nutrient mixture F12 are prepared following manufacturer's instructions and mixed (50:50 v:v). The pH is adjusted to 7.4 and the medium is sterilized by filtration.

3. α-MEM/F12 medium.

   Composition : α-Minimum Essential Medium (α-MEM) and DMEM/F12, 15 mM HEPES, 17 nM insulin, 1% FBS and antibiotics (100,000 units/L penicillin, 100 mg/L streptomycin). Prepare mediums following manufacturer's instructions and mix at equal parts. For 1 L, add: 3.75 g HEPES, 10 μL insulin (stock 1.75 mM, *see* **Note 2**), 10 mL FBS, and antibiotics. The pH is adjusted to 7.4 and the medium is sterilized by filtration.

2.2 Total RNA Isolation and Purification

4. Precellys 24 Lysing kit (sterile tubes with small beads, Bertin Technologies).
5. Precellys 24 lysis and homogenization machine (Bertin Technologies).
6. TRIzol® Reagent (Invitrogen) for WAT and isolated mature adipocytes.
7. Chloroform.
8. 100 % isopropanol.
9. 70 % ethanol (in RNase-free water).
10. DNase I kit (supplied with RNase-free DNase Set; Ambion). Store at −20 °C (*see* **Note 3**).

2.3 Reverse Transcription

11. High Capacity cDNA Reverse Transcription Kit (Applied Biosystems).
12. Sterile 96 PCR well-plates.
13. Thermal cycler.

2.4 Real-Time PCR

14. Fast SYBR Green PCR reaction master mix: PCR Master Mix (2×; Applied Biosystems).
15. PCR primers designed with Primer3 software or other similar software.
16. Real-time PCR plate and cover: Thermo-Fast 384 barcoded PCR well-plates (Thermo Scientific), and Optical clear adhesive seal sheets (Thermo Scientific). Other similar instrument is also suitable.
17. Real-time PCR machine: ABI PRISM 7900HT Sequence Detection System (Applied Biosystems). Other similar instrument is also suitable.

3 Methods

3.1 Adipocytes Isolation

1. Visceral adipose tissue situated on the abdominal cavity will be removed and washed with Krebs Ringer bicarbonate buffer (KRBH) without BSA and glucose and with 100 U/mL penicillin and 100 mg/mL streptomycin. After washing, the adipose tissue will be placed in a falcon tube containing around 10–15 mL of medium DMEM/F12 (*see* **Note 4**).

2. Clean the adipose tissue of fibrous material and visible blood vessels under the dissecting microscope.
3. Weight the adipose tissue (*see* **Note 5**) and put the adipose tissue in a clean sterile petri dish. In the laminar flow hood, add clean sterile DMEM/F12 medium to the adipose tissue. The volume of medium added will depend on the weight of the adipose tissue. In general, add the same amount of mL than the adipose tissue weight in grams. For example, if adipose tissue weights 0.5 g, add 0.5 mL of medium (*see* **Note 6**).
4. Mince the adipose tissue into very small pieces using sterile scissors and thumb forceps. The smallest the pieces, the more efficient the enzymatic digestion will be.
5. Dissolve collagenase type I in Krebs-Ringer HEPES Buffer containing 1 % BSA. The final concentration in the solution containing adipose tissue plus collagenase should be 1 mg/mL. Add the same volume of collagenase solution than the volume of medium added in **step 3**. For example, if we have previously added 500 μL of medium, we should now add 500 μL of collagenase solution (*see* **Note** 7). Take all the small pieces of adipose tissue from the dish and put them in a falcon tube.
6. Digest the adipose tissue at 37 °C for 20–30 min with gentle shaking. Keep constant checking of the solution. Digestion should be finished when most of the adipose tissue pieces are broken without apparent cell death (recognized by big amounts of oil in the solution) (*see* **Notes 8** and **9**).
7. After digestion, the digested tissue suspension will be filtered with a sterile 200 μm filter mesh on a 50 mL falcon tube. Add 5–10 mL of medium DMEM/F12 to wash the filter (*see* **Note 10**).
8. Centrifuge the solution at 50 × *g* during 5 min (*see* **Note 11**).
9. Carefully take the mature adipocytes (*white ring*) from the upper part of the solution and transfer to a clean tube. Add 5 mL of medium DMEM/F12 to wash the adipocytes and centrifuge again at 50 × *g* during 5 min. Repeat this step one more time.
10. Carefully take the mature adipocytes and put it in a 24-wells plate containing 500 μL of medium α-MEM/F12 plus Insulin plus FBS (*see* **Note 12**). Incubate at 37 °C for 24 h (*see* **Note 13**).
11. The next day, collect the medium for any concentration measurements in a separate tube and take the adipocytes and put them in a microcentrifuge tube containing 250 μL of TRIzol® Reagent (for RNA extraction) (*see* **Note 14**). Freeze at −80 °C.

For WAT, add up to 300 mg of mouse WAT to 750 μL of TRIzol® Reagent in Precellys 24 Lysing kit.

3.2 Total RNA Isolation and Purification from WAT and Mature Adipocytes

12. Homogenize the WAT with Precells-Lysis at medium speed for 15 s two times. For the mature adipocytes, mix them thoroughly by pipetting up and down, and incubate for 2 min at room temperature to allow complete dissociation of nucleoprotein complexes.
13. Add 200 μL of chloroform, and cap the tubes tightly. Shake tubes vigorously by hand for 15 s. Do not vortex. Incubate at room temperature for 2 min (until separation of the phases).
14. Centrifuge at 12,000 × *g* for 15 min at 4 °C. After centrifugation, we can distinct three different phases (*see* **Note 15**): a lower, red phenol–chloroform phase, interphase, and the colorless upper aqueous phase. RNA remains exclusively in the aqueous phase, whereas DNA and proteins are in the interphase and organic phase, respectively. The volume of the aqueous phase is about 60% of the volume of TRIzol Reagent used for homogenization. Transfer the upper aqueous phase that contains RNA into a new tube.
15. Add an equal volume of 100% isopropanol (500 μL) to the aqueous phase (step of nucleic acids precipitation). Incubate at room temperature for 10 min. Then, centrifuge at 12,000 × *g* for 10 min at 4 °C. A light pale pellet should be formed in the tube. Discard the supernatant with a pipette.
16. Add an equal volume of 70% ethanol (500 μL) to the pellet (wash). Centrifuge at 7500 × *g* for 5 min at 4 °C. Discard the supernatant without throwing away the pellet that can de-attach easily.
17. Dry the pellet at 37 °C (tubes opened, heating block) for 5 min.
18. Resuspend the pellet with a certain volume of RNase-free water (depending of the size of the pellet, generally 20–30 μL). Leave for 1 h on ice.
19. Denaturate at 65 °C for 5 min.
20. Dilute the total RNA by 250 (2 μL in 500 μL RNase-free water). The concentrations of total RNA are assessed by UV absorbance spectrophotometry at 260 nm. Standard agarose gel electrophoresis is also performed to check the quality and integrity (any degradation) of total RNA (*see* **Note 16**).
21. Prepare up to 5 and 10 μg of total RNA (for the mature adipocytes and the WAT respectively) in a final volume of 20 μL for the DNase I treatment to remove genomic DNA. Add 2 μL of 10× DNase Buffer and 1 μL of DNase I and complete with RNase-free water (qsp 17 μL). The final concentration will be 0.25 μg/μL and 0.5 μg/μL for the mature adipocytes and the WAT, respectively.
22. Incubate at 37 °C for 1 h. Stop reaction by incubating at 70 °C for 10 min.

23. For short-term storage, RNA can be stored at −20 °C; for long-term storage, it should be stored at −80 °C.

3.3 Reverse Transcription (RT)

The High Capacity cDNA Reverse Transcription Kit contains all components necessary for the quantitative conversion of up to 2 μg of total RNA to single stranded cDNA.

24. Prepare 2× RT Master Mix (for 1 reaction) as follows:

RNase-free water	3.2 μL
10× RT buffer	2 μL
10× random primers (*see* **Note 17**)	2 μL
25× dNTP mix (100 mM)	0.8 μL
MultiScribe™ Reverse Transcriptase	1 μL
RNase Inhibitor	1 μL
DNase treated-RNA	10 μL

25. Prepare up to 2 μg of total RNA in 10 μL of RNase-free water in a sterile 96 well-plate, and add 10 μL of 2× RT master mix (final reaction volume: 20 μL). Mix gently and spin the plate briefly.
26. Place the plate in a thermal cycler and run RT reactions with the following program (based on the manufacturer's instructions): 10 min at 25 °C, 2 h at 37 °C, and 5 min at 85 °C. After retro-transcription, transfer the content of each well in individual new tubes and store RT (cDNA) at −20 °C.

3.4 Real-Time PCR

27. Primers are used at 10 μM initial concentration (*see* **Note 17**). cDNA templates are diluted by 5 or 10 depending on the amount of material.
28. Set up negative controls: Two different negative controls should be prepared for each assay; one is no template control (RNase-free water), and the other is no reverse transcriptase control (−RT) (*see* **Note 18**). However, this last one is not necessary if the primers have been designed in order to be in two different exons.
29. Choose appropriate reference genes (*see* **Note 19**): Common reference genes, also known as housekeeping genes, include 18S rRNA, ubiquitin C (Ubc), hypoxanthine phosphoribosyltransferase (Hprt), and glyceraldehyde-3-phosphate (Gapdh).
30. Construct standard curves (*see* **Note 20**): Using a known starting concentration of template from one of a variety of sources, a dilution series is performed (arbitrary). The standard curve should consist of at least five dilutions in duplicate or triplicate.

31. Prepare PCR Master Mix (without cDNA templates). The following compositions are based on a 10-μL reaction volume per well in duplicate for 384-well plates. Assuming that 3 μL of RT products will be used per well, the total volume of PCR Master Mix for each sample will be 7 μL. For one tube, the following solutions are added per well, but a mix is prepared into a sterile 1.5 or 2.0 mL tube with everything, but the cDNA template:

Products	1 tube	Final concentration
Sterile ddH_2O	1.4	–
Fast SYBR Green PCR 10× Master mix	5 μL	2×
Primer forward (10 μM)	0.3 μL	300 nM
Primer reverse (10 μM)	0.3 μL	300 nM
cDNA template	3	

32. Cover with one Optical Adhesive Cover onto the plate. Mix gently by vortexing, and spin briefly. Keep on ice until the run on an ABI PRISM 7900HT Sequence Detection System (*see* **Note 21**).
33. At the end of PCR, select Analyze from the Analysis menu, and examine the semi-log view of the amplification plots. Then, adjust the default baseline setting to accommodate the earliest amplification plot, and select a threshold above the noise close to the baseline, but still in the linear region of the semi-log plot. Upon completion of the Analysis (*see* **Notes 22** and **23**), export data to Excel for further analysis.

4 Notes

1. A 10× Krebs-Ringer bicarbonate HEPES buffer can be prepared and stored at −20 °C. Weight: 14.6 g NaCl, 0.7 g KCl, 0.12 g NaH_2PO_4, 0.58 g $MgSO_4$, 0.764 g $CaCl_2$, 11.9 g Hepes in a final volume of 200 mL ultrapure water. Make 20–30 mL aliquots and freeze at −20 °C if desired. Take 10 mL of 10× solution and add 90 mL water. Supplement with 0.0168 g $NaHCO_3$ + 0.099 g glucose + 1 g BSA.
2. Prepare insulin stock at a concentration of 1.75 mM. Weight 10 mg/mL in 0.01 N HCl.
3. Mix by gently inverting the tube. Do not vortex, because DNase I is sensitive to physical denaturation.
4. Depending on the amount of adipose tissue the volume might change. This is just for the adipose tissue to be submerged in DMEM/F12 during transport until starting the adipocytes isolation.

5. For weighing, carefully dry against a tissue paper to remove the excess of medium within the tissue. This will avoid weight overestimation.
6. If there is a big amount of fat, it might be needed to add more medium to the tissue. Just remember the volume added to take it into account when adding collagenase in **step 5**.
7. This is a very important step. The collagenase solution should be freshly prepared and sterilized by filtration. Prepare the collagenase at 2 mg/mL: remember that there is some volume in contact with the adipose tissue already. If we add 500 μL of collagenase solution at a concentration of 2 mg/mL to the 500 μL of medium containing the adipose tissue, the final concentration of the solution will be 1 mg/mL.
8. It is better to stop the digestion before cell death occurs even if some small pieces still stay.
9. In some circumstances (particularly depending on the different adipose tissues), lower or higher concentrations of collagenase or some variations in digestion time might be needed. For example, if the enzymatic digestion takes too long, collagenase concentration can be increased. Conversely, if the enzymatic digestion takes too short or it is too aggressive, collagenase concentration should be decreased.
10. Depending on the amount of adipose tissue digested higher volumes of DMEM/F12 for washing might be needed in order to recover the biggest amount of adipocytes.
11. Do not stop the centrifugation with an aggressive break. Leave the rotor to stop by itself to prevent adipocytes rupture.
12. The amount of α-MEM/F12 and the plate will depend on the amount of adipocytes. This amount is appropriate for adipocytes obtained from adipose tissue (≈0.3–0.5 g) from one mouse. For big amounts of mature adipocytes the amount of plating medium should be increased.
13. Mature adipocytes might live longer in the incubator. It is recommended to check for cell death by evaluating visually oil presence in the cell culture.
14. The amount of TRIzol® Reagent will depend on the amount of adipocytes present in our cell culture. This amount is suitable for adipocytes obtained from adipose tissue (≈0.3–0.5 g) from one mouse. For big amounts of mature adipocytes the amount of TRIzol® Reagent should be increased.
15. After centrifugation, there should be three layers:
    (a) Top layer: solution containing RNA, which should be collected.
    (b) Middle layer: light pink color containing excess lipid, which should be discarded.

(c) Bottom layer: pellet containing extracellular membranes, polysaccharides, and high molecular weight DNA, which should be discarded.

However, in some cases, the aqueous phase containing the RNA and the pink color phase can be inverted when the amount of fat is high, and the phase that has to be collected will be the intermediate one.

16. The concentration of RNA is first estimated by UV absorption spectrophotometry. A relatively pure RNA sample should yield an optical density (O.D.) ratio of 1.80–2.0 at 260–280 nm. Samples diluted in water may give lower A260/280 O.D. ratios. Before gene expression analysis, RNA integrity should be checked by standard agarose gel electrophoresis. We routinely run 2 μL of total RNA on a 0.8 % agarose gel containing ethidium bromide. Intact total RNA will show two distinct and sharp bands representing 28S and 18S rRNA. The 28S rRNA band should be approximately twice as intense as the 18S rRNA band. This 2:1 ratio (28S:18S rRNA) is a good index of intact and non degraded RNA. Partially degraded RNA will have a smeared appearance, and will lack the sharp rRNA bands, or will have a lower 28S:18S rRNA ratio. Highly degraded RNA will appear as a very low molecular weight smear.
17. Although oligo-dT primers can also be used for RT, we recommend the use of random primers, because this will allow you the freedom of choosing whatever internal control you may wish to utilize in subsequent real-time PCR assays, including 18S rRNA and 28S rRNA as well as other housekeeping genes (e.g., Gapdh, Hprt, or Ubc). Based on our experience, the optimal concentration of primers for housekeeping genes and genes of your interest is 300 nM. When optimizing primers for SYBR Green I assays, it is crucial to analyze the melting curve data for each primer concentration pair to ensure a single homogenous product is being generated (for all the samples, one peak for one melting temperature (Tm)).
18. At least two negative controls (RNAse-free water and −RT) are used for quality control purposes. Ideally, signal amplification should not be observed in the RNase-free water wells, and when observed, C_T values should be at least five and preferably more than ten cycles from the C_T values of your least concentrated samples. RT serves as an indicator of genomic DNA contamination, and their C_T values should be at least five cycles more than those of your least concentrated samples.
19. Although using the same amount and quality of input RNA in each sample ensures that equivalent amounts of RNA are compared, it cannot compensate for variations in the efficiency of

reverse transcription, which is required to produce cDNA for subsequent PCR. Therefore, it is imperative that researchers normalize expression levels of genes of interest to that of a reference gene [14, 15]. This step can remove inaccuracies due to variations in reverse transcription efficiency because RNA of the reference gene is reverse transcribed along with that of the gene of interest. Housekeeping genes such as 18S rRNA, ubiquitin C (Ubc), hypoxanthine phosphoribosyl-transferase (Hprt), and glyceraldehyde-3-phosphate (Gapdh) have often been used as reference genes for normalization [16], with the assumption that the expression of these genes is constitutive and that a given treatment will not change their expression. However, this assumption must be validated empirically, as the expression of housekeeping genes can vary under certain conditions [17–19]. In any case, it is crucial to select a reference or even multiple reference genes whose expression has been empirically tested to be constant across all experimental conditions in your study.

20. Samples for constructing standard curves are chosen based on their anticipated levels of mRNA. Ideal samples should contain higher levels of the mRNA. If it is not possible to make a prediction, a small portion of cDNA from a few samples may be pooled, or cDNA from untreated control may be used. Alternatively, a separate RT reaction may be set up specifically for standard curves. The dilution series should encompass a large range of concentrations, ideally covering the expected levels of target in experimental samples. To accomplish this objective, a three- to tenfold dilution series over several orders of magnitude should be generated. For example, a typical serial dilution would consist of five points of a tenfold serial dilution, starting with 50–100 ng of cDNA per reaction.
21. PCRs are run with a standard program: incubation at 50 °C for 2 min, activation at 95 °C for 10 min, and 40 cycles of denaturation at 95 °C for 15 s and annealing/extension (detection) at 72 °C for 1 min. For SYBR Green I assays, a dissociation/melting curve should be run at the end of your amplification reaction. The purpose of the dissociation curve is to determine if anything other than the gene of interest is amplified in the PCR. Because SYBR green I will bind to any double-stranded DNA, nonspecific amplifications in your unknown wells will artificially increase fluorescence signal and make it impossible to accurately quantitate your sample. In addition, to facilitate post-PCR analyses, such as sequencing and restriction enzyme digestions, add a 5-min extension at 72 °C at the end of PCR program.
22. The slope and R squared (Rsq) values of the standard curve help determine the sensitivity and efficiency (E_{PCR}) of a given

assay. PCR cycles that generate a linear fit with a slope approximately −3.32 ($E_{PCR} = [1-10^{-(1/slope)}] \times 100$). PCR efficiency between 95 and 105 % are considered acceptable. The linearity is denoted by the Rsq value (correlation coefficient), which should be very close to 1 (>0.985). Another quality indicator of your assay is that there should be a difference of approximately 3.3 in C_T values between two standard curve points with a tenfold dilution.

23. Most PCR products will melt somewhere in the range of 80–90 °C, although this melting point can vary with the size and sequence of your specific target. Ideally, the experimental samples should yield a single sharp peak within this temperature range, and the melting temperature should be the same for all the samples. Furthermore, both water and −RT should not generate significant fluorescent signal. If the dissociation curve reveals a series of peaks, it indicates that there is not enough discrimination between specific and nonspecific reaction products (for example, due to dimerization of primers), which would render optimization of the qRT-PCR necessary.

Acknowledgement

A.M.B. is supported through the Ramón y Cajal program (RYC-2010-06473).

A.N.D.C. was supported by CIHR and by University of Glasgow.

References

1. Berg AH, Scherer PE (2005) Adipose tissue, inflammation, and cardiovascular disease. Circ Res 96:939–949
2. Ouchi N, Parker JL, Lugus JJ, Walsh K (2011) Adipokines in inflammation and metabolic disease. Nat Rev Immunol 11:85–97
3. Nguyen Dinh Cat A, Jaisser F (2012) Extrarenal effects of aldosterone. Curr Opin Nephrol Hypertens 21:147–156
4. Aghamohammadzadeh R, Heagerty AM (2012) Obesity-related hypertension: epidemiology, pathophysiology, treatments, and the contribution of perivascular adipose tissue. Ann Med 44:S74–S84
5. Rodbel M (1964) Metabolism of isolated fat cells. Effects of hormones on glucose metabolism and lypolisis. J Biol Chem 239: 375–380
6. Zhang HH, Kumar S, Barnett AH, Eggo MC (2000) Ceiling culture of mature human adipocytes: use in studies of adipocyte functions. J Endocrinol 164:119–128
7. Fernyhough ME, Vierck JL, Hausman GJ, Mir PS, Okine EK, Dodson MV (2004) Primary adipocyte culture: adipocyte purification methods may lead to a new understanding of adipose tissue growth and development. Cytotechnology 46:163–172
8. Van Harmelen V, Skurk T, Hauner H (2005) Primary culture and differentiation of human adipocyte precursor cells. Human Cell Cult Protoc 107:125–135
9. Carswell KA, Lee MJ, Fried SK (2011) Culture of isolated human adipocytes and isolated adipose tissue. Methods Mol Biol 806:203–214
10. Armani A, Mammi C, Marzolla V, Calanchini M, Antelmi A, Rosano GM, Fabbri A, Caprio M (2010) Cellular models for understanding adipogenesis, adipose dysfunction, and obesity. J Cell Biochem 110:564–572

11. Poulos SP, Dodson MV, Hausman GJ (2010) Cell line models for differentiation: preadipocytes and adipocytes. Exp Biol Med (Maywood) 235:1185–1193
12. Lafontan M (2012) Historical perspectives in fat cell biology: the fat cell as a model for the investigation of hormonal and metabolic pathways. Am J Physiol Cell Physiol 302:C327–C359
13. Fleige S, Pfaffl MW (2006) RNA integrity and the effect on the real-time qRT-PCR performance. Mol Aspects Med 27:126–139
14. Thellin O, Zorzi W, Lakaye B, De Borman B, Coumans B, Hennen G, Grisar T, Igout A, Heinen E (1999) Housekeeping genes as internal standards: use and limits. J Biotechnol 75:291–295
15. Vandesompele J, De Preter K, Pattyn F, Poppe B, Van Roy N, De Paepe A, Speleman F (2002) Accurate normalization of real-time quantitative RT-PCR data by geometric averaging of multiple internal control genes. Genome Bio 3, RESEARCH0034
16. Suzuki T, Higgins PJ, Crawford DR (2000) Control selection for RNA quantitation. Biotechniques 29:332–337
17. Zhong H, Simons JW (1999) Direct comparison of GAPDH, beta-actin, cyclophilin, and 28 S rRNA as internal standards for quantifying RNA levels under hypoxia. Biochem Biophys Res Commun 259:523–526
18. Schmittgen TD, Zakrajsek BA (2000) Effect of experimental treatment on housekeeping gene expression: validation by real-time, quantitative RT-PCR. J Biochem Biophys Methods 46:69–81
19. Murphy RM, Watt KK, Cameron-Smith D, Gibbons CJ, Snow RJ (2003) Effects of creatine supplementation on housekeeping genes in human skeletal muscle using real-time RT-PCR. Physiol Genomics 12:163–174

Chapter 23

Isolation and Differentiation of Murine Macrophages

Francisco J. Rios, Rhian M. Touyz, and Augusto C. Montezano

Abstract

Macrophages play a major role in inflammation, wound healing, and tissue repair. Infiltrated monocytes differentiate into different macrophage subtypes with protective or pathogenic activities in vascular lesions. In the heart and vascular tissues, pathological activation promotes cardiovascular inflammation and remodeling and there is increasing evidence that macrophages play important mechanisms in this environment. Primary murine macrophages can be obtained from: bone marrow by different treatments (granulocyte-macrophage colony-stimulating factor—GM-CSF, macrophage colony-stimulating factor—M-CSF or supernatant of murine fibroblast L929), peritoneal cavity (resident or thioglycolate elicit macrophages), from the lung (alveolar macrophages) or from adipose tissue. In this chapter we describe some protocols to obtain primary murine macrophages and how to identify a pure macrophage population or activation phenotypes using different markers.

Key words Macrophage, Murine, Peritoneum, Bone marrow, Resident, Thioglycollate, L929 supernatant

1 Introduction

Macrophages play a central role in inflammatory response and host defense, contributing the establishment of the innate immunity. Additionally these cells participate in homeostatic functions, including fibrosis, lipid metabolism, and tissue remodeling [1].

The most known process involved in macrophage activation is the phagocytosis. Monocytes from the blood vessels migrate to the tissue, where they encounter and engulf microorganisms. This process is followed by production and secretion of several mediators that increase the inflammatory response, such as tumor necrosis factor-α (TNF-α) and nitric oxide. On the other hand, in some situations, macrophages participate in tissue remodeling, secreting anti-inflammatory substances, such as interleucin-10 (IL-10) and transforming growth factor beta (TGFβ), that will control the inflammatory response, contributes to collagen production and tissue remodeling [2].

Rhian M. Touyz and Ernesto L. Schiffrin (eds.), *Hypertension: Methods and Protocols*, Methods in Molecular Biology, vol. 1527, DOI 10.1007/978-1-4939-6625-7_23, © Springer Science+Business Media LLC 2017

Macrophages have an extraordinary plasticity to change their phenotype according to the receptors that have been activated and the microenvironment where they are located. These cells can be polarized to classical activated phenotype (M1 macrophages), involved in the pro-inflammatory response or to an alternative activated phenotype (M2 macrophages) that are mostly involved in anti-inflammatory mechanism, fibrosis, and wound healing. M1 macrophages have high expression of Fc receptors and produce pro-inflammatory cytokines (MCP-1, IL-6, TNF, IL-12) and nitric oxide. Inversely, M2 macrophages have high expression of mannose receptor, arginase-1 and produce IL-10 and TGF-β. Although some studies have found the presence of both phenotypes in cardiovascular diseases, the main role of M1 and M2 macrophages in this context remains unclear [1, 2].

Macrophages in the tissue produce reactive oxygen species and metalloproteinases that will increase the inflammatory response and activate smooth muscle and endothelial cells, contributing to the cardiovascular disease [3]. In fact, it has been show that the activation of mineralocorticoid receptor in macrophages is related to oxidative stress and inflammation, playing a role in cardiac hypertrophy and blood pressure [4].

In this chapter we describe protocols to obtain murine macrophage in vitro. Depending on the method used, it can be obtained from different macrophage populations, which have different properties in the inflammatory response.

2 Murine Macrophage Identification

Murine macrophages can be identified by expressing F4/80 and CD11b (Mac1), MOMA-1 [5]. The antibodies required for these markers are supplied by different companies, they are well acceptable among the scientists and can be used for flow cytometry, immunohistochemistry, and immunofluorescence.

3 Culture of Murine Bone Marrow Derived Macrophages

This is a saving cost method to obtain macrophage population from murine bone marrow (Fig. 1). Macrophages can be differentiated from the bone marrow by treatment with murine recombinant M-CSF (10 ng/mL). However, several studies have demonstrated that L929 supernatant promotes differentiation of macrophages by producing M-CSF [6]. This is well accepted as a pure macrophage population model. It has been described that bone marrow derived macrophages are an important model to study reactive oxygen species production and endothelial cell adhesion [7].

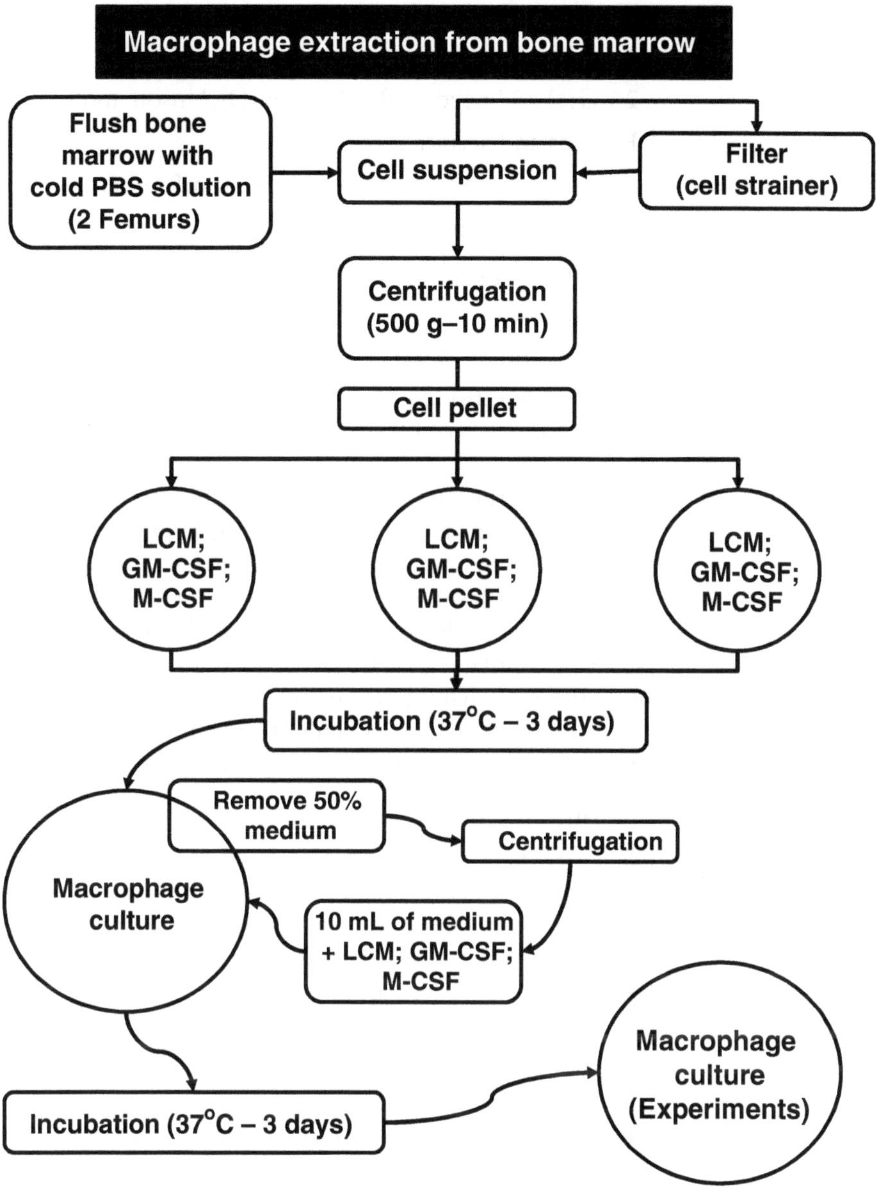

Fig. 1 Macrophage differentiation from the bone marrow. This is a simplified flowchart of the murine bone marrow isolation and macrophage differentiation from two femurs. *PBS* phosphate buffered saline, *LCM* L929 cell conditioned medium, *GM-CSF* granulocyte-macrophage colony-stimulating factor, *M-CSF* macrophage colony-stimulating factor

With this protocol it is possible to obtain $2–3 \times 10^7$ macrophages using two femurs. However, the cell number increases by using the tibias.

3.1 Materials

DMEM (containing 4.5 g glucose, L-glutamine, 20 mM HEPES, and penicillin and streptomycin).

- Endotoxin-free heat-inactivated fetal calf serum (FCS).

- Phosphate buffered saline (PBS), pH 7.2
- 10-mL syringe.
- 26 G×1/2″ needle (BD Becton, Dickinson and Company).
- Forceps and scissors.
- Centrifuge at 4 °C with rotor for 50 mL tube.
- 100×15-mm sterile bacterial plastic petri dishes.
- 50-mL polypropylene tubes.
- Cell strainers, 70 μm (BD Falcon™).
- 70% ethanol in water.
- L-Cell Conditioned Medium (LCM): DMEM (prepared as in **item 3.1**), 20% of L929 cell culture supernatant, 15% of FCS).

3.2 Methodology

Supernatant of the murine fibroblast L929 is obtained by growing 1×10^5 cells/mL in DMEM (fresh medium prepared according to **item 3.1**, supplemented with 10% FCS, 50 μM 2-Mercaptoethanol). Usually we add 60 mL of the cell suspension in a 150 cm² flask. Let the cells grow in a humidified incubator 5% CO_2 at 37 °C for 7 days, to accumulate growth factor in the supernatant. At day 7, remove the supernatant, wash the cells monolayer with PBS and harvest them using cell scraper. Centrifuge the supernatant at 5000×*g*, 10 min, filter at 0.22 μm and freeze at −80 °C (**Note 2**).

1. Sacrifice the mouse according to the ethical permission from your research institute.
2. Rub a piece of cotton embedded in alcohol along the abdomen of the mouse. Make an incision in the abdomen and with scissor remove the muscles from the bones to be able to expose the femur head. Be careful you do not break the femur. Soak the cleaned bone in ice-cold PBS until the extraction of the other bones has finished. Until this step the work can be performed in normal laboratory bench.
3. From this step the work must be done in a laminar flow hood. Sterilize the bones by soaking in alcohol for 10 s and keep them in ice-cold sterile PBS.
4. Carefully take the bone with a forceps and with a scissor, cut a small piece of both extremities. Using a 26 G×1/2″ needle in a 10 mL syringe, flush the bones with cold PBS. Repeat the flush until the bone change the color to white.
5. With a 10 mL pipette, do movement up and downs to be able to dissolve the cells aggregates.
6. Pass the cell suspension through a cell strainer (70 μm) to get a single cell suspension. After, wash the cell strainer with 5 mL of cold PBS.
7. Centrifuge the cell suspension at 400×*g* for 10 min.

8. Resuspend the cells in 10 mL of L-Cell conditioned Medium, count and adjust the cell concentration to 2×10^6 cells/mL.
9. Plate 10 mL of the cell suspension in a 100 × 15-mm sterile bacterial plastic Petri dishes. Incubate the plates in a humidified incubator with 5 % CO_2 at 37 °C. At day 3, add 15 mL of the L-Cell conditioned Medium.
10. At day 6, the cells are already differentiated in bone marrow derived macrophages and are strongly attached to the plastic (**Note 1**).
11. To detach the cells. Remove the LCM and add 10 mL of cold PBS. Place the plates with cells and PBS on ice for 30 min. By using a cell scraper, gently scrape the cells off the plate.
12. Centrifuge the cells at 300 × *g* for 5 min. Resuspend in DMEM/5 % FCS and plate according to the protocol required for the experiment. Stimulate the cells after 24 h (**Note 3–4**).

4 Culture of Resident Peritoneal Macrophages

4.1 Materials

- RPMI1640 (containing L-glutamine, 20 mM HEPES, and penicillin and streptomycin).
- Endotoxin-free heat-inactivated fetal calf serum (FCS).
- Phosphate buffered saline (PBS), pH 7.2.
- 10-mL syringe.
- 26 G × 1/2″ and 21 G needles (BD Becton, Dickinson and Company).
- Forceps and scissors.
- Centrifuge at 4 °C with rotor for 50 mL tube.
- 50-mL polypropylene tubes.
- 70 % ethanol in water.

4.2 Methodology (Fig. 2)

1. Sacrifice the mice according to the ethical permission from your research institute.
2. Sterilize the mouse, by placing it in 70 % ethanol for 5 s.
3. Using a forceps, delicately pitch up the skin of the inferior ventral abdomen and make an incision with a scissors to expose all peritoneum. Be careful you do not injure the peritoneal membrane.
4. Pull up the peritoneal membrane using a forceps and with 26 G × 1/2″ inject 6 mL of ice-cold PBS in the peritoneal cavity. Do not pierce the visceral organs or will contaminate the macrophages.

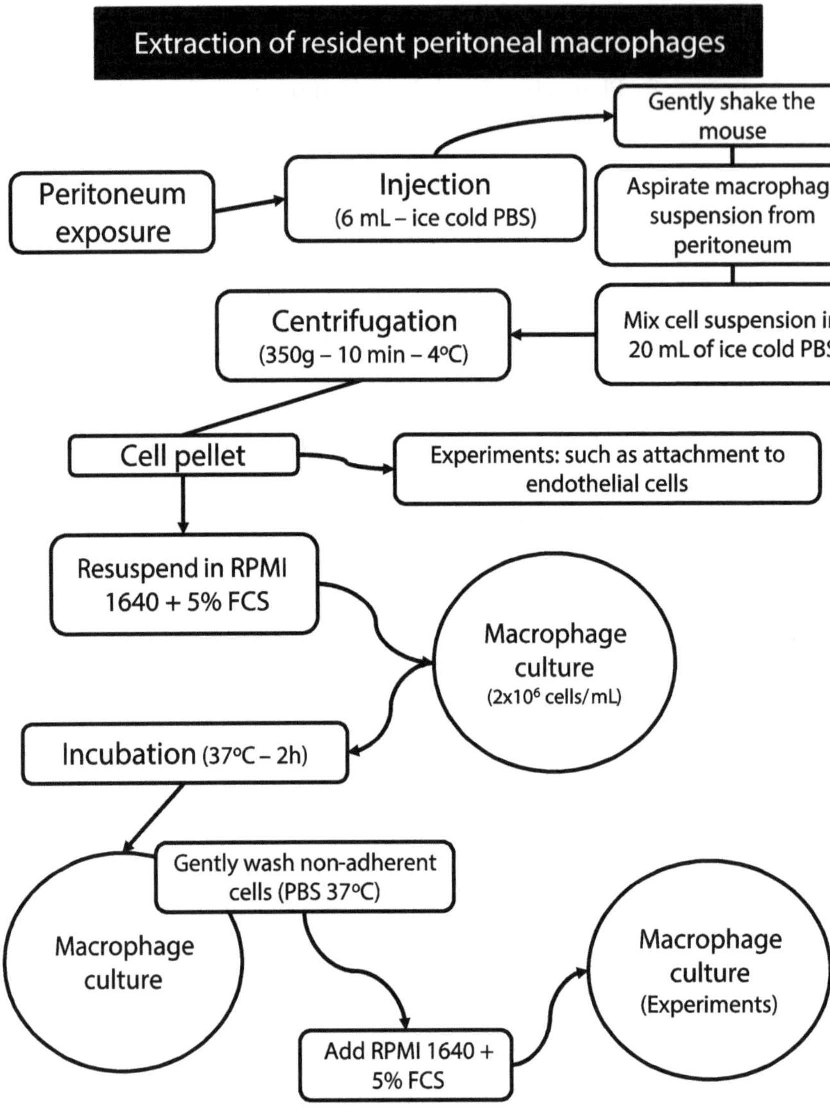

Fig. 2 Extraction of resident peritoneal macrophages. This is a simplified flowchart for the isolation of resident peritoneal macrophages. *PBS* phosphate buffered saline, *RPMI* Roswell Park Memorial Institute medium

5. Shake the mouse for 10 s. This step will detach macrophage from the peritoneal cavity and get a cell suspension.
6. Using the 21 G needle in a 10 mL syringe, remove the macrophages suspension from the peritoneal cavity. Insert the needle with beveled end facing down in the opposite side of the liver and distant from the fatty tissue. The needle might gets stack with the fat, to solve this problem removed the needle and insert it again.

7. Collect the cell suspension in a 50 mL tube containing 20 mL of ice-cold PBS and placed on ice.
8. Centrifuge the cells suspension at $350 \times g$ at 4 °C for 5 min.
9. Resuspend the cell pellet with RPMI 1640 supplemented with 5 % of FCS. Count the cells, plate then at 2×10^6 cells/mL and incubate for 2 h at 37 °C.
10. Gently, wash the non-adherent cells with PBS at 37 °C. Wash gently because resident peritoneal macrophages do not attach strongly.
11. Add RPMI 1640 with 5 % FCS to the adherent macrophages and proceed with your experiments. Usually with this protocol you might obtain $4–6 \times 10^6$ peritoneal cells and approximately 50 % are macrophages.

5 Thioglycollate Elicited Macrophages

Thioglycollate medium is often used to increase the amount of macrophages recruited to the peritoneal cavity. This procedure can be used to obtain activated inflammatory macrophages from mice, or it can be used as an analytical procedure to compare rates of leukocyte accumulation by different treatments. This protocol might results approximately 2×10^7 of inflammatory macrophages.

5.1 Materials

- RPMI1640 (containing L-glutamine, 20 mM HEPES, and penicillin and streptomycin).
- Endotoxin-free heat-inactivated fetal calf serum (FCS).
- Phosphate buffered saline (PBS), pH 7.2.
- 10-mL syringe.
- 26 G×1/2″ and 21 G needles (BD Becton, Dickinson and Company).
- Forceps and scissors.
- Centrifuge at 4 °C with rotor for 50 mL tube.
- 50 mL polypropylene tubes.
- 70 % ethanol in water.
- 3 % brewer modified thioglycollate medium (3 % w/v of an autoclaved stock prepared from dehydrated thioglycollate medium and sterile water).

5.2 Methodology

1. Using a 26 G×1/2″ needle, inject 1 mL of 3 % thioglycollate medium into the peritoneal cavity of the mouse.

2. After 4 days, thioglycollate elicited macrophages might be obtained from the peritoneal cavity (follow the protocol in Subheading 4.2, **steps 1–8**).
3. Plate the peritoneal cells in a concentration 1×10^6 cells/mL and incubate for 2 h at 37 °C.
4. Wash the non-adherent cells with PBS at 37 °C. Thioglycolate elicited macrophages attach strongly to the plate.
5. Add RPMI 1640 with 5 % FCS to the adherent macrophages and proceed with your experiments.

6 Alveolar Macrophages

Typically, a total of ~3–5 × 10^5 alveolar macrophages cells can be obtained per mouse. Therefore this procedure is often performed on groups of ten mice or more to provide sufficient alveolar macrophages for functional assays (Fig. 3).

6.1 Materials

- RPMI 1640 (containing L-glutamine, 20 mM HEPES, and penicillin and streptomycin).
- Endotoxin-free heat-inactivated fetal calf serum (FCS).
- Anesthetics: Cocktail of ketamine-HCl 100 mg/kg and xylazine-HCl 10 mg/kg in PBS.
- PBS containing 0.5 mM EDTA and without calcium and magnesium.
- Forceps and scissors.
- 18 G needles and 10-mL syringes.
- 50-mL polypropylene tubes.

6.2 Methodology

1. Anesthetize mice by injecting 100–200 μL of the Anesthetics Cocktail ketamine–xylazine cocktail. Do not sacrifice the mouse by cervical dislocation, because it might injure and contaminate the cells with blood. Also, do not use CO_2 asphyxia, because it might change the alveolar macrophage response.
2. In a laminar flow hood. Rub a piece of cotton embedded in alcohol along the neck and abdomen of the mouse. Make a small incision in the neck and expose the trachea on the ventral side. Insert a18 G needle in the trachea (just below the larynx) and tie up with a threat.
3. Hold a 5-mL syringe in the needle and slowly inject sterile 2–3 mL of PBS/EDTA at 37 °C under gentle massage of the lungs.
4. Gently pull the plunger of the syringe back to withdraw the cell suspension and collect it in a 50 mL tube containing

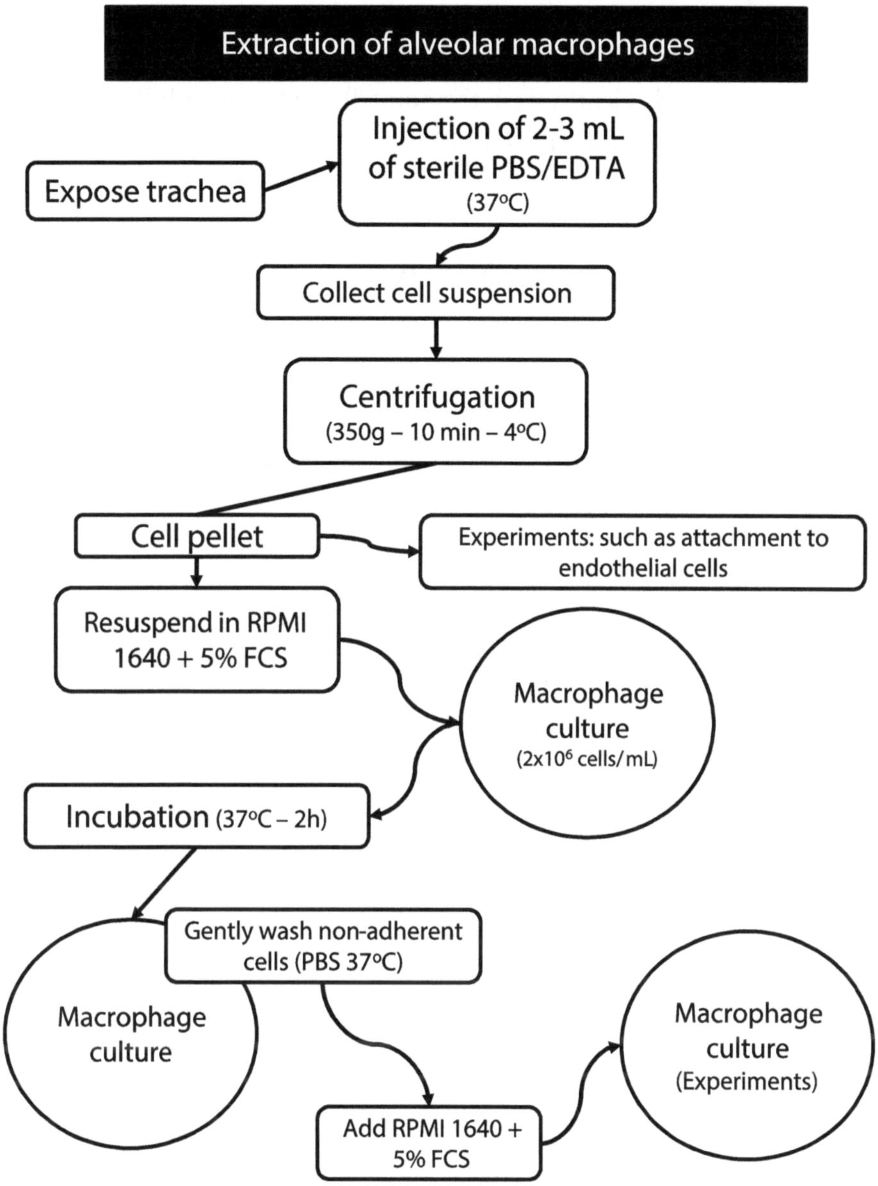

Fig. 3 Extraction of alveolar macrophages. This is a simplified flowchart for the isolation of alveolar macrophages. *PBS* phosphate buffered saline, *EDTA* ethylenediaminetetraacetic acid, *RPMI* Roswell Park Memorial Institute medium, *FCS* fetal calf serum

15 mL of cold sterile PBS and placed on ice. Repeat this step 3–4 times.

5. Centrifuge the cell suspension for 10 min at 350×*g*, 4 °C.
6. Resuspend the cell in pellet with RPMI1640, supplemented with 5% FCS for counting.

7. Plate the cells and incubate in a humidified incubator with 5% CO_2 at 37 °C for 2 h.
8. Gently, wash the non-adherent cells with PBS at 37 °C.
9. Add RPMI 1640 with 5% FCS to the adherent macrophages and proceed with your experiments.

7 Isolation of Macrophages from Adipose Tissue

7.1 Materials

- RPMI1640 (containing L-glutamine, 20 mM HEPES, and penicillin and streptomycin).
- Endotoxin-free heat-inactivated fetal calf serum (FCS).
- PBS, pH 7.2 at room temperature.
- Forceps and scissors.
- 15 and 50-mL polypropylene tubes.
- Collagenase type 1 (1 mg/mL in PBS).
- Water bath at 37 °C.
- P1000 pipette.
- CD11b MicroBeads for mouse samples (MACS Cell Separation System; Miltenyi Biotec).

7.2 Methodology (Fig. 4)

1. Sacrifice the mice according to the ethical permission from your research institute.
2. Rub a piece of cotton embedded in alcohol along the abdomen of the mouse. Make an incision in the abdomen and in the peritoneal cavity to expose the abdominal fatty tissue.
3. With forceps and scissor remove the fatty tissue from the abdominal cavity and place it in a 15 mL tube containing collagenase. Digest for 30 min in a water bath at 37 °C and in constant agitation. If you have to extract the adipose tissue from several mice, the fatty can be collected in PBS until the extraction of the samples have finished.
4. Homogenize the digested samples with P1000 pipette by up and down movements.
5. Transfer the digested sample to a 50 mL tube and immediately add 30 mL of cold RPMI 1640 supplemented with FCS 10% to inactivate the collagenase.
6. Centrifuge the samples at 350×*g* at 4 °C for 10 min. Macrophages will be on the cell pellet and the floating fraction is enriched in adipocytes.
7. Resuspend the cell pellet in 5 mL of cold PBS and filter through the cell strainer. After, wash the cell strainer with 5 mL of cold PBS.

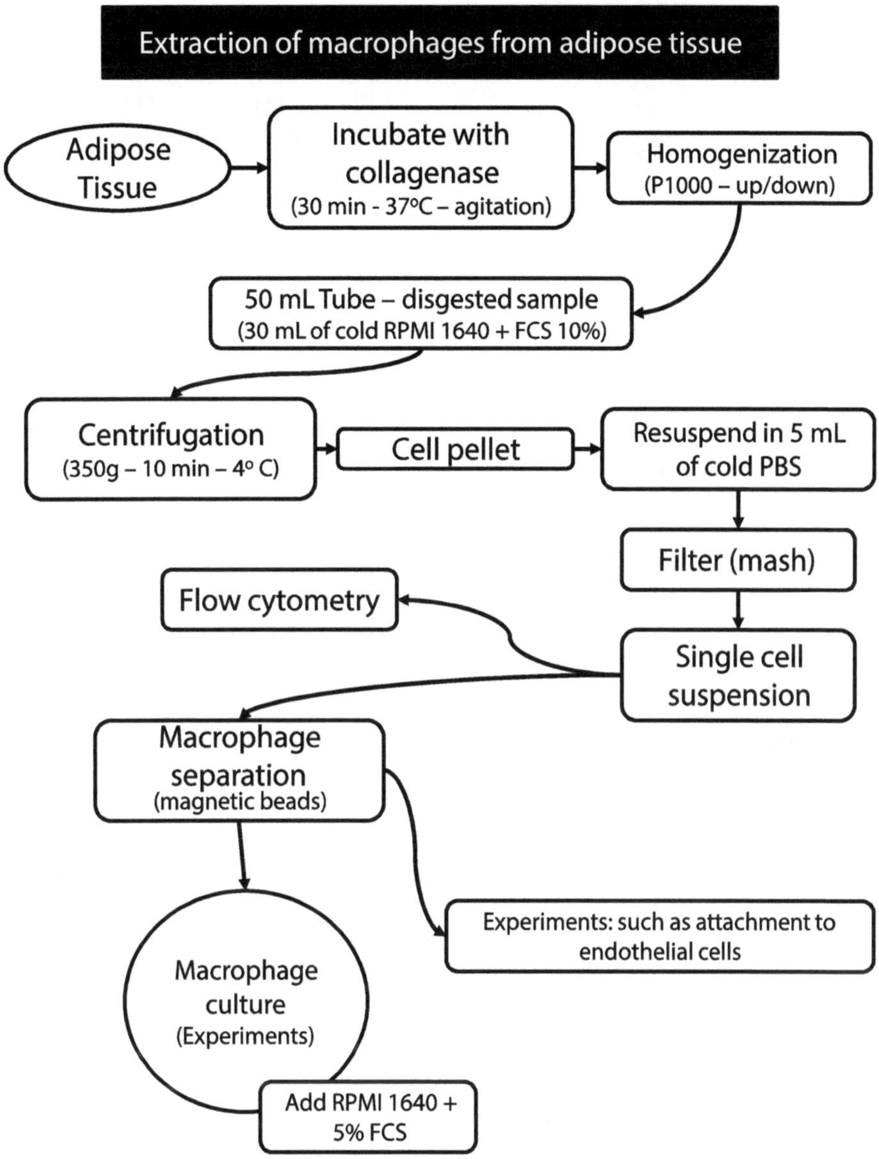

Fig. 4 Isolation of macrophages from adipose tissue. This is a simplified flowchart for the extraction of macrophages from adipose tissue. *RPMI* Roswell Park Memorial Institute medium, *FCS* fetal calf serum, *PBS* phosphate buffered saline

8. The single cell suspension might be stained for flow cytometry or be collected to isolate the macrophages.
9. Isolate macrophages using magnetic beads CD11b MicroBeads, according to manufacturer's instruction.
10. Plate the macrophages in RPMI 1640/ 5% FCS and perform the experiments

Table 1
Murine macrophage phenotype markers

	M1	M2	References
FIZZ1	↓	↑	[8]
Mannose receptor (CD206)	↓	↑	[9]
Arginase 1	↓	↑	[10]
Yml	↓	↑	[8]
Galectin 3	↓	↑	[1]
IL-10	↓	↑	[2]
TNFα	↑	↓	[12]
iNOS	↑	↓	[13]
IL-12	↑	↓	[12]
IL-6	↑	↓	[14]
IL-1β	↑	↓	[14]

8 Macrophage Markers

M1 and M2 macrophages can be obtained in vitro by treatment with different cytokine combination. After macrophage differentiation according to **item 3**, M1 macrophages are obtained by treatment with LPS 50 ng/mL and 5 U/mL of interferon-γ for 24. M2 macrophages are obtained by treatment with IL-4 (20 ng/mL) for 24 h.

M1 and M2 macrophages might be identified according to Table 1:

9 Notes

1. Trypsin can be used instead of cell scraper; however, in our experience, cells stand more passages by using cell scraper. Save the supernatant at −80 °C. Try to test each batch of supernatant and after collect the supernatants in the same flask for the macrophages differentiate with the same concentration of growth factors. Constantly test the L929 cell for mycoplasma contamination.
2. Differentiated macrophages attach strongly to the tissue culture. Common sterile plastic Petri dishes will allow the macrophages to detacheasier and get high number of viable cells than the plates treated for cell culture.

3. Different mouse strains can result in different cell proliferation. Try to optimize the cell concentration for your protocol.
4. After the differentiation from the bone marrow, macrophages appear clean cells. The presence of vacuole or low viability indicates contamination.

References

1. Gordon S, Martinez FO (2010) Alternative activation of macrophages: mechanism and functions. Immunity 32(5):593–604
2. Mosser DM, Edwards JP (2008) Exploring the full spectrum of macrophage activation. Nat Rev Immunol 8(12):958–969
3. Scholtes VP, Johnson JL, Jenkins N, Sala-Newby GB, de Vries JP, de Borst GJ et al (2012) Carotid atherosclerotic plaque matrix metalloproteinase-12-positive macrophage subpopulation predicts adverse outcome after endarterectomy. J Am Heart Assoc 1(6):e001040
4. Rickard AJ, Morgan J, Tesch G, Funder JW, Fuller PJ, Young MJ (2009) Deletion of mineralocorticoid receptors from macrophages protects against deoxycorticosterone/salt-induced cardiac fibrosis and increased blood pressure. Hypertension 54(3):537–543
5. Lai L, Alaverdi N, Maltais L, Morse HC III (1998) Mouse cell surface antigens: nomenclature and immunophenotyping. J Immunol 160(8):3861–3868
6. Tomida M, Yamamoto-Yamaguchi Y, Hozumi M (1984) Purification of a factor inducing differentiation ofmouse myeloid leukemic M1 cells from conditioned medium of mouse fibroblast L929 cells. J Biol Chem 259(17):10978–82
7. Cunnick J, Kaur P, Cho Y, Groffen J, Heisterkamp N (2006) Use of bone marrow-derived macrophages to model murine innate immune responses. J Immunol Methods 311(1–2):96–105
8. Raes G, De Baetselier P, Noel W, Beschin A, Brombacher F, Hassanzadeh GG (2002) Differential expression of FIZZ1 and Ym1 in alternatively versus classically activated macrophages. J Leuk Biol 71(4):597–602
9. Stein M, Keshav S, Harris N, Gordon S (1992) Interleukin 4 potently enhances murine macrophage mannose receptor activity: a marker of alternative immunologic macrophage activation. J Exp Med 176(1): 287–292
10. Loke P, Nair MG, Parkinson J, Guiliano D, Blaxter M, Allen JE (2002) IL-4 dependent alternatively-activated macrophages have a distinctive in vivo gene expression phenotype. BMC Immunol 3:7
11. MacKinnon AC, Farnworth SL, Hodkinson PS, Henderson NC, Atkinson KM, Leffler H et al (2008) Regulation of alternative macrophage activation by galectin-3. J Immunol 180(4):2650–2658
12. Mantovani A, Sica A, Locati M (2005) Macrophage polarization comes of age. Immunity 23(4):344–346
13. Martinez FO, Helming L, Gordon S (2009) Alternative activation of macrophages: an immunologic functional perspective. Annu Rev Immunol 27:451–483
14. Sica A, Mantovani A (2012) Macrophage plasticity and polarization: in vivo veritas. J Clin Invest 122(3):787–795

Chapter 24

Isolation and Differentiation of Human Macrophages

Francisco J. Rios, Rhian M. Touyz, and Augusto C. Montezano

Abstract

Macrophage subtypes display protective or pathogenic activities in vascular lesions. They recognize and engulf modified lipids, accumulate in the arterial intima, contributing to the atherosclerosis development. In the heart, vascular tissues and perivascular adipose tissues, there is increasing evidence that macrophages play a role in endothelial dysfunction, vascular inflammation and remodeling. In this chapter we describe protocols to isolate human monocytes from peripheral blood mononuclear cell and how to differentiate them into macrophages by using growth factors (granulocyte-macrophage colony-stimulating factor—GM-CSF or colony-stimulating factor—M-CSF) or by different cell culture medium concentration. We also describe how to indentify different macrophage activation phenotypes.

Key words Macrophage, Monocyte, Human, Culture, GM-CSF, M-CSF

1 Introduction

Macrophages are long-lived cells derived from the circulating monocytes that differentiate as they leave the blood vessels. They play a major role in the activation of the innate immune system, contributing to the inflammation, wound healing, and tissue repair. Macrophages express a variety of different receptors able to interact with several and different stimuli, including microbial ligands, endogenous danger signals, lipid mediators, and cytokines. Once activated, they acquire microbicidal competence that usually leads to effective immunity. However, several bacterial ligands may also interfere with activation process and modulate host responses [1].

Macrophages have been described as phagocytes that secrete pro-inflammatory and antimicrobial mediators. However, the current knowledge describes a more complex model involving multiple macrophage phenotypes carrying out different effect on the inflammatory response and innate immunity. In response to cytokines or microbial products present in the microenvironment, macrophages can change their phenotype and be polarized to M1 or M2 macrophages (Fig. 1). M1 are the classically activated macrophages and are induced by microbial stimuli (e.g., lipopolysaccharide-LPS), pro-inflammatory

Rhian M. Touyz and Ernesto L. Schiffrin (eds.), *Hypertension: Methods and Protocols*, Methods in Molecular Biology, vol. 1527, DOI 10.1007/978-1-4939-6625-7_24,

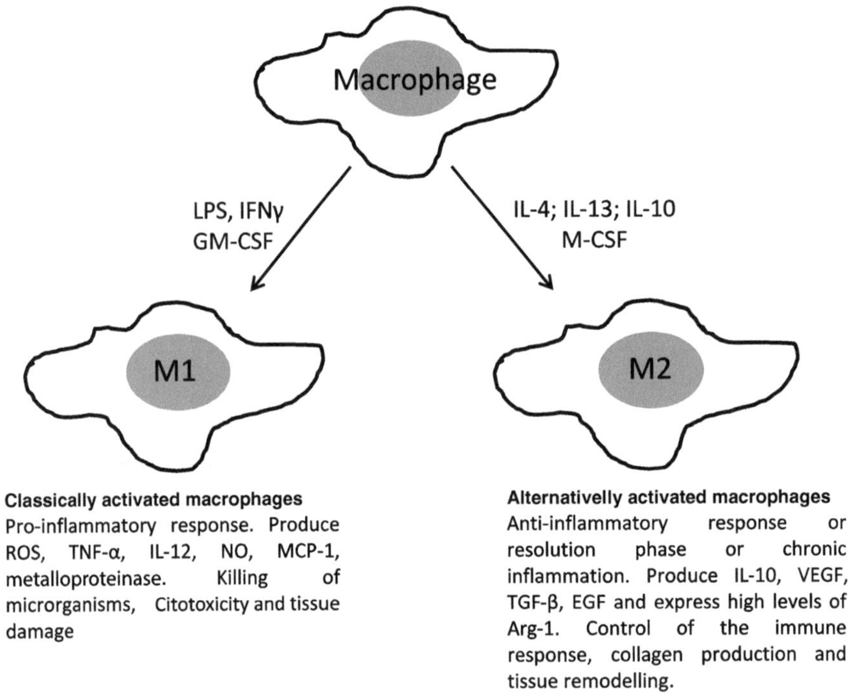

Fig. 1 Macrophage activation phenotype. By treatment with different stimuli or cytokines present in the microenvironment, macrophages can be polarized to M1 or M2 macrophages. *ROS* reactive oxygen species, *IL* interleukin, *NO* nitric oxide, *MCP-1* monocyte chemotactic protein-1, *VEGF* vascular endothelial growth factor, *TGFβ* transforming growth factor-beta, *EGF* epidermal growth factor, *Arg-1* arginase -1

cytokines [interferon-γ (IFNγ); tumor necrosis factor-α (TNF-α)]. Classically activated macrophages exhibit pro-inflammatory and microbicidal properties, promote extracellular matrix degradation and tissue injury. On the opposite side, M2 or alternatively activated macrophages are induced by stimulation with interleukin-4 (IL-4), IL-13, glucocorticoids, and peroxisome proliferator-activated receptor-gamma (PPARγ) activation [2]. M2 macrophages produce transforming growth factor beta (TGFβ) and IL-10 that are involved in the resolution process of the inflammatory response and wound healing by extracellular matrix construction, cell proliferation, angiogenesis, and stimulation of collagen production [3].

Macrophages play a central role in the atherosclerosis development by interfering with the lipid metabolism and production of inflammatory mediators, such as cytokines and reactive oxygen species that increase the inflammatory cell infiltration and contribute to the lesion progression [4]. New studies have been addressed the importance of the presence of inflammatory macrophages in the adipose tissue that might affect the obesity and the insulin resistance [5]. Additionally, inflammatory mechanisms related to pulmonary hypertension and vascular remodeling have been found to be dependent on macrophage activation [6]

In this chapter we describe protocols to differentiate human macrophages in vitro. Depending on the method used, it can be obtained from different macrophage population, which have different properties in the inflammatory response.

2 Isolation of Peripheral Blood Mononuclear Cell from Buffy Coat

2.1 Materials

Human buffy coat or a conical shape blood filter.

- 50-mL polypropylene tubes.
- Ficoll-Hypaque 1077 (Sigma-aldrich or GE healthcare) or Lymphoprep™ (Axis-Shield PoC AS) at room temperature.
- PBS, Ca^{2+}- and Mg^{2+}-free, pH 7.2. One flask at room temperature and other at 4 °C.
- 10-mL pipette.
- Centrifuge with rotor for 50 mL tube.
- Pasteur pipette.

2.2 Methodology (Fig. 2)

1. The conical blood filter and the buffy coat have approximately 10 and 70 mL respectively.
2. Collect the samples to a 50 mL tube. If you are using the conical blood filter, dilute the sample by adding 10 mL of PBS at room temperature.
3. In a 50-mL centrifuge tube, add 10 mL of Ficoll-Hypaque-1077 (or Lymphoprep) at room temperature.
4. Carefully layer 3 mL of the blood onto the Ficoll-Hypaque-1077. The blood will stay in the upper layer and the Ficoll-Hypaque 1077 in the lowest one.
5. Centrifuge at 400 × *g* for 30 min at room temperature. Set the centrifuge for 0 (zero) acceleration and 0 (zero) break (*see* **Note 1**).
6. After centrifugation you might be able to see three layers. The upper layer containing plasma and the Ficoll-Hypaque. One opaque interface containing the mononuclear cells, and the red lowest layer.
7. Using a Pasteur pipette, aspirate carefully the upper layer until close to the opaque phase containing the mononuclear cells. Discard the upper layer.
8. Aspirate carefully the interface opaque and transfer to a 50 mL tube.
9. Fill up the 50-mL tube with cold PBS.
10. Centrifuge at 250 × *g* for 10 min at 4 °C. Set the centrifuge to full acceleration and break 5.

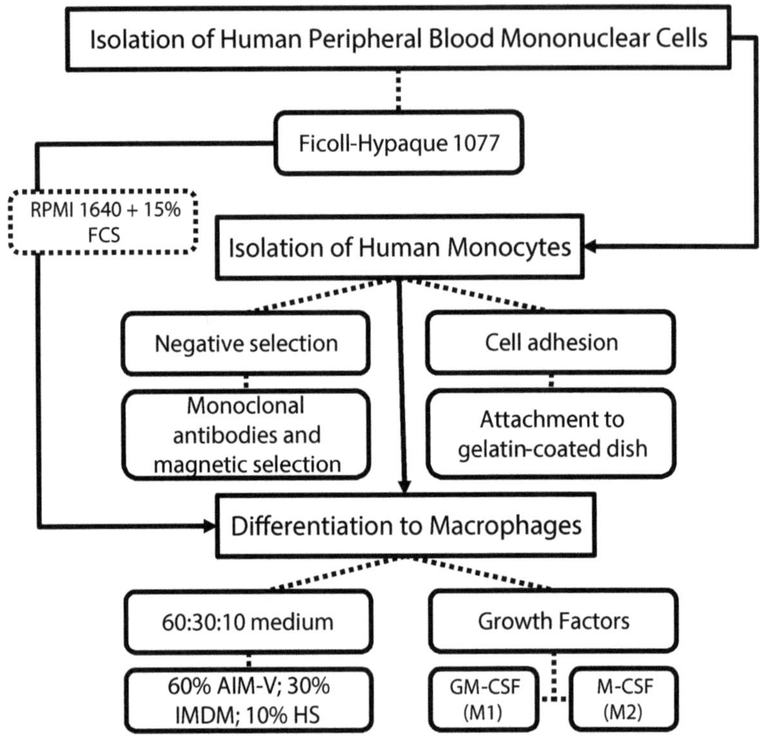

Fig. 2 Isolation and differentiation of macrophages from human blood samples. This is a simplified flowchart for the isolation and differentiation of human macrophages. Once human blood samples are obtained, the isolation of peripheral blood mononuclear cells is performed by gradient centrifugation using Ficoll-Hypaque 1077. After centrifugation, the interface between the plasma (*top*) and red (*bottom*) layer, is carefully collected and used for the isolation of monocytes. The monocytes isolation can be performed by negative selection (monoclonal antibodies and magnetic selection) or cell adhesion protocols. The differentiation of monocytes to macrophages can be done by either the 60:30:10 medium protocol or exposure of these cells to growth factors, such as granulocyte-macrophage colony-stimulating factor (GM-CSF), which will generate M1 macrophages, and macrophage colony-stimulating factor (M-CSF), which will generate M2 macrophages. Human macrophages can also be obtained by incubation of isolated peripheral blood mononuclear cells with RPMI 1640 containing 15% fetal calf serum (FCS)

11. At the end of the first washing, the supernatant will appears turbid due to presence of platelets. Aspirate the supernatant and resuspend the pellet with cold PBS. Centrifuge at 250 × *g* for 10 min at 4 °C. Repeat these washing steps 3–4 times, until you get a clear supernatant.

3 Isolation of Human Monocytes by Negative Selection

Human macrophages can be isolated by negative selection, using the Monocyte Isolation Kit II for human samples from MACS Cell Separation System; Miltenyi Biotec (cat number 130-091-153). This kit has a cocktail of monoclonal antibodies to CD3, CD7, CD16, CD19, CD56, CD123, and glycophorin A. It permits the isolation of untouched monocytes from human peripheral blood mononuclear cells (PBMCs). The protocol may be performed according to manufacturer's instruction.

4 Isolation of Human Monocytes by Cell Adhesion

In order to coast saving, human monocytes can be isolated by adhesion to tissue culture plastic. However, the cell number increases if you use gelatin-coated surfaces.

4.1 Materials

Gelatin sterile Solution, 2 % (Sigma-Aldrich cat number #G1393).

- Tissue culture petri dishes P100.
- RPMI1640 (containing l-glutamine, 20 mM HEPES, penicillin, and streptomycin).
- Cell scraper.
- 50 mL tubes.

4.2 Methodology

1. Pre-coat the tissue culture petri dishes. Add 2–3 mL of the gelatin solution 2 % in the plate in order to coat the whole surface. Remove the gelatin solution. If more plates needed to be coated, you can transfer the gelatin from one to another. Leave the plates to dry at 37 °C.
2. After PBMC isolation, as described in **item 2** resuspend the cells in serum free RMP1 1640, count and adjust the cell concentration to 1×10^7 cells/mL.
3. Add 10 mL of the cells suspension in a tissue culture petri dishes P100.
4. Incubate the plates in a humidified incubator with 5 % CO_2 at 37 °C.
5. After 1 h, the cells are already attached to the plates. Carefully wash the non-adherent cells with warm PBS (*see* **Note 2**).
6. Add 10 mL of RMPI 1640 supplemented with 10% FCS to the plates and incubate them at 5 % CO_2 at 37 °C.
7. After 1 day, most part of the cells are detached or easy to detach. Remove the cells from the plate using the cell scraper and transfer to a 50 mL tube.

8. Centrifuge the cells at 250 × *g* for 10 min at 4 °C.
9. Resuspend the cells with the medium that you will use for differentiation. Count and adjust the cell concentration to 1×10^6 cells/mL.

5 Macrophages Differentiation by 60:30:10 Medium

Performing this protocol, about 10–15 % of the whole PBMC will be differentiated to macrophages.

5.1 Materials

- AIM V® Medium (Life Technologies), containing penicillin and streptomycin.
- Iscove's Modified Dulbecco's Medium (IMDM) (Life Technologies), containing penicillin and streptomycin.
- Heat-inactivated AB-Human Serum (HS) (Life Technologies) (*see* **Note 3**).

5.2 Methodology

1. Prepare the 60:30:10 medium. In a sterile flask add 60 % of AIM-V; 30 % IMDM and 10 % of HS.
2. After isolation step as described in **items 2–3**, add 10 mL of the 60:30:10 medium to the plates and incubate in a humidified incubator with 5 % CO_2 at 37 °C.
3. At day 3, remove 5 mL of the supernatant and centrifuge at 250 × *g* for 10 min at 4 °C.
4. Remove the supernatant and resuspend the pellet in 7 mL of 60:30:10 medium. Back the plates to the humidified incubator with 5 % CO_2 at 37 °C.
5. At day 7, the cells are already differentiated in macrophages and are strongly attached to the plastic.
6. To detach the cells. Remove the medium and add 10 mL of cold PBS. Place the plates on ice for 30 min. By using a cell scraper, gently scrape the cells off the plate (*see* **Note 4**).
7. Centrifuge the cells at 250 × *g* for 5 min. Resuspend in RPMI/5 % FCS and plate according to the protocol required for the experiment.

6 Macrophages Differentiation by Growth Factors (GM-CSF or M-CSF)

Human macrophages can be differentiated from monocytes by using GM-CSF or M-CSF. However, the treatment with GM-CSF or M-CSF may generate different macrophage phenotype. The use of GM-CSF will differentiate macrophages to M1 phenotype and M-CSF to M2 phenotype [7, 8].

6.1 Materials

- RPMI 1640 (containing penicillin, streptomycin, and 2 mM glutamine).
- Human recombinant GM-CSF or human recombinant M-CSF.
- Heat-inactivated FCS.

6.2 Methodology

1. After isolation protocol according to **items 2–3**, add 10 mL of RPMI 1640 supplemented with 10% FCS and GM-CSF (10 ng/mL) for M1 or M-CSF (10 ng/mL) for M2.
2. At day 3, remove 5 mL of the supernatant and centrifuge at 250 ×*g* for 10 min at 4 °C.
3. Resuspend the pellet in 7 mL of RPMI 1640 supplemented with FCS and GM-CSF (10 ng/mL) or M-CSF (10 ng/mL) and transfer to the plate.
4. At day 7, the cells are already differentiated in macrophages and are strongly attached to the plastic.
5. To detach the cells. Remove the medium and add 10 mL of cold PBS. Place the plates on ice for 30 min. By using a cell scraper, gently scrape the cells off the plate (*see* **Note 4**).
6. Centrifuge the cells at 250 ×*g* for 5 min. Resuspend in RPMI/5 % FCS and plate according to the protocol required for the experiment.

7 Macrophages Differentiation Using Total PBMC

7.1 Materials

- RPMI 1640 (containing penicillin, streptomycin, and 2 mM glutamine).
- Heat-inactivated FCS.
- tissue culture petri dishes P100.
- PBS, pH 7.2.
- Cell scraper.

7.2 Methodology

1. After the PBMC isolation protocol, according to **item 2**, add 10 mL of RPMI 1640 supplemented with 15% FCS. Count and adjust the cell concentration to 1×10^7 cells/mL.
2. Place 10 mL of the cell suspension in tissue culture petri dishes P100. Do not remove the non-adherent cells.
3. Incubate the plates in a humidified incubator with 5 % CO_2 at 37 °C.
4. Change the medium for a new fresh RPMI/15 % FCS after 2 and 4 days.
5. At day 6, the cells are already differentiated into macrophages and are strongly attached to the plastic.

6. To detach the cells. Remove the medium and add 10 mL of cold PBS. Place the plates with cells and PBS on ice for 30 min. By using a cell scraper, gently scrape the cells off the plate (*see* **Note 4**).
7. Centrifuge the cells at 250×*g* for 5 min. Resuspend in RPMI/5 % FCS and plate according to the protocol required for the experiment.

8 Macrophage Polarization to M1 or M2

M1 and M2 macrophages can be obtained in vitro by differentiation according to **item 6** or by treatment with different cytokines.

1. Differentiate the macrophages according to one of the protocols described above (**item 5 or 6**).
2. Change the medium for a new fresh RMPI 1640 supplemented with FCS 10 %.
3. M1 macrophages can be obtained by treatment with LPS 10 ng/mL and 5 U/mL of human recombinant interferon-γ (IFN-γ).
4. M2 macrophages are obtained by treatment with human recombinant IL-4 (20 ng/mL).
5. Incubate the cells for 24 h, at 37 °C, 5 % CO_2.
6. Remove the supernatant and change the medium for new fresh RPMI160/5 % FCS.
7. After 24 h start the experiments according to your protocol.

Human macrophages can be identified by specific expression of a number of proteins including CD14, CD11b, CD68, and MAC-1/MAC-3 by flow cytometry or by immunohistochemistry.

M1 or M2 macrophages might be identified according to Table 1:

9 Notes

1. The centrifugation temperature is very important to the gradient formation.
2. The monocytes will attach to the plates in approximately 1 h. After this time they will detach spontaneously. After isolation, you can proceed to one of the differentiation protocols described here. However, if you want to differentiate the cells in small plates (e.g., 6- or 24-well plates), after washing the cells with warm PBS, add 10 mL of RPMI1640/FCS 10 % and incubate at 37 °C and 5 % CO_2 overnight. After this time, the monocytes are floating in the supernatant. Using a cell

Table 1
Human macrophage phenotype markers

	M1	M2	References
CD163	↓	↑	[2, 9]
Mannose receptor (CD206)	↓	↑	[2, 9]
AMAC1 (CCL-18)	↓	↑	[2, 9]
IL-10	↓	↑	[2, 3]
TNFα	↑	↓	[10]
iNOS	↑	↓	[11]
IL-12	↑	↓	[10]
IL-6	↑	↓	[12]
MCP-1 (CCL2)	↑	↓	[2]

scraper, detach the cells that remained attached. Centrifuge at 250 × *g* for 5 min, 4 °C. Count the cells, plate and proceed according to the differentiation protocol of your choice.

3. The human serum can be acquired from different companies. However if you get human serum from blood donors, try to make a pool of different donors to avoid differences between differentiated cells. Before use, heat it in a water bath at 56 °C for 30 min.
4. Try to move the cell scraper in only one direction. Movements in several directions may decrease the cell viability.

References

1. Auffray C, Sieweke MH, Geissmann F (2009) Blood monocytes: development, heterogeneity, and relationship with dendritic cells. Annu Rev Immunol 27: 669–692
2. Bouhlel MA, Derudas B, Rigamonti E, Dievart R, Brozek J, Haulon S et al (2007) PPARgamma activation primes human monocytes into alternative M2 macrophages with anti-inflammatory properties. Cell Metab 6(2):137–143
3. Mosser DM, Edwards JP (2008) Exploring the full spectrum of macrophage activation. Nat Rev Immunol 8(12):958–969
4. Yan ZQ, Hansson GK (2007) Innate immunity, macrophage activation, and atherosclerosis. Immunol Rev 219:187–203
5. Koppaka S, Kehlenbrink S, Carey M, Li W, Sanchez E, Lee DE et al (2013) Reduced adipose tissue macrophage content is associated with improved insulin sensitivity in thiazolidinedione-treated diabetic humans. Diabetes 62(6):1843–1854
6. Savai R, Pullamsetti SS, Kolbe J, Bieniek E, Voswinckel R, Fink L et al (2012) Immune and inflammatory cell involvement in the pathology of idiopathic pulmonary arterial hypertension. Am J Respir Crit Care Med 186(9):897–908
7. Sierra-Filardi E, Vega MA, Sanchez-Mateos P, Corbi AL, Puig-Kroger A (2010) Heme oxygenase-1 expression in M-CSF-polarized M2 macrophages contributes to LPS-induced IL-10 release. Immunobiology 215(9-10):788–795
8. Martinez FO, Gordon S, Locati M, Mantovani A (2006) Transcriptional profiling of the human monocyte-to-macrophage differentiation and polarization: new molecules and patterns of gene expression. J Immunol 177(10):7303–7311

9. Mantovani A, Sica A, Sozzani S, Allavena P, Vecchi A, Locati M (2004) The chemokine system in diverse forms of macrophage activation and polarization. Trends Immunol 25(12):677–686
10. Mantovani A, Sica A, Locati M (2005) Macrophage polarization comes of age. Immunity 23(4):344–346
11. Martinez FO, Helming L, Gordon S (2009) Alternative activation of macrophages: an immunologic functional perspective. Annu Rev Immunol 27:451–483
12. Sica A, Mantovani A (2012) Macrophage plasticity and polarization: in vivo veritas. J Clin Invest 122(3):787–795

Chapter 25

Isolation of Immune Cells for Adoptive Transfer

Tlili Barhoumi, Pierre Paradis, Koren K. Mann, and Ernesto L. Schiffrin

Abstract

Adoptive transfer of T lymphocytes is a useful technique to characterize the role of the immune system in hypertension and vascular disease. Here we describe as an example the isolation of splenic T regulatory cells from donor mice processed to obtain a single cell suspension, followed by negative and positive selection to obtain $CD4^+$ T cells and $CD4^+CD25^+$ Treg cells, respectively. Treg cells can be subsequently transferred to recipient animals.

Key words Adoptive transfer, $CD4^+CD25^+$ Treg cells, T Cells, Magnetic beads, Flow cytometry, Intravenous injection, Immunofluorescence

1 Introduction

Low-grade inflammation plays an important role in the pathogenesis of cardiovascular disease including hypertension [1–3]. Both innate and adaptive immune responses have been shown to participate in mechanisms that contribute to low-grade inflammation associated with the development of hypertension and vascular injury [4–11]. Many of the advances in our understanding of the role of the adaptive immune system in the development of hypertension and vascular damage were made possible through the use of adoptive transfer of immune cells such as T and B lymphocytes into *recombination activating gene 1* knockout (*Rag1−/−*) mice that are deficient in T and B cells or T regulatory lymphocytes (Treg) into wild-type mice [4, 6, 7, 11]. Adoptive transfer of T, but not B lymphocytes, restored angiotensin II- and deoxycorticosterone acetate (DOCA)/salt-induced hypertension and vascular injury [6]. Adoptive transfer of Treg into mice prevented angiotensin II and aldosterone-induced hypertension or vascular injury [4, 7, 11].

In this chapter, we present the method used to prepare and perform adoptive transfer of Treg into mice. $CD4^+CD25^+$ lymphocytes highly enriched in Treg can be isolated from the spleen of wild-type C57BL/6 mice with magnetic beads using a $CD4^+$ T

Rhian M. Touyz and Ernesto L. Schiffrin (eds.), *Hypertension: Methods and Protocols*, Methods in Molecular Biology, vol. 1527, DOI 10.1007/978-1-4939-6625-7_25, © Springer Science+Business Media LLC 2017

lymphocyte negative selection, followed by a $CD25^{+}$ T lymphocyte positive selection (Fig. 1). $CD4^{+}CD25^{-}$ lymphocytes can also be collected from the spleen and used as control cells for the adoptive transfer. Purity of isolated Treg is confirmed by flow cytometry (Fig. 2). Mice are injected via the tail vein with the vehicle, Treg or $CD4^{+}CD25^{-}$ control cells. The efficiency of the Treg adoptive transfer is confirmed by determining the number of cells positive for forkhead box P3 (FOXP3), a marker of Treg, in the renal cortex by immunofluorescence.

2 Materials

2.1 Instruments

1. Small animal anesthesia machine.
2. Dissecting tools.
3. Tissue culture hood.
4. Sterile forceps.
5. Pipet Aid Xp (Falcon).
6. Centrifuge 5804 with swinging bucket rotor A-4-44 and adapter for 5 and 50 mL Eppendorf tubes.
7. A set of 10, 20, 200, and 1000 μL pipettes.
8. Improved Bright-line Neubauer Hemocytometer (La Fontaine).
9. Mini Spin plus centrifuge with fixed angle rotor (Eppendorf).
10. Purple *EasySep* Magnet (STEMCELL Technologies).
11. Basic flow cytometer: FACS *Calibur* flow cytometer (Becton Dickinson), equipped with 488 and 633 nm excitation lasers and appropriate bandpass filters.
12. Multicolor flow cytometer: BD LSR Fortessa (Becton Dickinson), equipped 405, 488, 561, and 640 nm lasers and appropriate bandpass filters.
13. FlowJo V7 (Tree Star) flow cytometry analysis software.
14. Mouse cages with wire bar lids.
15. Infrared heat lamp.
16. Mouse restrainer for tail vein injection.
17. Wheaton staining dish.
18. Shandon Sequenza™ Slide Rack (Thermo Scientific, Anatomical Pathology).
19. Shandon coverplate™ (Thermo Scientific, Anatomical Pathology).
20. Fluorescent microscope with appropriate filters, camera, and capture software.
21. ImageJ software (National Institutes of Health, http://rsbweb.nih.gov/ij/index.html).

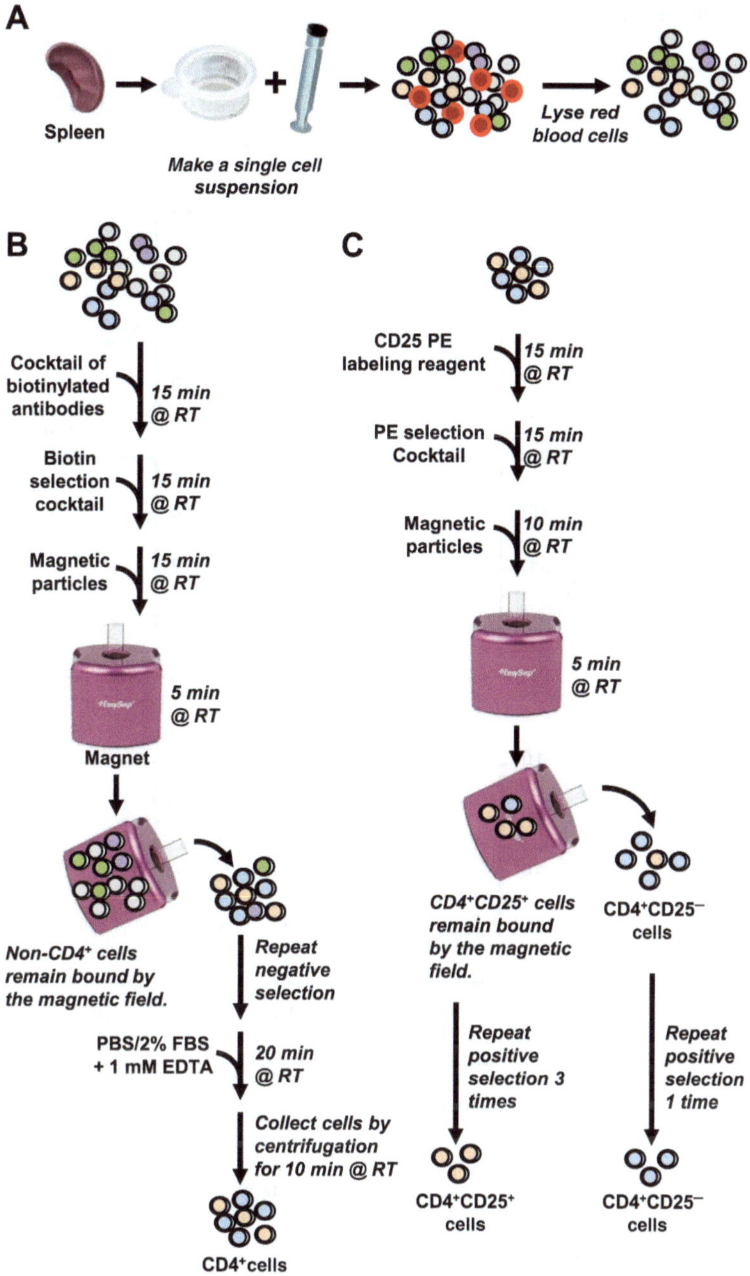

Fig. 1 Isolation of $CD4^+CD25^+$ highly enriched in T regulatory cells (Treg) and $CD4^+CD25^-$ lymphocytes. (**a**) Single splenocytes are obtained by releasing the splenocytes by forcing fragments of spleen through a 70 μm nylon mesh cell strainer with the back of a sterile 3 mL syringe plunger. Red blood cells are eliminated using the Red Blood Cell lysis buffer. (**b**) $CD4^+$ cells are obtained by negative selection by incubating splenocytes sequentially with the cocktail of biotinylated monoclonal antibodies directed against cell surface antigens on mouse cells of hematopoietic origin, with the biotin selection cocktail constituted of bispecific Tetrametric Antibody Complexes recognizing both dextran and biotin following with magnetic dextran iron particles. Magnetically labeled cells are separated from the $CD4^+$ cells using a magnet. The $CD4^+$ cells are collected by centrifugation and resuspended in PBS/5 % FBS. (**c**) $CD4^+CD25^+$ cells are purified by positive selection by incubating sequentially $CD4^+$ cells with phycoerythrin (PE)-conjugated anti-CD25 antibody, with the PE selection cocktail constituted of bispecific tetrameric antibody complexes recognizing both dextran and PE following with magnetic dextran iron particles. Magnetically labeled $CD4^+CD25^+$ cells are separated from the $CD4^+CD25^-$ cells using a magnet. $CD4^+CD25^+$ cells are collected by removing the tube from the magnet and $CD4^+CD25^-$ cells by centrifugation

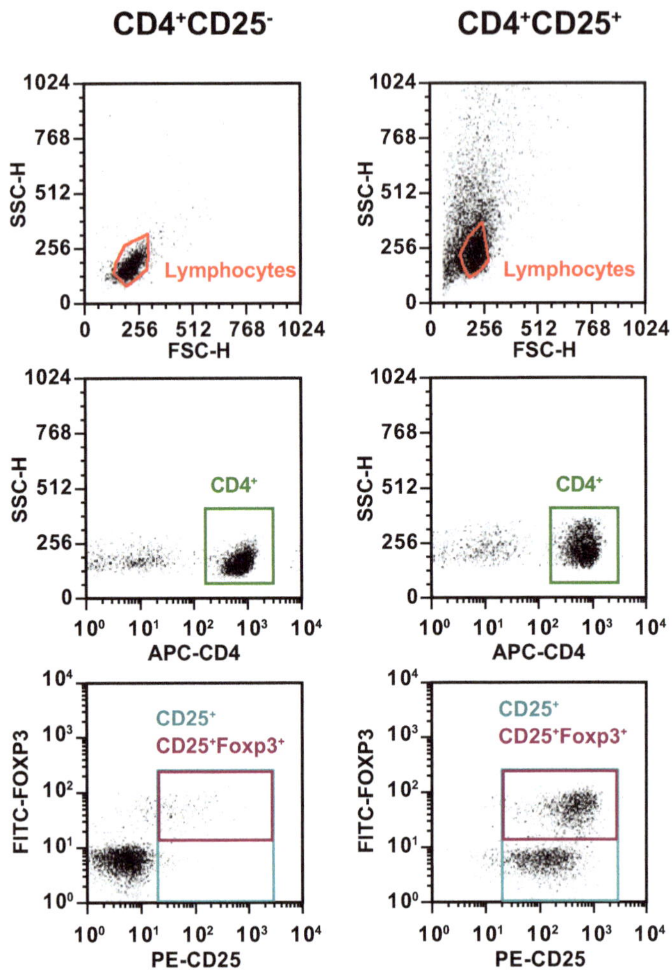

Gate	CD4+CD25+	CD4+CD25-	Reference gate
	(% of gated)		
CD4+	82.3	86.5	Lymphocytes
CD4+CD25+	96.6	5.3	CD4+
CD4+CD25+Foxp3+	44.2	4.0	CD4+

Fig. 2 Flow cytometry profile of CD4+CD25− and CD4+CD25+ cells. Cells are separated using CD4+ T cell negative selection followed by CD25+ T cell positive selection of splenocytes, stained with APC-conjugated anti-mouse CD4, PE-conjugated anti-mouse CD25 and FITC-conjugated anti-mouse Foxp3 antibodies, and analyzed by flow cytometry. APC are analyzed using a 633 nm excitation laser with a 661/16 bandpass filter; PE was excited with a 488 nm laser with 585/42 bandpass filter and FITC signal are excited at 488 nm and collected with a 530/30 bandpass filter. Lymphocytes are gated in the side scatter-height (SSC-H)/forward scatter (FSC)-H plot. Using the SSC-H/CD4 plot, CD4+ cells are gated. Gated CD4+ cells are further characterized for CD25 and FOXP3 expression. A representative flow cytometry gating procedure and the % of CD4+ cells in lymphocytes, % of CD4+CD25+ cells in CD4+ cells and % of CD4+CD25+FOXP3+ cells in CD4+ cells are presented for CD4+CD25− and CD4+CD25+ cells

2.2 Reagents

1. Isoflurane.
2. Oxygen gas (O_2).
3. Fifty mL Falcon tubes.
4. Phosphate buffered saline pH 7.4, Ca^{2+} and Mg^{2+} free (PBS, Life Technologies).
5. Fetal bovine serum, Qualified, Canada origin (FBS, Life Technologies).
6. PBS supplemented with 5 % FBS (PBS/5 % FBS).
7. Sterile 100 mm petri dish.
8. Feather disposable scalpel (Fisher Scientific).
9. BD Falcon cell strainer, 70 μm nylon mesh (Fisher Scientific).
10. Sterile 0.5 and 3 mL syringe.
11. Five and ten mL serological pipette (Falcon).
12. Ten, 20, 200 and 1000 μL pipette tips.
13. Red Blood Cell Lysing Buffer Hybri-Max (RBC lysis buffer, Sigma-Aldrich).
14. Trypan Blue Stain 0.4 % (Life Technologies).
15. *EasySep®* mouse $CD4^+CD25^+$ regulatory T cell isolation Kit (Stem Cell Technologies) that is constituted of two kits: *EasySep®* mouse $CD4^+$ T cell pre-enrichment kit and the *EasySep®* mouse $CD25^+$ Positive Selection Kit. *EasySep®* mouse $CD4^+$ T cell pre-enrichment kit contains Mouse $CD4^+$ T cell pre-enrichment cocktail, biotin selection cocktail, D magnetic particles, blocking solution and normal rat serum (NRS). The *EasySep®* mouse $CD25^+$ Positive Selection Kit contains PE selection cocktail, Special Application (SA) magnetic nanoparticles and mouse CD25 PE labeling reagent.
16. PBS supplemented with 5% FBS and 2% NRS (PBS/5% FBS/5 % NRS).
17. Five mL 12×75 mm polystyrene round-bottom tubes (BD Falcon).
18. Antibodies for flow cytometry with basic or multicolor flow cytometer are presented in Table 1 and 5, respectively. Determine the dilution of antibodies in a previous experiment (*see* **Note 1**). A representative example of antibody titration is show in Fig. 3. Prepare stocks of pre-diluted antibodies in PBS/5 % FBS and store at 4 °C in the dark.
19. Fc blocking reagent: rat anti-mouse CD16/CD32 Fc-Block (clone 2.4G2, 0.5 mg/mL, BD Biosciences) diluted 1/50 in FBS/5 % FBS.
20. FOXP3 Fixation/Permeabilization Concentrate and Diluent Kit (eBiosciences). This kit contains two components: Fixation/Permeabilization Concentrate (4×) and Fixation/Permeabilization Diluent. The Fixation/Permeabilization

Table 1
Antibodies for flow cytometry with basic equipment

Antibodies	Description	Clone, company
CD4	APC-conjugated rat anti-mouse CD4 antibody	RM4-5, BD Bioscience
CD4 isotype	APC-conjugated rat IgG2a κ isotype control antibody	R35-95, BD Bioscience
CD25	PE-conjugated rat anti-mouse CD25 antibody	PC61, BD Bioscience
CD25 isotype	PE-conjugated rat IgG1 κ isotype control antibody	A110-1, BD Bioscience
FOXP3	FITC-conjugated rat anti-mouse Foxp3 antibody	FJK16s, BD Bioscience
FOXP3 isotype	FITC-conjugated rat IgG2a κ isotype control antibody	A95-1, eBioscience

APC allophycocyanin, *BD* Becton Dickinson, *FITC* Fluorescein, *FOXP3* PE, transcription factor X-linked forkhead/winged helix, *PE* phycoerythrin

working solution is prepared by diluting one part of Fixation/Permeabilization Concentrate in three part of Fixation/Permeabilization diluent.

21. Live/dead dye: Dilute enough Fixable Viability Dye eFluor® 506 (eBioscience) 1:50 in PBS to stain cells of all tubes except the unstained tube.
22. BD PrecisionGlide needles, 26 G × 5/8 in (BD).
23. Polypropylene micro tubes, 0.5 mL (Sarstedt).
24. Sterile 2 × 2 gauzes.
25. Microscope Slides VWR® Superfrost Micro Slides 75 × 25 mm (VWR international).
26. Coverslips. Fisherbrand cover glasses no. 1, rectangle 50 × 24 mm (Fisher Scientific).
27. Fisherbrand Foam-lined 100-place slide Boxes (Fisher Scientific).
28. Acetone–methanol (1:1) mixture, −20 °C. At least 1 h before doing immunostaining, combine one part of acetone with one part of methanol in a bottle resistant to acetone. Bring down the mixture temperature to −20 °C by storing the bottle in a freezer for at least 1 h.
29. PBS containing 0.1 % Tween 20 (PBST).
30. Normal goat serum (NGS, Jackson Immuno Research).
31. PBST/10 % NGS is PBST containing 10 % normal goat serum.
32. Rabbit anti-Foxp3 antibody (1.3 mg/mL, Abcam). The antibody is diluted 1:500 in PBST/10 % NGS.
33. Alexa Fluor 555-conjugated goat anti-rabbit antibody (Invitrogen Corp). The antibody is diluted 1:200 in PBST/10 % NGS.
34. Vectashield mounting medium containing 4′,6-diamidino-2-phenylindole (DAPI, Vector Laboratories).

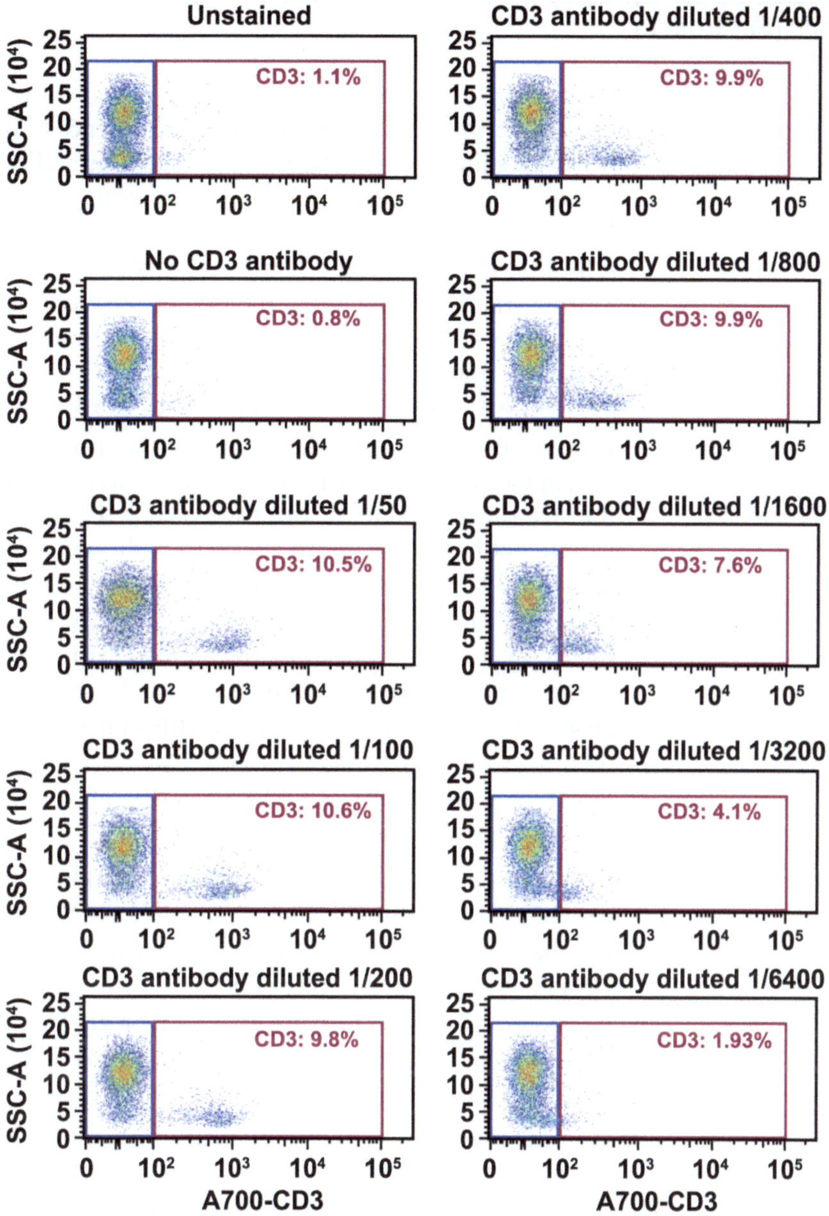

Fig. 3 Example of antibody titration. Splenocytes stained with Fixable Viability Dye eFluor® 506 (e506) without or with serial dilution of Alexa Fluor® 700 (A700)-conjugated anti-mouse CD3 antibody, are analyzed by flow cytometry. Fluorophores are respectively excited and analyzed with appropriate laser and bandpass filter (BP) (e506: 405 nm with 525/50 BP, A700: 640 nm with 730/45 BP). The lymphocyte gate is identify by the side scatter (SSC)/forward scatter (FSC) plot. Singlet lymphocytes are gated using FSC height (FSC-H) over FSC area (FSC-A). Live lymphocytes are gated on the viability dye/FSC-A plot. $CD3^+$ cells are gated on the SSC-A/CD3 plot. The A700-CD3 antibody titration indicates that the optimal antibody dilution is 1/400. Optimal staining is found at the lowest dilution giving a distinct separate population of positively stained cells

3 Methods (*See* Note 2)

3.1 Single Splenocyte Suspension

1. Anesthetize a mouse with 3% isoflurane mixed with O_2 at 1 L/mL and verify depth of anesthesia by the absence of reaction to rear foot squeezing (*see* **Note 3**). Dissect out and transfer the spleen to a sterile 50 mL Falcon tube containing 30 mL of PBS/5% FBS stored on ice. Kill the mouse by exsanguination. Repeat the operation with another mouse (*see* **Note 4**).
2. Transfer the tube containing the two spleens to a sterile tissue culture hood. Transfer the spleens to a 100 mm sterile petri dish using a sterile forceps. Remove necrotic tissues with a scalpel (*see* **Note 4**) and cut each spleen into 3–4 fragments.
3. Place a 70 μm nylon mesh cell strainer over a 50 mL Falcon tube, pipette 0.5 mL of PBS/5% FBS to wet the strainer and transfer the fragments of the two spleens to the cell strainer with a sterile forceps. Wash the Petri dish with 0.5–1 mL of PBS/5% FBS and transfer the liquid to the cell strainer.
4. Using up and down motion, gently press the fragments of spleen against the bottom of the strainer with the back of a sterile 3 mL syringe plunger to macerate the spleen pieces and push cells through the nylon mesh. It is important to be careful not to damage the cells (*see* **Note 5**).
5. Pipette 0.5 mL of PBS/5% FBS onto the cell strainer to flush the cells through the nylon mesh.
6. Repeat the two previous steps until only the splenic connective tissue remains in the cell strainer. Remove the strainer.
7. Fill the tube with PBS/5% FBS and centrifuge at $300\times g$ for 10 min at room temperature (RT).
8. Resuspend the pellet in 5 mL/spleen of RBC lysis buffer (*see* **Note 6**) and incubate at RT for 3 min with occasional gentle mixing by tilting the tube 3–4 times.
9. Stop the reaction by diluting the RBC lysis buffer with 3 volumes (30 mL) of PBS/5% FBS.
10. Filter the cells through a 70 μm nylon mesh cell strainer placed over a 50 mL tube.
11. Centrifuge the cells at $300\times g$ for 5 min at RT, carefully decant the supernatant and resuspend the pellet in 2 mL of PBS/5% FBS.
12. Count splenocytes using a hemacytometer with trypan blue to assess the percentage of live cells. Dilute 50 μL of cell suspension with 50 μL of trypan blue and incubate for 1 min at RT. Splenocytes are counted. Calculate the % of live white cells (*see* **Note 7**). The count of live white cells is used for the next step.
13. Save 2×10^6 splenocytes on ice for flow cytometry study.

3.2 Isolation of Treg

$CD4^+CD25^+$ cells (Treg) are isolated through $CD4^+$ T cell negative selection followed by a $CD25^+$ T cell positive selection of splenocytes using *EasySep*® Mouse $CD4^+$ T Cell Pre-Enrichment and CD25 Positive Selection Kits with minor changes as follows.

3.2.1 $CD4^+$ T Cell Negative Selection

1. Dilute the single white cell suspension to a concentration of $1–1.5 \times 10^8$ cells/mL with PBS/5 % FBS/5 % NRS in a sterile 5 mL polystyrene tube (*see* **Note 8**). The final volume should be between 0.5 and 1.2 mL.
2. Centrifuge the tube of *EasySep*® $CD4^+$ pre-enrichment cocktail of biotinylated monoclonal antibodies at $12{,}000 \times g$ for 20 s at RT before use to remove liquid stuck in the lid. Add 50 μL of *EasySep*® $CD4^+$ pre-enrichment cocktail per mL of cell suspension, mix by gently pipetting up and down 2–3 times, and incubate for 15 min at RT (*see* **Note 9**).
3. Add 150 μL of EasySep® biotin selection cocktail at per mL of cell suspension, mix by gently pipetting up and down 2–3 times and incubate for 15 min at RT. This cocktail contains antibodies directed against biotin and dextran (*see* **Note 10**).
4. Vortex the *EasySep*® D magnetic particles for 30 s to ensure uniform suspension of particles with no visible aggregates. Add 150 μL of *EasySep*® D magnetic particles per mL of cell suspension, mix by gently pipetting up and down 2–3 times and incubate at RT for 10 min (*see* **Note 11**).
5. Bring total volume of the cell suspension to 2.5 mL with PBS/5 % FBS. Mix the cells by gently pipetting up and down 2–3 times with a serological pipette (*see* **Note 12**).
6. Place the tube without lid into the purple *EasySep*® magnet and incubate for 5 min at RT.
7. Pick up the magnet, and in one continuous motion, invert the magnet and tube and pour off the cell suspension enriched in $CD4^+$ lymphocytes into a new 5 mL polystyrene tube. Keep the magnet and the tube inverted for 2–3 s, and then return to the upright position in one continuous motion. Do not shake or blot off any drops that may remain hanging from the mouth of the tube (*see* **Note 13**). Discard this tube containing unwanted non-$CD4^+$ cells.
8. Add 100 μL of *EasySep*® blocking solution to the $CD4^+$ enriched cell suspension, mix by gently pipetting up and down 2–3 times and place the tube inside the magnet to perform a second round of magnetic separation. Incubate for 5 min at RT and repeat the previous step (*see* **Note 14**).
9. Repeat **steps 5**–**7** one more time.
10. Wash the $CD4^+$ enriched cells as follows. Adjust the volume of the new tube to 4 mL with PBS/5 % FBS and centrifuge the $CD4^+$ enriched cells at $250 \times g$ for 10 min at RT.

11. Remove supernatant and resuspend the cells in 4 mL of PBS/5 % FBS and centrifuge again at 250 × *g* for 10 min at RT.
12. Remove the supernatant and resuspend cells in 4 mL of PBS/5 % FBS. Incubate for 20 min at RT.
13. Centrifuge at 250 × g for 10 min at RT. Resuspend the cells in 1 mL of PBS/5 % FBS.
14. Count the $CD4^+$ enriched cells using a hemacytometer with trypan blue to assess the percent of live cells. Dilute 50 μL of cell suspension with 50 μL of trypan blue and incubate for 1 min at RT. Alive and dead cells are counted. Calculate the percent of live cells (*see* **Note 7**). The count of live $CD4^+$ enriched cells is used for the next step.
15. Dilute $CD4^+$ enriched cells to a concentration of 5×10^7 cells/mL in PBS/5 % FBS and proceed to $CD25^+$ cell selection. The final volume should be between 0.5 and 1.2 mL.

3.2.2 $CD25^+$ T Cells Positive Selection

1. Add 50 μL of *EasySep®* CD25 PE labeling reagent per mL of cells, mix by gently pipetting up and down 2–3 times and incubate for 15 min at RT (*see* **Note 15**).
2. Add 33 μL of *EasySep®* PE selection cocktail per mL of cells, mix by gently pipetting up and down 2–3 times and incubate at RT for 15 min (*see* **Note 16**).
3. Mix *EasySep®* special application (SA) magnetic nanoparticles by pipetting vigorously up and down 5–6 times to ensure uniform suspension (*see* **Note 17**). Add 50 μL of SA magnetic nanoparticles at per mL of cells, mix by gently pipetting up and down 2–3 times and incubate at RT for 10 min.
4. Adjust the total volume of the cell suspension to 2.5 mL with PBS/5 % FBS. Mix the cells by gently pipetting up and down 2–3 times, then place the tube without lid into the magnet and incubate for 5 min at RT.
5. Pick up the magnet and in one continuous motion, invert the magnet and the tube, and pour off the supernatant fraction containing the $CD4^+CD25^-$ cells into a new 5 mL polystyrene tube. The magnetically labeled, $CD4^+CD25^+$ Treg cells remain inside the tube held by the magnetic field of the magnet. Keep the magnet and the tube inverted for 2–3 s and then return to the upright position in one continuous motion. Do not shake or blot off any drops that may remain hanging from the mouth of the tube. Save the collecting tube containing $CD4^+CD25^-$ enriched cells (*see* **Note 18**).
6. Remove the tube from the magnet and add 2.5 mL of PBS/5 % FBS and mix the cell suspension by gently pipetting up and down 2–3 times and place the tube containing back in the magnet and incubate for 5 min at RT.

7. Repeat the two previous steps twice and **step 6** once more.
8. Remove the tube from the magnet and resuspend cells in 500 μL of PBS/5 % FBS.
9. Purifiy further the $CD4^+CD25^-$ cells obtained at **step 5** by placing the tube containing the $CD4^+CD25^-$ cells into the magnet and incubate for 10 min at RT.
10. Pick up the magnet and in one continuous motion, invert the magnet and the tube, and pour off the supernatant fraction containing the $CD4^+CD25^-$ cells into a new 5 mL polystyrene tube. The cells are ready to use.
11. Count the $CD4^+CD25^+$ and $CD4^+CD25^-$ enriched cells using a hemacytometer with trypan blue to assess percent live cells. Dilute 50 μL of cell suspension with 50 μL of trypan blue and incubate for 1 min at RT. Count live and dead cells and calculate the percent of live cells (*see* **Note 7**). The count of live $CD4^+CD25^+$ and $CD4^+CD25^-$ cells is used for the next step. It is expected to obtain between $5–6 \times 10^5$ $CD4^+CD25^+$ and up to 2×10^6 $CD4^+CD25^-$ cells from the two spleens.
12. The $CD4^+CD25^+$ and $CD4^+CD25^-$ cells are ready for flow cytometry or tail vein injection.

3.3 Confirmation of the Purity of Isolated Treg by Flow Cytometry

The purity of *EasySep®* prepared $CD4^+CD25^+$ and $CD4^+CD25^-$ cells is assessed by flow cytometry. The protocol described in Subheading 3.3.1 is designed for the average user of flow cytometry with basic equipment. However, if a multicolor flow cytometer is available, it is recommended to perform the more detailed analysis of the Treg population described in Subheading 3.3.2. This can be accomplished using dyes for live/dead, incorporating a more extensive panel of antibodies and using fluorescence minus one (FMO) gating protocols .

3.3.1 Protocol for Flow Cytometry with Basic Equipment

Preparation of Cells for Flow Cytometry with Basic Equipment

Several flow cytometry control tubes should be prepared: unstained, isotype, and compensation controls (*see* **Note 19**). Unstained samples containing unlabelled splenocytes and isotype controls containing splenocytes stained with isotype-matched, nonspecific antibodies are run to determine the background fluorescence. Compensation tubes stained with a single fluorophore are used to correct for fluorescence spillover. In addition, two other tubes are prepared with one tube containing $CD4^+CD25^+$ cells and one tube containing $CD4^+CD25^-$ cells. Table 1 presents the list of antibodies. The distribution of cells is described in Table 2. The distribution of antibodies is presented in Tables 3 and 4.

1. Distribute 2×10^5 cells per 0.5 mL micro tubes as follows.
   (a) Prepare five control tubes using splenocytes obtained as in Subheading 3.1 as follows. Dilute splenocytes to 4×10^7 mL^{-1} in PBS/5 % FBS. Mix gently by pipetting up

and down 2–3 times and distribute 5 μL of splenocytes to the unstained, isotype, and compensation control tubes (Table 2).

(b) Prepare suspensions of 4×10^7/mL of *EasySep®* separated $CD4^+CD25^+$ and $CD4^+CD25^-$ as above and distribute 5 μL of cell suspension to their respective microtubes (Table 1).

2. Add 25 μL of Fc blocking reagent to each tube. Mix gently by pipetting up and down 2–3 times.
3. Block Fc-gamma receptors by incubating the tubes for 30 min at 4 °C (*see* **Note 20**).
4. Prepare enough mixture of antibodies for all experiments of the week by combining pre-diluted CD4 and/or CD25 antibodies and isotype antibodies with PBS/5 % FBS respecting the proportions depicted in Table 3 (*see* **Note 1**). Store the antibody mixtures at 4 °C in the dark. *For this step and all the following steps, it is important to protect tubes from light (see* Note 15*).*
5. Add 25 μL of PBS/5 % FBS or mixture of antibodies to appropriate tubes as indicated in Table 3 (*see* **Note 21**).
6. Mix gently by pipetting up and down 2–3 times and incubate for 30 min at 4 °C.
7. Transfer the cells to 5 mL polystyrene tubes.
8. Wash the cells by adding 1 mL of PBS/5 % FBS and centrifuge at 300 × *g* for 5 min at RT.
9. Aspirate the supernatant and resuspend the cells in 100 μL of PBS/5 % FBS.

Table 2

Cells to prepare for flow cytometry with basic equipment

	Tubes						
			Compensation			Samples	
Cells	Unstained	Isotypes	1	2	3	$CD4^+CD25^+$	$CD4^+CD25^-$
Splenocytes (μL)	5	5	5	5	5		
$CD4^+CD25^+$ (μL)						5	
$CD4^+CD25^-$ (μL)							5

Prepare a splenocyte suspension containing 4×10^7 mL^{-1} of splenocytes, $CD4^+CD25^+$ and $CD4^+CD25^-$ lymphocytes (2×10^5 cells/5 μL). Distribute 5 μL splenocytes suspension to the tubes shaded in gray and $CD4^+CD25^+$ and $CD4^+CD25^-$ lymphocyte suspension to the $CD4^+CD25^+$ and $CD4^+CD25^-$ sample tubes, respectively

Table 3
Anti-CD4 and CD25 antibodies and isotype antibody mixtures for the flow cytometry with basic equipment

	Tubes						
Reagents	Unstained	Isotypes	Compensations			Samples	
			1	2	3	$CD4^+CD25^+$	$CD4^+CD25^-$
APC-anti-CD4 antibody (μL)			1			1	1
APC-CD4 isotype antibody (μL)		1		1	1		
PE-anti-CD25 antibody (μL)				1		1	1
PE-CD25 isotype antibody (μL)		1	1		1		
PBS/5 % FBS (μL)	25	23	23	23	23	23	23

This table presents the volume of PBS/5 % FBS and pre-diluted isotypes, anti-CD4 and/or CD25 antibodies to combine per tube. Prepare enough mixtures of antibodies for all the experiments of the week. Store these antibody mixtures at 4 °C in the dark. After blocking Fc-gamma receptors, distribute 25 μL of appropriate antibody mixture according to the table above

10. Fix and permeabilize the cells by adding 900 μL of Foxp3 Fixation/Permeabilization working solution to each tube. Mix gently up and down 2–3 times and incubate for 30 min at 4 °C.
11. Add 2 mL of PBS/5 % FBS and mix gently up and down 2–3 times. Centrifuge at 300 × *g* for 5 min at RT.
12. Aspirate the supernatant and resuspend the cells with 100 μL of PBS/5 % FBS.
13. Add 2 μL of 2 % NRS to block intracellular background staining. Incubate for 15 min at RT.
14. Add the 2 μL of PBS/5 % FBS, isotype antibody or anti-FOXP3 antibody to the tubes as described in Table 4 and incubate for 30 min at 4 °C.
15. Wash the cells by adding 2 mL of PBS/5 % FBS to the cells suspension and mix gently up and down 2–3 times. Centrifuge at 300 × *g* for 5 min at RT.
16. Aspirate the supernatant and resuspend the cells with 300 μL of PBS/5 % FBS and analyze for flow cytometry.

Flow Cytometry with Basic Equipment

The profile of Treg ($CD4^+CD25^+$) and $CD4^+CD25^-$ cells was determined using a *FACSCalibur*™ flow cytometer and the data are analyzed using FlowJo V7 software.

Table 4
FOXP3 antibody and isotype antibody for the flow cytometry with basic equipment

	Tubes						
			Compensations			Samples	
Reagents	Unstained	Isotypes	1	2	3	$CD4^+CD25^+$	$CD4^+CD25^-$
FOXP3 antibody (μL)					2	2	2
FOXP3 isotype antibody (μL)		2	2	2			
PBS/5 % FBS (μL)	2						

After blocking with FOXP3 Fixation/Permeabilization working solution, distribute 2 μL of PBS/5 % FBS, FOXP3 isotype antibody, and anti-FOXP3 antibody according to the table above

1. Using the unstained sample, adjust the side scatter (SSC) and forward scatter (FSC) voltages to locate the cell population and define the lymphocyte population gate. Adjust the photomultiplier tube (PMT) voltage of fluorescence parameters so that the negative populations of CD4, CD25 and FoxP3 are at about first decade (between 10^0 and 10^1 on a 4- to 5-log scale).
2. Run the isotype control tube to determine antibody specificity.
3. Run the CD4, CD25 and FoxP3 single-stained compensation control tubes and correct for spill over (*see* **Note 19**).
4. Acquire samples.
5. Record a minimum of 10^5 events within the lymphocyte gate.
6. Export FCS files and analyze the data with FCS Express software. A representative analysis is presented in Fig. 2.

3.3.2 Protocol for Flow Cytometry with a Multicolor Flow Cytometer

Several flow cytometry control tubes should be prepared: unstained, FMO controls for each fluorophore and compensation controls (*see* **Note 19**). Unstained samples containing unlabelled splenocytes and a series of FMO controls containing splenocytes stained alternatively with the isotype-matched, nonspecific antibody for one of the fluorophores and all the other antibodies are run to determine the background fluorescence. Compensation tubes stained with a single fluorophore are used to correct for fluorescence spillover. In addition, two sample tubes are prepared with one tube containing $CD4^+CD25^+$ cells and one tube containing $CD4^+CD25^-$ cells. Table 5 presents the list of antibodies. The distribution of the cells is described in Table 6. The distribution of antibodies is presented in Tables 7 and 8.

Preparation of Cells for Flow Cytometry a Multicolor Flow Cytometer

1. Distribute 2×10^5 cells per 0.5 mL micro tubes as follows.

Table 5
Antibodies for flow cytometry with a multicolor flow cytometer

Antibodies	Description	Clone, company
CD3	A700-conjugated rat anti-mouse CD3 antibody	17A2, eBioscience
CD3 isotype	A700-conjugated rat IgG2b κ Isotype Control antibody	eB149/10H5, eBioscience
CD4	PerCP-e710-conjugated rat anti-mouse CD4 antibody	RM4-5, eBioscience
CD4 isotype	PerCP-e710-conjugated rat IgG2a κ isotype control antibody	eBR2a, eBioscience
CD8a	APC-e780-conjugated rat anti-mouse-CD8a antibody	53-6.7, eBioscience
CD8a isotype	APC-e780-conjugated rat IgG2a κ isotype control antibody	eBR2a, eBioscience
CD25	e450-conjugated rat anti-mouse-CD25 antibody	PC61.5, eBioscience
CD25 isotype	e450-conjugated rat IgG1 κ isotype control antibody	eBRG1, eBioscience
FOXP3	APC-conjugated rat anti-mouse-FOXP3 antibody	FJK-16s, eBioscience
FOXP3 isotype	APC-conjugated rat IgG2a κ isotype control antibody	eBR2a, eBioscience

A700 Alexa Fluor® 700, *PerCP-e710* PerCP-eFluor® 710, *APC-e780* allophycocyanin-eFluor® 780, *e450* eFluor® 450, *APC* allophycocyanin, *FOXP3* PE, transcription factor X-linked forkhead/winged helix

Table 6
Cells to prepare for flow cytometry with a multicolor flow cytometer

	Tubes												
		FMO					Compensations					Samples	
Cells	Unstained	1	2	3	4	5	1	2	3	4	5	$CD4^{+}CD25^{+}$	$CD4^{+}CD25^{-}$
Splenocytes (μL)	5	5	5	5	5	5	5	5	5	5	5		
$CD4^{+}CD25^{+}$ (μL)												5	
$CD4^{+}CD25^{-}$ (μL)													5

Prepare a splenocyte suspension containing 4×10^7 mL^{-1} of splenocytes, $CD4^{+}CD25^{+}$ and $CD4^{+}CD25^{-}$ lymphocytes (2×10^5 cells/5 μL). Distribute 5 μL of splenocytes suspension to the tubes shaded in gray and $CD4^{+}CD25^{+}$ and $CD4^{+}CD25^{-}$ lymphocyte suspension to the $CD4^{+}CD25^{+}$ and $CD4^{+}CD25^{-}$ sample tubes, respectively

(a) Prepare 11 control tubes using splenocytes obtained in Subheading 3.1 as follows. Dilute splenocytes to 4×10^7 mL^{-1} in PBS (*see* **Note 22**). Mix gently by pipetting up and down 2–3 times and distribute 5 μL of splenocytes to the unstained, FMO, and control tubes (Table 1).

(b) Prepare suspensions of 4×10^7/mL of *EasySep*® separated $CD4^{+}CD25^{+}$ and $CD4^{+}CD25^{-}$ as above and distribute 5 μL of cell suspension to their respective microtubes (Table 6).

Table 7
Anti-CD4 and CD25 antibodies and isotype antibodies mixtures for flow cytometry with a multicolor flow cytometer

	Tubes												
		FMO					Compensations					Samples	
Reagents	Unstained	1	3	3	4	5	1	2	3	4	5	$CD4^{+}CD25^{+}$	$CD4^{+}CD25^{-}$
A700-anti-CD3 antibody (μL)			1	1	1	1	1					1	1
A700-CD3 isotype antibody (μL)		1						1	1	1	1		
PerCP-e710-anti-CD4 antibody (μL)		1		1	1	1		1				1	1
PerCP-e710-CD4 isotype antibody (μL)			1				1		1	1	1		
APC-e780-anti-CD8a antibody (μL)		1	1		1	1			1			1	1
APC-e780-CD8a isotype antibody (μL)				1			1	1		1	1		
e450-anti-CD25 antibody (μL)		1	1	1		1				1		1	1
e450-CD25 isotype antibody (μL)			1		1		1	1	1		1		
PBS/5% FBS (μL)	25	21	21	21	21	21	21	21	21	21	21	21	21

This table presents the volume of PBS/5% FBS and pre-diluted isotypes, anti-CD3, CD4, CD8, and/or CD25 antibodies to combine per tube. Prepare enough mixtures of antibodies for all the experiments of the week. Store these antibody mixtures at 4 °C in the dark. After blocking Fc-gamma receptors, distribute 25 μL of appropriate antibody mixture according to the table above

2. Add 25 μL of PBS to the unstained tube and 25 μL of Live/dead dye to all other tubes. *For this step and all the following steps, it is important to protect the tubes from light (see* Note 15*)*.
3. Incubate for 30 min on ice.
4. Add 100 μL of PBS to each tube and centrifuge at 300 × *g* for 5 min at 4 °C.
5. Aspirate the supernatant and add 25 μL of Fc blocking reagent to each tube. Mix gently by pipetting up and down 2–3 times.

Table 8
FOXP3 antibody and isotype antibody for flow cytometry with a multicolor flow cytometer

	Tubes												
		FMO					Compensations					Samples	
Reagents	Unstained	1	2	3	4	5	1	2	3	4	5	$CD4^+CD25^+$	$CD4^+CD25^-$
APC-anti-FOXP3 antibody (μL)		2	2	2	2						2	2	2
APC-FOXP3 isotype antibody (μL)						2	2	2	2	2			
PBS/5 % FBS (μL)	2												

After blocking with FOXP3 Fixation/Permeabilization working solution, distribute 2 μL of PBS/5 % FBS, FOXP3 isotype antibody, and anti-FOXP3 antibody according to the table above

6. Block Fc-gamma receptors by incubating the tubes for 30 min at 4 °C (*see* **Note 20**).
7. Prepare enough mixtures of antibodies for all the experiments of the week by combining pre-diluted CD3, CD4, CD8, and/or CD25 antibodies and isotype antibodies with PBS/5 % FBS by respecting the proportion described in Table 7 (*see* **Note 1**). Store the antibody mixtures at 4 °C in the dark.
8. Add 25 μL of PBS/5 % FBS to the unstained tube and mixture of antibodies to appropriate tubes as indicated in Table 7 (*see* **Note 21**).
9. Mix gently by pipetting up and down 2–3 times and incubate for 30 min at 4 °C.
10. Transfer the cells to 5 mL polystyrene tubes.
11. Wash the cells by adding 1 mL of PBS/5 % FBS and centrifuge at 300 × *g* for 5 min at RT.
12. Aspirate the supernatant and resuspend the cells in 100 μL of PBS/5 % FBS .
13. Fix and permeabilize the cells by adding 900 μL of Foxp3 Fixation/Permeabilization working solution to each tube. Mix gently up and down 2–3 times and incubate for 30 min at 4 °C.
14. Add 2 mL of PBS/5 % FBS and mix gently up and down 2–3 times. Centrifuge at 300 × *g* for 5 min at RT.
15. Aspirate the supernatant and resuspend the cells with 100 μL of PBS/5 % FBS.
16. Add 2 μL of 2 % NRS to block intracellular background staining. Incubate for 15 min at RT.

17. Add the 2 μL of PBS/5% FBS, FOXP3 isotype antibody or anti-FOXP3 antibody to appropriate tubes as described in Table 8 and incubated for 30 min at 4 °C.
18. Wash the cells by adding 2 mL of PBS/5% FBS to the cells suspension and mix gently up and down 2–3 times. Centrifuge at 300 × *g* for 5 min at RT.
19. Aspirate the supernatant and resuspend the cells with 300 μL of PBS/5% FBS and analyze for flow cytometry.

Flow Cytometry with Multicolor Flow Cytometer

The profile of Treg ($CD4^+CD25^+$) and $CD4^+CD25^-$ cells is determined using a *BD LSR Fortessa* multicolor flow cytometer and the data are analyzed using FlowJo software.

1. Using the unstained sample, adjust the side scatter (SSC) and forward scatter (FSC) voltages to locate the cell population and define the lymphocyte population gate. As for fluorescence channels, PMT voltages are set to leave the negative population at least at three standard deviation above the noise of the instrument for each channel.
2. Run compensation controls to correct for spillover (*see* **Note 19**).
3. Run the FMO control tubes. FMOs are used as gating controls (*see* **Note 19**).
4. Acquire samples.
5. Record a minimum of 10^5 events within the lymphocyte gate.
6. Export FCS files and analyze the data with FlowJo software. A representative analysis of splenocytes is presented in Fig. 4.

3.4 Adoptive Transfer of Treg and $CD4^+CD25^-$ Cells

1. Dilute the $CD4^+CD25^+$ and $CD4^+CD25^-$ cells to 3×10^5 cells per 100 μL of PBS in a sterile tissue culture hood.
2. Prepare syringes for injection as follows. Load a 0.5 mL syringe with ~150 μL of cell suspension. Add a 26 G needle to each syringe, remove the protective cap and eliminate the bubble trap inside the syringes with caution not to damage the cells and lose too much liquid (*see* **Note 23**). Put the cap back on each needle.
3. Prepare the mice to inject by putting one mouse per cage with a wire bar lid without food.
4. Warm up the mouse by putting its cage under an infrared lamp for 5 min (*see* **Note 24**).
5. Place the mouse inside a mouse restrainer and position the tail close and perpendicular to the person who will do the injection.
6. Dilate the tail vein of the mouse by massage. The dilatation of the tail vein can be enhanced by warming the tail using an infrared heat lamp or by immersion in warm water to increase blood flow. A supplemental 3–4 min of heating may be necessary for optimal dilation (*see* **Note 24**).

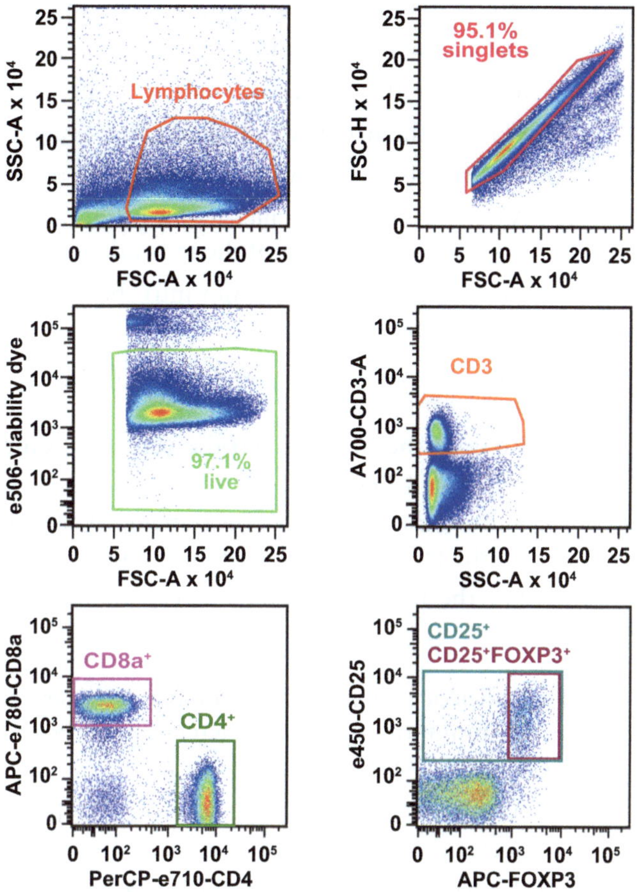

Gate	(% of gated)	Reference gate
$CD3^+$	24.0	Lymphocytes
$CD3^+CD4^+$	51.5	$CD3^+$
$CD3^+CD8a^+$	36.6	$CD3^+$
$CD3^+CD4^+CD25^+$	13.4	$CD4^+$
$CD3+CD4^+CD25^+Foxp3^+$	10.1	$CD4^+$

Fig. 4 Flow cytometry profile of splenocytes. Splenocytes are stained with Fixable Viability Dye eFluor® 506 (e506), Alexa Fluor® 700 (A700)-conjugated anti-mouse CD3, PerCP-eFluor® 710 (PerCP-e710) anti-mouse CD4, APC-eFluor® 780 (e780) anti-mouse CD8a, eFluor® 450 (e450)-conjugated anti-mouse CD25 and APC-conjugated anti-mouse Foxp3 antibodies, and analyzed by flow cytometry. Fluorophores are respectively excited and analyzed with appropriate laser and bandpass filter (BP) (e450: 405 nm with 450/50 BP, e506: 405 nm with 525/50 BP, A700: 640 nm with 730/45 BP, PerCP-eFluor® 710: 488 nm with 695/40 BP, APC-e780: 640 nm with 780/60 BP, APC: 640 nm with 670/14 BP). Lymphocytes are gated in the side scatter (SSC)/forward scatter (FSC) plot. Singlet lymphocytes are gated using FSC height (FSC-H) over FSC area (FSC-A). Live lymphocytes are gated in the viability dye/FSC-A plot. $CD3^+$ cells are gated in the CD3/SSC-A plot. $CD3^+CD4^+$ and $CD3^+CD8^+$ are gated in the CD8/CD4 plot from the $CD3^+$ cells population. Gated $CD3^+CD4^+$ cells are further characterized for CD25 and FOXP3 expression in the CD25/FOXP3 plot. A representative flow cytometry gating procedure and the % of singlet cells, % live cells, % of $CD3^+$ cells in lymphocytes, % of $CD4^+$ and $CD8^+$ cells in $CD3^+$ cells, % of $CD4^+CD25^+$ cells in $CD4^+$ cells and % of $CD4^+CD25^+FOXP3^+$ cells in $CD4^+$ cells are presented for splenocytes

7. Visualize both left and right lateral tail veins. Select the vein that appears easier to inject.
8. Make sure that there is no bubble in the syringe (*see* **Note 23**).
9. Remove the needle cap and take the syringe.
10. Position the needle with the bevel hole up.
11. Align the needle parallel to the vein and localize the site of injection at one-third of the tail end (*see* **Note 25**).
12. Insert the needle ~3–4 mm into the vein using a continuous movement.
13. Pull on the syringe plunger and stop as soon as blood is visualized in the syringe and inject the cells.
14. Remove the needle from the vein and compress the tail vein with sterile gauze.
15. Remove the mouse from the restrainer while keeping compression on the tail and hold the mouse head down for 5 s.
16. Put the mouse back into its cage and verify that there is no bleeding.

3.5 Confirmation of the Efficiency of Treg Adoptive Transfer

The efficiency of the Treg adoptive transfer can be determined using immunofluorescence detection of Foxp3 for example in sections of renal cortex (*see* **Note 26**).

1. At least 1 h before the immunostaining, prepare −20 °C acetone–methanol (1:1) mixture.
2. Air-dry for 30 min, 5 μm-thick cryostat sections of renal cortex in a slide box at RT.
3. Fix the tissue sections in the acetone–methanol (1:1) mixture prechilled at -20 °C in a Wheaton staining dish for 5 min at RT.
4. Rehydrate and wash the tissue sections as follows.
   (a) Transfer the slides to a new staining glass jar with PBST and incubate for 10 min at RT.
   (b) Repeat the previous step.
5. The following steps are performed using a Sequenza™ slide rack holding slide with a coverplate™ (*see* **Note 27**). Put a coverplate™ on each slide and insert the assembly into the Sequenza™ slide rack.
6. Add 100–150 μL of PBST/10% NGS per slide and incubate for 1 h at RT to block the tissue sections.
7. Add 100–150 μL of rabbit anti-Foxp3 antibody diluted 1:500 in PBST per slide and incubate overnight at 4 °C (*see* **Note 28**).
8. Wash the tissue sections by adding three times 2 mL of PBST to the slide/coverplate assemblies.

9. Add 100–150 μL of Alexa Fluor® 555-conjugated, goat anti-rabbit diluted 1:200 in PBST/10% NGS and incubate for 1 h at RT.
10. Wash the tissue sections by adding three times 2 mL of PBST to the slide/coverplate assemblies.
11. Remove a slide and Coverplate™ assembly from the Sequenza™ slide rack. Remove the PBST contained within the capillary gap by applying the edge of the assembly on a paper stack and remove the Coverplate™.
12. Dry the edge of the slide without touching the tissue sections with a Kimwipes task Wipers and add one drop of Vectashield mounting media containing 4′,6-diamidino-2-phenylindole (DAPI) and then cover with coverslip.
13. Repeat the two previous steps until all slides are processed.
14. Wait for at least 15–20 min until dry and proceed to imaging. Slides could be stored for up to 3 days in a slide box in the dark at 4 °C.
15. Images are captured using a fluorescent microscope.
16. The number of $Foxp3^+$ cells per μm^2 is determined using ImageJ software.

4 Notes

1. Use of too high an antibody concentration results in an overestimation or inaccurate determination of the number of cells due to elevated background or bad separation of labeled cells in the flow cytometer. The appropriate dilution for each antibody used for flow cytometry study is determined in a separate experiment. This is done by comparing 8 twofold dilutions starting with the dilution recommended by the company. An example of antibody titration is shown in Fig. 3. Using the right antibody dilution provides good results and can also save money. Diluted dye conjugated antibody dilutions are stored at 4 °C in the dark for up to 6 months.
2. All the procedures are done using a sterile technique.
3. Ten to 12-week old mice are used to isolate Treg for adoptive transfer. It is important that the donor mice be of the same strain as the recipient mice. Due to some variation in the strains between suppliers, it is preferable to get donor and recipient mice from the same supplier.
4. In general, two spleens are sufficient to isolate enough $CD4^+CD25^+$ Treg to inject 3×10^5 Treg into one mouse. However, if the spleens are small or have some necrosis, more

spleens may be required to isolate enough Treg. CD4+CD25− lymphocytes are not limiting as we routinely isolate more than a million cells per spleen.

5. It is important not to use a grinding motion as this will damage cells.
6. RBC lysis buffer is formulated for optimal lysis of erythrocytes in single-cell suspensions of hematopoietic tissues such as spleen or whole blood. RBC lysis buffer contains 8.3 g/L ammonium chloride in 0.01 M Tris–HCl buffer, which lyses red cells with minimal effect on lymphocytes when used as recommended. Nucleated red cells are not effectively lysed with ammonium chloride. RBC lysis buffer has been developed for removal of mouse red blood cells. The RBC lysis buffer may not be optimal for the lysis of red blood cells of other species.
7. The percent of live cells is calculated using the number of alive and dead cells. This percentage is used to assess the efficiency of the preparation. In general, the percent of live cells should be ≥90%.
8. Cells must be placed in a 5 mL (12×75 mm) polystyrene tube to properly fit into the purple EasySep® Magnet.
9. The EasySep® CD4+ pre-enrichment cocktail is a combination of biotinylated monoclonal antibodies directed against cell surface antigens on mouse cells of hematopoietic origin (CD8, CD11b, CD19, CD24, CD45R, CD49b) to remove non-CD4+ T lymphocytes.
10. The Easysep® biotin selection cocktail is a combination of two mouse IgG1 monoclonal antibodies against biotin and dextran that are bound in bispecific tetrameric antibody complexes by rat monoclonal antibodies against mouse IgG1 [12].
11. The EasySep® D magnetic particles solution is a suspension of magnetic dextran iron particles in TRIS buffer.
12. Gently pipetting up and down when mixing avoids damaging cells.
13. The non-CD4+, unwanted cells are bound to the magnetic particles and are retained by the magnet inside the original tube.
14. The EasySep® blocking solution is required for subsequent CD25+ cell selection from CD4+ T cell pre-enriched cell populations.
15. Protect from light by not exposing directly to fluorescent light or daylight. Aluminum foil can be used to cover the tubes.
16. The Easysep® PE selection cocktail contains a combination of mouse monoclonal IgG1 antibodies bound in bispecific tetrameric antibody complexes (TAC) which are directed against PE (phycoerythrin) and dextran.

17. The EasySep® SA magnetic nanoparticles are supplied as a suspension of magnetic dextran iron particles in water.
18. $CD4^+CD25^-$ cells are used as negative control for adoptive transfer.
19. In the protocol for flow cytometry with basic equipment, unstained and conjugated isotype antibodies are used to assess background staining to Fc receptors, and are also used as a gating control. Single fluorophore-stained cells are used to correct for fluorescence spillover. In the protocol for flow cytometry with multicolor flow cytometer, unstained and fluorescence minus one (FMO) controls are used to assess background staining to Fc receptors and to correct for fluorescence spillover. FMO are generated by staining cells with all the antibodies minus one. Single fluorophore stained cells are used to correct for fluorescence spillover.
20. BD Fc-Block is used to decrease nonspecific binding to mouse Fc-gamma receptors.
21. Anti-CD25 antibody is added to the sample tube containing $CD4^+CD25^+$ cells, even if the cells are stained with PE-conjugated anti-mouse CD25 antibody during the CD25 positive selection step (*see* Subheading 3.2.2).
22. Cells are diluted in PBS because FBS interferes with live/dead staining.
23. Monitor carefully the loading of the prepared syringe and make sure to eliminate bubbles as they can harm the mouse.
24. Be careful not to burn or overheated the animal with the infrared lamp.
25. The site of injection can be closer to the tail end. This will allow a second injection if the injection does not succeed at the first site.
26. The efficiency of Treg adoptive transfer can be determined by counting the number of immunofluorescently labeled Foxp3 cells in the renal cortex. Treg number is determined in the renal cortex because the renal cortex because number of $Foxp3^+$ cells in the aorta for example is too low. We have shown that adoptive transfer of Treg increases $Foxp3^+$ cells twofold in the renal cortex compared with control mice [4]. Treg number can also be determined in immune organs such as the spleen and lymph nodes.
27. Immunostaining is performed using the Sequenza™ Slide Rack that holds slides with a Coverplate™. This assembly forms a capillary gap between the slide and the coverplate, which greatly reduces the volume of antibody needed. It is also possible to do the immunostaining with a humid chamber and Parafilm coverslips. The humid chamber could be made by wetting a piece of paper towel and putting it in the bottom of a plastic slide box.

The blocking and antibody solutions are pipetted directly on the tissue section and covered with a small coverslip made by cutting a section of Parafilm. The coverslips are removed from the slide by immersing the slide in PBST in a vertical staining jar. Slides are washed in a Wheaton staining dish on a rocking platform agitator such as a VariMix platform (Thermolyne).

28. The new solution pushes the previous solution down out of the capillary gap.

Acknowledgments

We are grateful to Christian Young for excellent technical assistance and suggestions. The work of the authors was supported by Canadian Institutes of Health Research grants 82790 and 102606, a Canada Research Chair on Hypertension and Vascular Research from Canadian Institutes of Health Research/Government of Canada, and the Canada Fund for Innovation (all to E.L.S.). K.K.M is supported by CIHR grant 115000 and is a Junior 2 Chercheur Boursier of the FRQ-S.

References

1. Schiffrin EL (2008) The flame that lights the fire: oxidative stress, inflammation, and renal damage in angiotensin II-induced hypertension. Hypertension 52:205–206
2. Schiffrin EL (2010) T lymphocytes: a role in hypertension? Curr Opin Nephrol Hypertens 19:181–186
3. Schiffrin EL (2013) The immune system: role in hypertension. Can J Cardiol 29(5):543–548
4. Barhoumi T, Kasal DA, Li MW, Shbat L, Laurant P, Neves MF, Paradis P, Schiffrin EL (2011) T Regulatory lymphocytes prevent angiotensin II-induced hypertension and vascular injury. Hypertension 57:469–476
5. De Ciuceis C, Amiri F, Brassard P, Endemann DH, Touyz RM, Schiffrin EL (2005) Reduced vascular remodeling, endothelial dysfunction, and oxidative stress in resistance arteries of angiotensin II-infused macrophage colony-stimulating factor-deficient mice: evidence for a role in inflammation in angiotensin-induced vascular injury. Arterioscler Thromb Vasc Biol 25:2106–2113
6. Guzik TJ, Hoch NE, Brown KA, McCann LA, Rahman A, Dikalov S, Goronzy J, Weyand C, Harrison DG (2007) Role of the T cell in the genesis of angiotensin II induced hypertension and vascular dysfunction. J Exp Med 204:2449–2460
7. Kasal DA, Barhoumi T, Li MW, Yamamoto N, Zdanovich E, Rehman A, Neves MF, Laurant P, Paradis P, Schiffrin EL (2012) T regulatory lymphocytes prevent aldosterone-induced vascular injury. Hypertension 59:324–330
8. Ko EA, Amiri F, Pandey NR, Javeshghani D, Leibovitz E, Touyz RM, Schiffrin EL (2007) Resistance artery remodeling in deoxycorticosterone acetate-salt hypertension is dependent on vascular inflammation: evidence from m-CSF-deficient mice. Am J Physiol Heart Circ Physiol 292:H1789–H1795
9. Kvakan H, Kleinewietfeld M, Qadri F, Park JK, Fischer R, Schwarz I, Rahn HP, Plehm R, Wellner M, Elitok S, Gratze P, Dechend R, Luft FC, Muller DN (2009) Regulatory T cells ameliorate angiotensin II-induced cardiac damage. Circulation 119:2904–2912
10. Leibovitz E, Ebrahimian T, Paradis P, Schiffrin EL (2009) Aldosterone induces arterial stiffness in absence of oxidative stress and endothelial dysfunction. J Hypertens 27:2192–2200
11. Matrougui K, Zakaria AE, Kassan M, Choi S, Nair D, Gonzalez-Villalobos RA, Chentoufi AA, Kadowitz P, Belmadani S, Partyka M (2011) Natural regulatory T cells control coronary arteriolar endothelial dysfunction in hypertensive mice. Am J Pathol 178:434–441
12. Peters CE, Woodside SM, Eaves AC (2005) Isolation of subsets of immune cells. Methods Mol Biol 302:95–116

Chapter 26

Isolation and Culture of Endothelial Cells from Large Vessels

Augusto C. Montezano, Karla B. Neves, Rheure A.M. Lopes, and Francisco Rios

Abstract

The endothelium, which is at the interface between circulating blood and the vascular wall, comprises a simple squamous layer of cells that lines the inner surface of all blood vessels. Endothelial cells are highly metabolically active and play an important role in many physiological functions, including control of vasomotor tone, blood cell trafficking, vascular permeability, and maintenance of vascular integrity (Mensah, Vascul Pharmacol 46(5):310–314, 2007; Yetik-Anacak and Catravas, Vascul Pharmacol 45(5):268–276, 2006). Endothelial cells are characteristically 'quiescent' in that they do not actively proliferate, with the average lifespan of an endothelial cell being >1 year. The endothelium is very sensitive to mechanical stimuli (stretch, shear stress, pressure), humoral agents (angiotensin II (Ang II), endothelin-1 (ET-1), aldosterone, bradykinin, thromoxane) and chemical factors (glucose, reactive oxygen species (ROS)) and responds by releasing endothelial-derived mediators, such as nitric oxide (NO), prostacyclin (PGI2), platelet-activating factor (PAF), C-type atrial natriuretic peptide (ANP), and ET-1 to regulate vascular tone, prevent thrombosis and inflammation, and maintain structural integrity. Primary culture of endothelial cells is an important tool in dissecting the role of the endothelium in many physiological or pathological responses. This chapter describes the explant method for culture of endothelial cells from large vessels. Cells derived by the protocol described here can be used for cell biology and molecular biology studies in hypertension and other cardiovascular diseases where endothelial function may be impaired.

Key words Endothelial cells, Primary culture, Large vessels

1 Introduction

Endothelial cells (ECs) are the inner layer of cells of all blood vessels becoming the unique interface between the blood and the vessel wall. ECs form a continuous monolayer which plays a crucial role in the immune response, coagulation, growth regulation, production of extracellular matrix components, and it is an essential modulator of blood vessel tone [1–5].

The endothelium plays a key role in vascular homeostasis [6]. ECs produce and release several vasoactive molecules that modulate vascular smooth muscle cells tone. Furchgott and Zawadzki

Rhian M. Touyz and Ernesto L. Schiffrin (eds.), *Hypertension: Methods and Protocols*, Methods in Molecular Biology, vol. 1527, DOI 10.1007/978-1-4939-6625-7_26, © Springer Science+Business Media LLC 2017

were the first to demonstrate an endothelium-derived relaxing factor, nitric oxide (NO) [7], a molecule converted from L-arginine by of endothelial NO synthase (eNOS) [8]. NO leads to cGMP-mediated vasodilatation when diffuses to the vascular smooth muscle cells and activates guanylate cyclase. The endothelium also can sustain vasodilator tone mediating hyperpolarization of vascular smooth muscle cells in a NO-independent manner, which promotes increase in potassium conductance and consequent propagation of depolarization of vascular smooth muscle cells [9]. Alterations in endothelial function strongly regulate pathological processes such as atherosclerosis, thrombosis, inflammation, or vascular wall remodeling [4, 6]. Over recent years, the understanding of the endothelial cell biology has increased with the possibility to grow endothelial cells in vitro [10]. In this chapter we describe methods to isolate endothelial cells by the explant technique. Cells isolated by this protocol can not only be used for molecular biology techniques but also for electrophysiology studies [11].

2 Materials

1. Ham's F12 nutrient mix (pH 7.2) containing: penicillin/streptomycin (1×), HEPES (15 mM), L-glutamine (1 mM), sodium bicarbonate (14 mM).
2. Endothelial Cell Medium: Dulbecco's Modified Eagle Medium (DMEM) (pH 7.2) containing: low D-glucose (5.5 mM), penicillin/streptomycin (1×), HEPES (25 mM), L-glutamine (4 mM), sodium bicarbonate (44 mM), sodium pyruvate (1 mM), fetal bovine serum (10%). Add to 1 L of DMEM: 10 mL of nonessential amino acids solution (MEM—10 mM—100×), 1 mL of heparin (10,000 U.S.P. units/mL), 30 mg of endothelial cell growth supplement from bovine neural tissue (ECGS).
3. Matrigel.
4. Dispase (use 0.2 mL/10 cm^2—10 U) (*see* **Note 1**).
5. 6-well plate.
6. Surgical material: toothed forceps, straight fine forceps, angled fine forceps, small sharp scissors, microdissecting scissors.

3 Methods

1. Prior to the vessel collection, prepare the Matrigel in a 6-well plate. Dilute the Matrigel, following manufacturer's instructions, in endothelial cell medium and make a layer of Matrigel in each well spreading it evenly.

2. Carefully dissect the vessel from anesthetized and heparinized mice and place it in complete Ham's F12 nutrient mix.
3. In a petri dish, carefully clean the vessels of periadventitial fat and connective tissue (*see* **Note 2**).
4. Open the vessel longitudinally and cut it into squares of 2–3 mm length each (*see* **Note 3**).
5. Place each piece of vessel with the intima side facing the Matrigel layer in each well.
6. Place the 6-well plate with the vessel pieces in a 37 °C incubator for 24 h (*see* **Note 4**).
7. After the 24 h, add carefully (through the side of the well), 300–400 μL of endothelial cell medium, avoiding that the Matrigel dries up.
8. Change medium every second day. Be careful to not remove the vessel pieces from the Matrigel.
9. After 6–8 days, remove the vessel pieces with a pipette.
10. Allow cells to grow on the Matrigel until the 12th day.
11. Remove cells from the Matrigel with dispase (10 U). Remove excess of endothelial cells medium and add dispase. Incubate for 60 min at 37 °C. With a P1000, pipette up and down to remove cells and disperse them from the Matrigel (*see* **Note 5**).
12. Add more endothelial cell medium and centrifuge the cell suspension at 300 × *g* for 5 min.
13. Aspirate the supernatant and remove as much Matrigel as possible.
14. Resuspend the cell pellet in endothelial cell medium (growth medium) and grow the cells as needed (*see* **Notes 6** and 7).

4 Notes

1. Concentration of dispase may differ accordingly to different manufacturers and vessel of choice (It may vary from 100 to 10 U). Trypsin will not work since the endothelial cell medium contains FBS.
2. Do not use pre-digestion protocols to facilitate the cleaning of adventitial and connective tissue. It may harm endothelial cells.
3. Smaller pieces are not stable in the Matrigel. Bigger pieces generate poor extraction of endothelial cells.
4. 24 h is the necessary time for the stabilization of the vessel pieces in the Matrigel layer.
5. This is a crucial step. If endothelial cells are not viable after this step, one should decrease the dispase concentration or incubation

times in order to a successful primary culture. Concentrations and incubation times suggested here were optimized for murine aortas.

6. After the cells are attached and growing, one should proceed with the endothelial cell characterization to ensure that the cells obtained are positive for endothelial cell markers, such as platelet endothelial cell adhesion molecule (PECAM) and von Willebrand's factor (vWF).
7. To ensure that the phenotype of cells is maintained with passaging, it is important to characterize cells at all passages. At some point in passaging (usually around passage 6–7 in our experience), the phenotype changes and expression of receptors and ion channels change. We suggest that cells beyond this point of passage are not used for further experiments.

References

1. Mensah GA (2007) Healthy endothelium: the scientific basis for cardiovascular health promotion and chronic disease prevention. Vascul Pharmacol 46(5):310–314
2. Yetik-Anacak G, Catravas JD (2006) Nitric oxide and the endothelium: history and impact on cardiovascular disease. Vascul Pharmacol 45(5):268–276
3. Manconi F, Markham R, Fraser IS (2000) Culturing endothelial cells of microvascular origin. Methods Cell Sci 22:89–99
4. Michiels C (2003) Endothelial cell functions. J Cell Physiol 196:430–443
5. Sumpio BE, Riley JT, Dardik A (2002) Cells in focus: endothelial cell. Int J Biochem Cell Biol 34(12):1508–1512
6. Vita JA, Keaney JF (2002) Endothelial function: a barometer for cardiovascular risk? Circulation 106:640–642
7. Furchgott RF, Zawadzki JV (1980) The obligatory role of endothelial cells in the relaxation of arterial smooth muscle by acetylcholine. Nature 288:373–376
8. Forstermann U, Munzel T (2006) Endothelial nitric oxide synthase in vascular disease: from marvel to menace. Circulation 113:1708–1714
9. Busse R, Edwards G, Feletou M, Fleming I, Vanhoutte PM, Weston AH (2002) EDHF: bringing the concepts together. Trends Pharmacol Sci 3:374–380
10. Garlanda C, Dejana E (1997) Heterogeneity of endothelial cells specific markers. Arterioscler Thromb Vasc Biol 17:1193–1202
11. Suh SH, Vennekens K, Manolopoulos VG, Freichel M, Schweig U, Prenen J, Flockerzi V, Droogmans G, Nilius B (1999) Characterisation of explanted endothelial cells from mouse aorta: electrophysiology and Ca2+ signalling. Eur J Physiol 438:612–620

Chapter 27

Isolation and Culture of Vascular Smooth Muscle Cells from Small and Large Vessels

Augusto C. Montezano, Rheure A.M. Lopes, Karla B. Neves, Francisco Rios, and Rhian M. Touyz

Abstract

Primary culture of vascular smooth muscle cells is an important in vitro model for the dissection of molecular mechanisms related to a specific physiological or pathological response at the cellular level. Cultured cells also provide an excellent model to study cell biology. This chapter describes a user-friendly and practical protocol for isolation of vascular smooth muscle cells from small and large vessels by enzymatic dissociation, which can be applied to vessels from different species, including rodents and humans.

Key words Vascular smooth muscle cells, Primary culture, Small vessels, Large vessels

1 Introduction

Smooth muscle cells (SMC) can be cultured from several human tissues such as placenta, bladder, umbilical cord and vessels (VSMCs). VSMCs cells are the major component of arteries, veins, and microvessels and are major regulators of vascular function. Primary culture of VSMCs represents an in vitro model, which retain a high degree of plasticity and can be used to study responses that range from contraction to proliferative or secretory responses. Interestingly, the phenotype of VSMC is heterogeneous and varies according to the vessel size, vessels type (conduit versus resistance), age, species and vascular bed. The layer from where the cells derive can also impact on phenotype. For example, intimal VSMC presents lower levels of contractile proteins and more organelles such as mitochondria and sarcoplasmic reticulum and gene expression may vary in different cell layers [1–4].

VSMC can be easily isolated from aorta by the explant technique and are mainly useful to study responses related to atherosclerosis. However, this isolation protocol may be selective to a specific type of VSMCs, and may not represent the whole content

Rhian M. Touyz and Ernesto L. Schiffrin (eds.), *Hypertension: Methods and Protocols*, Methods in Molecular Biology, vol. 1527, DOI 10.1007/978-1-4939-6625-7_27, © Springer Science+Business Media LLC 2017

of a vessel or part of it. On the other hand, cells isolated from small-resistance arteries, such as mesenteric arteries isolated by enzymatic digestion, are suitable to verify events that regulate arterial blood pressure, since those vessels contribute to control of total peripheral vascular resistance [5].

VSMCs, that are freshly isolated and in primary culture, can be used for electrophysiology experiments at early days (from 5 to 7 days). It is important take into consideration that VSMC have a finite number of divisions, after which they lose their phenotype, undergo growth arrest and become senescent [1, 6]. These observations raise an important aspect of working with cultured VSMCs, where one should always confirm that the process of culturing VSMCs does not affect the expression of receptors, channels, transporters, enzymes, or any other protein important to the study. As such characterizing cells at different passages is important to ensure that cells do not undergo dedifferentiation with loss of receptors, channels etc.

Once isolated by enzymatic digestion, primary culture VSMCs retain the original phenotype, providing an important in vitro model to study disease-associated signaling pathways. For this reason, this chapter only concentrates on the isolation of VSMCs by enzymatic dissociation. This protocol has been demonstrated to not alter the expression of smooth muscle specific marker α-actin, and has many advantages as described above. In addition, the protocol described in this chapter is relatively fast, reducing risks of cell contamination by other resident cells from the vasculature and microorganisms. VSMCs isolated by enzymatic dissociation have been successfully used in many experimental approaches such as RT-PCR, northern blot, immunoblotting, live cell microscopy and imaging protocols (i.e., immunofluorescence).

2 Materials

1. Ham's F12 nutrient mix (pH 7.2) containing: penicillin/streptomycin (1×), HEPES (15 mM), l-glutamine (1 mM), sodium bicarbonate (14 mM).
2. Pre-digestion mix: 30 mL of complete Ham's F12 nutrient mix containing 90 mg collagenase type I (≥125 U/mg) (*see* **Note 1**).
3. Digestion mix for small vessels: 12.5 mL of complete Ham's F12 nutrient mix containing 25 mg of bovine serum albumin (BSA, 2%), 25 mg of collagenase type I (≥125 U/mg), 1.5 mg of elastase (≥4 U/mg), 4.5 mg of soybean trypsin inhibitor (*see* **Note 2**).
4. Digestion mix for large vessels: 25 mL of complete Ham's F12 nutrient mix containing 50 mg of BSA, 50 mg of collagenase

type I (≥125 U/mg), 3 mg of elastase (≥4 U/mg), 9 mg of soybean trypsin inhibitor (*see* **Note 2**).

5. Dulbecco's Modified Eagle Medium (DMEM) (pH 7.2) containing: low d-glucose (5.5 mM), penicillin/streptomycin (1×), HEPES (25 mM), l-glutamine (4 mM), sodium bicarbonate (44 mM), sodium pyruvate (1 mM), fetal bovine serum (10%).
6. 100 mm petri dishes.
7. Syringes and needles (20 G, 18 G).
8. 100 μm nylon filter.
9. 50 mL or 15 mL centrifuge tubes.
10. Cell culture flasks (25 or 75 cm^2) or sterile coverslips inserted in a 6-well plate (*see* **Note 3**).
11. Surgical material: toothed forceps, straight fine forceps, angled fine forceps, small sharp scissors, microdissecting scissors.

3 Methods

3.1 VSMC Isolation from Small Vessels (i.e., Mesenteric Arteries from Rodents)

1. Isolate the whole mesenteric bed and place it in cold complete Ham's F12 nutrient mix (*see* **Note 4**).
2. Clean the mesenteric bed by carefully removing the fat with two fine forceps in a 100 mm petri dish containing Ham's F12 nutrient mix. First, identify the main mesenteric artery and with one of the fine forceps hold the mesenteric bed. Once the mesenteric bed is stably secured, with the help of the second fine forceps, remove the fat from the artery tree by gently pulling it (*see* **Note 1**).
3. Preheat the digestion mix at 37 °C for 5 min.
4. Once cleaned, incubate the mesenteric bed in a centrifuge tube containing the digestion mix for small vessels for 30 min, at 37 °C and under agitation. The digestion is complete when the vessels appearance is similar to cotton. Do not digest the vessels to a point where it is not possible to see the artery tree.
5. Syringe the vascular bed through a 20 G needle four times in order to obtain a homogenized solution.
6. Filter cells and tissue debris through a 100 μm nylon filter, collecting the cell solution in a centrifuge tube.
7. Centrifuge the cell solution for 3 min at 300 × *g*.
8. After the centrifugation it may be possible to see a cell pellet (it will depend on the amount of tissue available for the culture and the efficacy of the previous steps). Aspirate the supernatant and resuspend the cell pellet in 5 mL of DMEM (as described in Subheading 2, **item 5**).

9. Add the cell solution to a 25 cm^2 flask and keep it in a humidified 37 °C/5% CO_2 incubator (*see* **Note 5**).
10. Replace the medium after 24 h to a fresh 5 ml DMEM (*see* **Note 6**).
11. Keep changing the medium every 2 days until cells reach confluence and are ready for either further culture (passages) or the experimental protocol.

3.2 VSMC Isolation from Large Vessels (i.e., Aorta from Rodents or Humans)

1. Isolate the whole vessel, remove the perivascular tissue and remaining blood, and place it in cold Ham's F12 nutrient mix.
2. Incubate the large vessel in the pre-digestion mix for 15 min at 37 °C under agitation. This step will facilitate the removal of the adventia and intima layers.
3. In a 100 mm petri dish containing Ham's F12 nutrient mix, cut the large vessel longitudinally and remove the endothelial cells (intima layer) by gently scrapping the inner surface of the vessel.
4. Under a dissection microscope, turn the vessel with the inner surface down. With a fine forceps remove the adventitia layer by gently peeling it off the vessel wall. This step is important to decrease the contamination of the primary culture with fibroblasts.
5. Preheat the digestion mix for large vessels at 37 °C for 5 min.
6. Cut the vessel in small pieces to facilitate digestion. Pieces should range in size between 2 and 5 mm (*see* **Note 7**).
7. Incubate in a centrifuge tube containing the digestion mix for large vessels for 60–90 min, at 37 °C and under agitation (*see* **Note 8**). The digestion is complete when the vessel appearance is similar to cotton. Do not digest the vessel to a point where it is not possible to see it anymore (*see* **Note 9**).
8. Syringe the vascular bed through an 18 G needle (one time) and then through a 20 G needle (four times) in order to obtain a homogenized solution.
9. Filter cells and tissue debris through a 100 μm nylon filter, collecting the cell solution in a centrifuge tube.
10. Centrifuge the cell solution for 3 min at 300 × *g*.
11. After the centrifugation it may be possible to see a cell pellet (it will depend on the amount of tissue available for the culture and the efficacy of the previous steps). Aspirate the supernatant and resuspend the cell pellet in 5 mL of DMEM.
12. Add the cell solution to a 25 cm^2 flask and keep it in a humidified 37 °C/5% CO_2 incubator (*see* **Note 5**).
13. Replace the medium after 24 h to a fresh 5 ml DMEM (*see* **Note 6**).

14. Keep changing the medium every 2 days until cells reach confluence and are ready for either further culture (passages) or the experimental protocol.

4 Notes

1. The pre-digestion solution may be necessary to facilitate further cleaning of large vessels from rats and humans. Is also extremely useful for the cleaning of mesenteric beds from rats. It is not recommended to perform the pre-digestion step in vessels from mice, due to these vessels being very fragile. If necessary, the concentration of collagenase type I suggested here must be decreased.
2. Concentrations of collagenase type I and elastase may vary accordingly to the material available. Large vessels from humans may require higher concentrations of both. Moreover, collagenase type II may be used as well [2, 3].
3. The amount of material available for culture will determine if one will use a cell culture flask or a coverslip inserted in a 6-well plate, i.e., a pull of many vessels vs. a single vessel. If a coverslip is to be used, ensure that all instruments are properly sterile to avoid contamination.
4. Avoid damage of the intestine during the collection of the mesenteric bed, since this could be a major source of contamination. This protocol can also be used for the extraction and culture of VSMCs from the microvasculature of human material.
5. If one is culturing VSMCs from a single small vessel (usually the case for human material) or a single animal, the cell pellet should be resuspended in 500 μL of DMEM and transferred to the top of a sterile coverslip inserted in a 6-well plate. Cells will grow in the coverslip and migrate to the surface of the plate. Once cells are found in the surface of the plate, one should transfer the coverslip to another well by using a sterile fine forceps, allowing the primary culture to expand.
6. Cells may take a couple of days to adapt to the culture and acquire the appropriate shape of a VSMC. One should be aware that VSMCs in culture can be heterogeneous and display differences in shape, size, and growth.
7. Pieces that are too small may lead to a poor cell population, as the same for bigger pieces of vascular tissue (increasing the digestion time and efficiency)
8. Digestion time may vary accordingly to the nature of the material. Usually human large vessels require longer periods of digestion.
9. Cell viability will be affected by the digestion protocol.

References

1. Golovina VA, Blaustein MP (2006) Preparation of primary cultured mesenteric artery smooth muscle cells for fluorescent imaging and physiological studies. Nat Protoc 1(6):2681–2687
2. Karamariti E et al (2013) Smooth muscle cells differentiated from reprogrammed embryonic lung fibroblasts through DKK3 signaling are potent for tissue engineering of vascular grafts. Circ Res 112(11):1433–1443
3. Lu S et al (2013) Isolation and culture of smooth muscle cells from human acute type A aortic dissection. J Cardiothorac Surg 8:83
4. Schwartz SM, deBlois D, O'Brien ER (1995) The intima. Soil for atherosclerosis and restenosis. Circ Res 77(3):445–465
5. Davis MJ, Hill MA (1999) Signaling mechanisms underlying the vascular myogenic response. Physiol Rev 79(2):387–423
6. Bierman EL (1978) The effect of donor age on the in vitro life span of cultured human arterial smooth-muscle cells. In Vitro 14(11):951–955

Chapter 28

Evaluation of Endothelial Dysfunction In Vivo

Mihail Todiras, Natalia Alenina, and Michael Bader

Abstract

Vascular endothelial cells play a major role in maintaining cardiovascular homeostasis. Impairment of physiological properties of the endothelium, such as the promotion of vasodilation and anti-aggregation, leads to a condition called endothelial dysfunction. Endothelial dysfunction is an important early event in the pathogenesis of atherosclerosis and has been shown to have prognostic value in predicting vascular events including stroke and myocardial infarction.

Endothelial-dependent vasodilation is one of the most widely used methods for assessment of endothelial function in rodents. It includes pharmacological stimulation (for example by acetylcholine) of endothelial release of NO and other vasoactive compounds in comparison with vascular response to endothelium-independent dilators such as sodium nitroprusside. However, usually this technique is performed in anesthetized animals. Here we describe a method which allows evaluation of endothelial dysfunction in conscious, freely moving mice and rats.

Key words Blood pressure, Acetylcholine, Sodium nitroprusside, eNOS, Catheter, Endothelial function

1 Introduction

The great discoveries in the 1980s on the biology of the endothelium stimulated an enormous number of studies in the last three decades to elucidate its physiological and pathophysiological roles.

In the early 1980s it was shown that intra-arterial administration of acetylcholine (ACh) to canine femoral artery causes vasodilation and subsequent lowering in arterial pressure. This response was completely abolished by removal of the endothelium, suggesting that ACh requires an intact endothelium to elicit vasodilatation in vivo. Furthermore, in these circumstances ACh causes vasoconstriction [1]. Later studies revealed that ACh binds to specific endothelial muscarinic receptors and causes the release of endothelium-derived relaxing factors (EDRFs), which induce vascular relaxation. This endothelium-dependent vasodilatation has been shown to be mediated by multiple factors which are now identified as nitric oxide (NO), endothelium-dependent

Rhian M. Touyz and Ernesto L. Schiffrin (eds.), *Hypertension: Methods and Protocols*, Methods in Molecular Biology, vol. 1527, DOI 10.1007/978-1-4939-6625-7_28, © Springer Science+Business Media LLC 2017

hyperpolarizing factor (EDHF), prostaglandin I2 (prostacyclin), and other prostanoids [2]. A large body of work emerged emphasizing the importance of the endothelium in the control of arterial tone and its role in the development of cardiovascular diseases. The loss of adequate vascular function by endothelial damage is likely to be an early event in most if not all vascular disorders. Endothelial dysfunction has been implicated as a key factor in the development of a wide range of cardiovascular diseases from essential hypertension to vasospastic disorders such as systemic sclerosis.

Elevations of angiotensin II (Ang II) levels accompany many cardiovascular diseases. It has been suggested to be a key component contributing to the development of endothelial dysfunction by stimulation of AT1 receptors and increase in oxidative stress. On the contrary, the heptapeptide angiotensin-(1-7) (Ang-(1-7)) opposes many of Ang II actions. Ang-(1-7) is generated by angiotensin-converting enzyme 2 (ACE2) which metabolizes Ang II by the removal of a single carboxy-terminal amino acid, phenylalanine [3, 4]. Acting through the G protein-coupled receptor Mas, Ang-(1-7) swiftly upregulates eNOS and NO production through activation of Akt in endothelial cells [5–10]. Moreover, it was shown that chronic Ang-(1-7) infusion protects against a loss of endothelial function after stenting of various arterial beds [11].

Numerous methods have been developed over the past two decades to measure endothelial function as a predictor of cardiovascular events. Several distinct invasive and noninvasive clinical methodologies, such as venous occlusion plethysmography (VOP), brachial artery flow-mediated dilatation (FMD), iontophoresis in conjunction with laser Doppler imaging (LDI), and pulse-wave analysis are currently being used for in vivo endothelial function assessment in humans. Some of these approaches have been successfully adapted for use in small experimental animals, such as rats and mice. Hence, modern high-resolution ultrasound devices and plethysmography coupled with video-based intravital microscopy allow to study in vivo vascular structure and function in rodents [12–15]. Nevertheless, a majority of these techniques have to be performed in anesthetized animals.

We developed a method which allows to estimate endothelial function in conscious freely moving mice. This method is based on the changes in blood pressure produced by administration of the endothelium-dependent vasodilator ACh as well as the endothelium-independent vasodilator sodium nitroprusside (SNP) directly into the descending thoracic aorta by a very thin catheter inserted into the left carotid artery. Notably, the direct administration of ACh into the arterial system did not cause any direct cardiac effects attributable to its rapid degradation. This model was used to analyze endothelial function in our genetically modified rodents for ACE2 and Mas [8, 9, 16].

2 Materials

2.1 Anesthetics and Analgesics

1. Ketamine hydrochloride (100 mg/ml) (Ketavet, Pharmacia GmbH, Berlin, Germany).
2. Xylazine Hydrochloride 2% (Rompun, Bayer Vital GmbH, Leverkusen, Germany).
3. Isoflurane (Forene 100 ml, Abbott GmbH & Co., Wiesbaden, Germany).
4. Procaine hydrochloride (Procain 1%, Steigerwald, Arzneimittelwerk GmbH, Darmstadt, Germany).
5. Lidocaine hydrochloride, local anesthetic (Xylocain Gel 2%, AstraZeneca, Wedel, Germany).

2.2 Drugs

1. Acetylcholine chloride (Sigma-Aldrich Chemicals, Steinheim, Germany).
2. Sodium nitroprusside dihydrate (Sigma-Aldrich Chemicals, Steinheim, Germany).
3. NG-nitro-L-arginine methyl ester (Sigma-Aldrich Chemicals, Steinheim, Germany).

2.3 Other

1. Antibiotic ointment (Polyspectran Salbe: Polymyxin B sulfate—7500 IU + bacitracin—300 IU + neomycin sulfate—3500 IU; Alcon Pharma GmbH, Freiburg, Germany).
2. Heparin (Heparin-Natrium 25,000 I.E./5 ml, B. Braun Melsungen AG, Melsungen, Germany).
3. 0.9% Sodium Chloride Intravenous Infusion (B. Braun Melsungen AG, Melsungen, Germany).

2.4 Equipment

1. PowerLab/4sp with LabChart Software (AD Instruments Pty Ltd. Castle Hill, Australia).
2. Bridge Amp ML110 (AD Instruments Pty Ltd. Castle Hill, Australia).
3. Pressure transducers (model MLT1050) (AD Instruments Pty Ltd. Castle Hill, Australia).
4. Table top anesthesia unit (Univentor 400 Anaesthesia Unit, AgnTho, Lidingö, Sweden).
5. Stereo microscope (Zeiss Stemi SV6, Carl Zeiss, Gottingen, Germany).
6. Fiber optic light source (KL 1500, Schott, Wiesbaden, Germany).
7. Temperature-controlled surgical table (TKM-0903, FMI GmbH, Seeheim, Germany).
8. Vessel cannulation forceps (S&T 00608–11, Fine Science Tools, North Vancouver, BC, Canada).

9. Strabismus scissors, curved (Fine Science Tools, Art.-Nr. 14075-09).
10. Fine iridectomy scissors (Fine Science Tools, Art.-Nr. 14041-10).
11. Student halsted mosquito hemostat, straight (Fine Science Tools, Art.-Nr. 91308-12).
12. Ultra fine hemostat (Fine Science Tools, Art.-Nr. 13020-12).
13. Dumont #3C forceps (Fine Science Tools, Art.-Nr. 11231-20).
14. Dumont #45 forceps, dumoxel (Fine Science Tools, Art.-Nr. 11245-30).
15. Dumont #5/45 forceps (Fine Science Tools, Art.-Nr. 11251-35).
16. Student Halsted-Mosquito Hemostat, straight (Fine Science Tools, Art.-Nr. 91308-12).
17. Moria MC32/B forceps, smooth straight (Fine Science Tools, Art.-Nr. 11373-22).
18. Graefe forceps, straight (Fine Science Tools, Art.-Nr. 11050-10).
19. Graefe forceps, curved (Fine Science Tools, Art.-Nr. 11052-10).
20. Micro serrefine, straight (Fine Science Tools, Art.-Nr. 18052-01).
21. Halsey needle holder (Fine Science Tools, Art.-Nr. 12001-13).
22. Spinocan anesthesia needle 29 G × 3½ with red-coded stylet (Spinocan, B. Braun, Melsungen AG, Germany).
23. Hamilton microsyringe 50 μl (705 N, Hamilton Bonaduz AG, Bonaduz, Switzerland).
24. Mercury sphygmomanometer (Mercuro 300, Speidel & Keller, Juningen, Germany).

2.5 Consumables

1. Silicone tubing, Micro-Renathane type MRE-025 (Braintree Scientific Inc., Braintree, MA, USA).
2. Silicone tubing, Micro-Renathane type SIL-080 (Braintree Scientific Inc., Braintree, MA, USA).
3. Polyethylene tubing, type PE-50 (Portex, Hythe, UK).
4. Silk black 4/0, cassette pack 100 m (SMI AG, St. Vith, Belgium).
5. Silk black 6/0, cassette pack 100 m (RESORBA Medical GmbH, Nuremberg, Germany).
6. Silk suture 3/0 with needle SH-1 (Ethicon, Perma-Hand 3-0, Johnson & Johnson Ltd).

7. Surgical steel 5/0, cassette pack 50 m (SMI AG, St. Vith, Belgium).
8. Cotton-tipped applicators, sterile (Weisweiler GmbH & Co. KG, Münster Germany).
9. Biocompatible gel (276-0038-001—Re-gel, Data Science, International, St. Paul, USA).
10. Histoacryl tissue adhesive, blue (B. Braun Melsungen AG, Melsungen, Germany).

3 Methods

3.1 Catheter Design and Construction

1. The vascular catheters are made from Micro-Renathane silicone tubing (MRE-025) connected to polyethylene tubing (PE-50) (*see* **Notes 1** and **2**).
2. For carotid artery catheter we use a 25 mm long silicone tube bonded to a 15 mm polyethylene tube. The anchoring tip of the silicone tube is prepared by inserting a surgical stainless steel (size USP 5/0) and its end (the final 2.5–3 mm) is thinned under hot air blowing to a thickness of about 0.3 mm.
3. The femoral artery catheter is made from a 35 mm silicone tube connected to a 50 mm polyethylene tube. The tip of the silicone tube is prepared by insertion of a red-coded stylet from an anesthesia needle 29 G × 3½ (Spinocan). The end of the tube is elongated by heating until a thickness of approximately 0.3 mm (inner diameter) × 0.4 mm (outer diameter) is obtained for about 10 mm length. To produce a smooth end, the tip is cut straight with a scalpel.
4. To connect the silicone and polyethylene tubes the end of the polyethylene tubing is slightly dilated by heating and insertion of a blunted 22-G hypodermic needle up to 2 mm. Thereafter, the silicone tubing is inserted into the dilated part and the dead space between the walls is filled with Histoacryl tissue adhesive and allowed to dry for several days.
5. One day before surgery, the so formed catheters are sterilized for 2 h in 6% hydrogen peroxide and then placed in ethylene oxide.
6. Right before surgery, the catheters are filled with heparinized saline (20 U/ml). The tip of the femoral catheter is anointed with biocompatible gel (DSI) and a red-coded stylet hub (Spinocan) is inserted through the femoral artery to aid in catheter introduction. The void volume of the carotid cannula should be about 5 μl, and of the femoral catheter around 12 μl.

3.2 Anesthesia

1. Mice are weighed and anesthetized with a single intraperitoneal injection of a mixture of ketamine (100 mg/kg) and xylazine (10 mg/kg) (*see* **Note 3**).
2. The level of anesthesia is continuously monitored by inspection of the breathing rate and via toe or tail pinch and for an extended period of time deep anesthesia is achieved by inhalation of isoflurane with an anesthesia machine (Univentor 400).

3.3 Surgery

1. Once pain reflexes are absent, the frontal area, nape of the neck and inguinal regions are shaved and the mice are transferred to a temperature-controlled surgical table and fixed in a dorsal recumbency with a rectal thermometer probe attached to thermal feedback controller to maintain body temperature at 37 °C (*see* **Notes 4** to **6**).
2. After fixation of the maxillar incisors onto the pad by using a plastic rubber band, the skin is anointed with 70% ethanol and Betadine.

3.4 Carotid Artery Cannulation

1. Left of the midline, a ventral cervical skin incision of 10 mm length is made. Tissue is carefully separated and the left carotid artery is then isolated by a blunt dissection of the paratracheal muscles. Using fine tipped dissecting forceps the left vagus nerve is carefully separated from the carotid artery (*see* **Note 7**).
2. Approximately 2 mm proximal to the bifurcation, the common carotid artery is ligated with suture (4/0 silk) and then the suture is moved towards the head (*see* **Note 8**). A second suture (6/0 silk) is placed approximately 7 mm proximal to the bifurcation, and the blood flow is occluded by moving this suture towards the tail. A third suture (6/0 silk) is placed between proximal and distal sutures and together with a small micro serrefine clamp is used to prevent bleeding when the catheter is introduced.
3. A small incision is made with iris scissors just below the distal ligature, and the tip of the catheter is inserted into the artery lumen using vessel cannulation forceps. The clamp is taken off and the catheter is advanced so that the internalized tip gets located in the aortic arch.
4. With several knots at all three sutures the catheter is secured and the patency of the catheter is checked by heparinized saline infusion. Via subcutaneous tunnel the end of the catheter is externalized at the posterior side of the neck between the scapulae. The frontal wound is then closed with interrupted silk sutures.

3.5 Femoral Artery Cannulation

1. Over the femoral triangle a 10 mm incision is made. The inguinal fat pad overlying the femoral artery and vein is carefully removed from the vessels without causing bleeding. Using for-

ceps with two blunted tips the vessels are carefully cleaned from the surrounding tissue and the femoral artery is isolated from the neurovascular bundle.

2. Three loops of suture are placed around the artery. The first suture (4/0 silk) is placed on the distal end of the artery, close to where it branches, and using double knots the vessel is ligated to prevent backflow. This suture is retracted and stretched by taping the end of the suture. A second suture (6/0 silk) is placed underneath approximately 5 mm proximal to the first suture and is elevated with forceps to occlude blood flow during introduction of the catheter. A third suture is placed between the first two, and also in this region near the proximal suture a small clamp is placed.
3. To minimize vasospasm the femoral artery is irrigated with a 1 % procaine solution, for at least 2 min. With iris scissors a small incision is made 2 mm above the distal ligature. Using vessel cannulation forceps and a bent 27-G hypodermic needle as an introducer, the tip of the catheter is inserted into the artery lumen and advanced approximately 15 mm to reach the abdominal aorta. All three silk ligatures are then tied around the vessel and catheter to fix it at the right position relative to surrounding structures (*see* **Note 9**).
4. The catheter is clamped with padded forceps, the stylet is taken out from catheter and a 1 ml syringe filled with the heparinized/saline is connected to it. After the patency of the catheter is checked, the catheter is sealed with a 23-G stainless steel plug.
5. The catheter is then routed subcutaneously using 16-G stainless steel tubing to the posterior side of the neck and exteriorized near the other catheter.
6. The remainder of the fat pad are repositioned over the vessels and ligated with silk 6/0 suture.
7. The local anesthetic Xylocain 2 % gel and antibiotic ointment Polyspectran are applied and the wound is closed with interrupted silk 3/0 sutures.
8. The mouse is turned in the prone position and the ends of both catheters are introduced into 5 mm of Micro-Renathane silicone tubing (type SIL-080) and then altogether are secured under the skin with discontinuous sutures.
9. Patency of both catheters is confirmed by flushing a heparinized saline and then they are sealed with a plug.
10. For immediate recovery, the mouse is placed in a heated cage in a position with the head and chest slightly higher than the abdomen.

11. Once the mice have recovered fully from anesthesia, they are housed in individual cages for 3 days for postoperative recovery with food and water provided ad libitum. The catheters are flushed daily with heparinized saline (100 U/ml) to ensure patency.

3.6 Equipment Setup

Blood pressure and heart rate are recorded with pressure transducers (model MLT1050) connected via Bridge Amp (ML110) to a multichannel data acquisition system (PowerLab/4sp) and computed by LabChart 5.5.6 software with sampling frequency 200 Hz.

1. The pressure transducers are connected with a three-way stopcock and a 23-G blunted needle to a 50 cm long PE-50 polyethylene tubing with a 23-G stub adaptor on the proximal end required to access the port.
2. To the other way of the stopcock a 1 ml tuberculin syringe is attached with heparinized saline to fill the transducer and backfill the cannula.
3. Two-point calibration of the pressure transducers is performed using a precision mercury manometer.
4. The whole setup is allowed to stabilize for 30 min and zero balancing of the pressure transducers is done prior to each recording procedure.

3.7 Drugs for Intravascular Infusion

Acetylcholine chloride (ACh), sodium nitroprusside dihydrate (SNP), and NG-nitro-L-arginine methyl ester (L-NAME) are purchased from Sigma-Aldrich. ACh and SNP are dissolved in sterile distilled water and divided into small aliquots at concentrations (0.25, 0.5, 1, and 2 μg/ml for ACh; and 100 μg/ml for SNP) and stored frozen at −20 °C. For each injection a new aliquot is used.

3.8 Hemodynamic Measurements and Drug Infusion

1. Experiments are performed 3 days after surgical instrumentation.
2. Near the back incision, the catheter from femoral artery is secured and the stainless steel plug is quickly pulled out to build up negative pressure and to let the fluid to come out from the catheter (*see* **Note 10**).
3. At the moment when the first drop of blood appears, the catheter is clamped with padded hemostats and the stub adaptor from the pressure transducer is connected. The stopcock is turned towards the mouse and the catheter is backfilled with heparinized saline.
4. By turning back the stopcock the patency of the catheter is confirmed by visual analysis of the tracing amplitude. Subsequently, the catheter from the carotid artery is flushed with 30 μl of heparinized saline.

5. Following attachment of the pressure transducer, mice are left undisturbed for 60 min for continuous measurement of the baseline blood pressure. Twisting and knotting of the tubing should be prevented in this time (*see* **Note 11**).
6. To keep disturbance of the mouse to a minimum during intra-aortic injection of the substances an extended injector is used from outside of the cage. The injector consists of a 50 µl Hamilton syringe connected to 50 cm of PE-50 polyethylene tubing with a 23-G stub adaptor at the end. A drop of drug (0.1 µl/g body weight) is inserted into the syringe/injector assembly prefilled with saline and the stub adaptor is connected to the carotid catheter (*see* **Note 12**).

In an experiment using Mas-deficient and wild-type mice shown in Fig. 1, vehicle (15 µl of isotonic saline), ACh (25, 50, 100, and 200 ng/kg), and SNP (10 µg/kg) were injected in bolus separated by at least 5 min intervals [8]. A typical response of a wild-type animal to the highest dose of Ach is shown in Fig. 2. The data clearly show that the administration of ACh into the arterial system does not cause any direct cardiac effects, which is probably due to its rapid degradation. Between the last dose of ACh and SNP the catheter was flushed with additional 30 µl of saline. In control experiments, responses to ACh and SNP were tested in all mice 15 min after pretreatment with the NO synthase inhibitor L-NAME (30 mg/kg). In a previous study, we had tested responses to a range of doses of SNP (1, 3, 5, 10, 15, and 20 µg/kg) and found that a dose of 10 µg/kg induces significant falls in blood pressure and allows adequate recovery of mice from these experiments.

3.9 Data Analysis

1. Mean arterial pressure (MAP) and heart rate (HR) are calculated by Chart 5 Software using the blood pressure and pulse frequency data. To evaluate the response to the drug infusion ΔMAP is calculated as a difference between MAP (averaged from basal measurement 60 s before the infusion) and maximal responses to each dose of ACh and SNP.
2. To correct for differences in vascular smooth muscle reactivity, the response to ACh is normalized by the SNP response (10 µg/kg) according to the formula ΔMAP(ACh)/ΔMAP(SNP).

4 Notes

1. The catheter used for the carotid artery requires a shorter and much thinner end of the tip than the catheter used for the femoral artery, but, otherwise, they are similar. However, it should be noted that the connection between the silicone and the polyethylene tubings have to be well fixed and stabile. Stylet can be used for better fixation. The empty space between

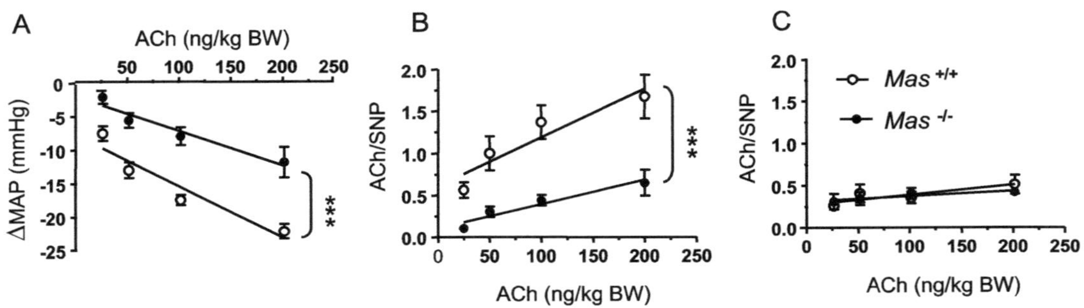

Fig. 1 Endothelial function in conscious *Mas*$^{-/-}$ mice. (**a**) Vascular response to increasing concentrations of ACh in conscious *Mas*$^{-/-}$ ($n=8$) and *Mas*$^{+/+}$ ($n=11$) mice. (**b**) Vascular response to ACh normalized by SNP. (**c**) Vascular response to ACh normalized by SNP after L-NAME treatment. Data represent means ± SEMs. ***$P<0.001$ (2-way ANOVA) (modified from ref. 8)

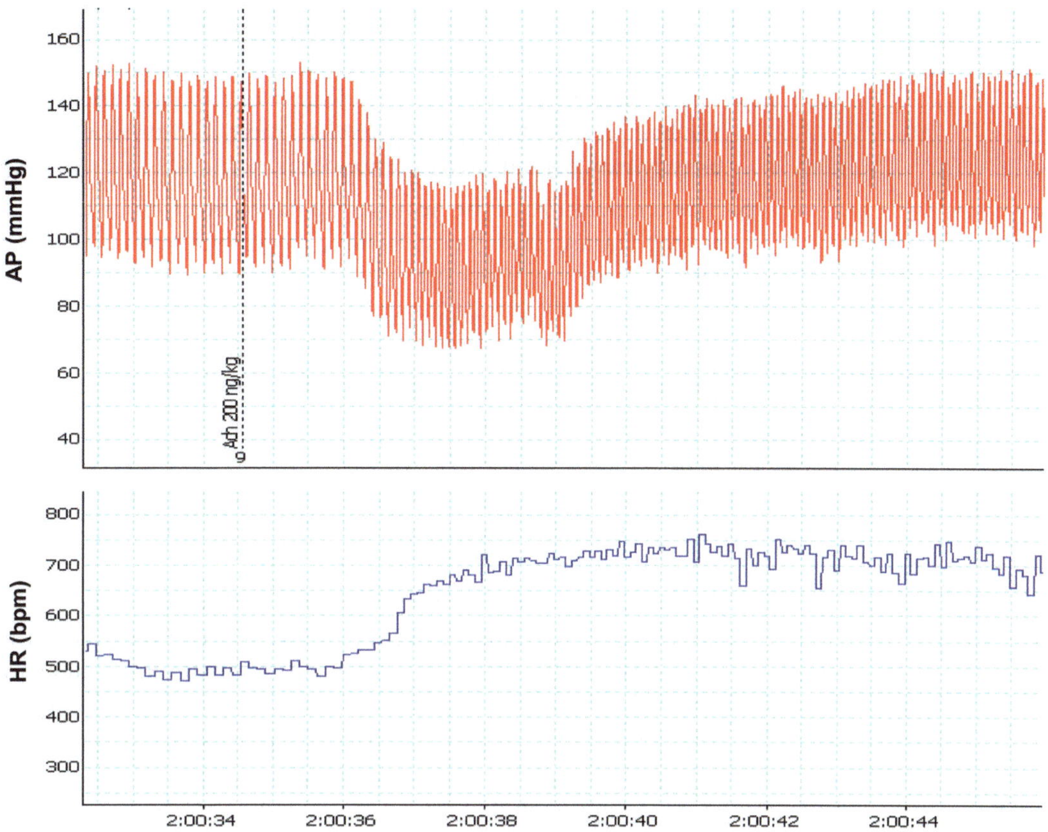

Fig. 2 Arterial pressure (AP, *upper panel*) and heart rate (HR, *lower panel*) of a wild-type mouse before and after administration of ACh (200 ng/kg). ACh induced a fall in AP causing a baroreflex-mediated increase in HR and not a decrease, which would be expected if ACh would directly affect the heart. *bpm* beats per minute

the two tubes has to be filled well with adhesive, and drying of the glue should not be forced. After the manufactured catheters are dried, they should be carefully checked to not drop, especially at the connection.

2. Do not insert the stylet until the end of the catheter. Around 2 mm of the tip should be flexible. Otherwise, during manipulations, the tip of the stylet can damage the aorta.
3. The femoral catheter must be positioned at the abdominal aorta. Never force the catheter, since this can perforate the vessels. If some resistance is encountered gently pull the catheter back and reposition the operated leg to be aligned with the axis of the body. Try to advance the catheter again until the tip of the catheter will be at least 5 mm above the aorta bifurcation.
4. Injectable anesthetics should be diluted before injection. We are using intraperitoneal injection of a ketamine/xylazine mixture in 1 ml of physiological saline solution. This will protect from rapid absorption of anesthetics which maybe lethal for

the mouse. Also, this volume will prolong anesthesia and will counteract dehydration.

5. Shave the surgery area and use adhesive or the paper to remove the hair pieces. Do not apply any hair removal lotion or cream, as they may contain toxic components.
6. The temperature of the heating pad has to be carefully adapted to the mouse body temperature, since overheating may be lethal.
7. Do not stretch too strong the silk suture attached to the upper incisors. This may lead to closure of the nostrils. Mice are obligate nose breathers, and therefore the nostrils of a mouse have to be not obstructed.
8. Damaging or excessively manipulating the vagus nerve during preparation of the carotid artery may lead to arrhythmia, respiratory abnormalities and a variety of other problems, which may impair the experimental procedure.
9. At least 2 mm of the catheter tip should be located in the aortic arch. The flow of blood may bend the flexible tip of the catheter downwards. In this case ACh will not enter into the heart or head.
10. During the recording the steel plug is pulled out to build up a negative pressure and to let the fluid to go out from the catheter. In case no fluid comes out after the stopper is removed, there may be a clot, do not inject the content of the catheter into a mouse. The catheter must be filled with clean heparinized saline by using a blunt Spinocan anesthesia needle 29 G×3½ connected to a 1 ml syringe. This needle is much thinner than the internal diameter of the catheter, it allows to clean the catheter. Then connect the syringe/injector assembly to the catheter and by creating a negative pressure absorb the content from the catheter.
11. Movements of the mouse during the injection of ACh can impair the recording. In this case the tested dose should be repeated.
12. After the last dose of ACh, the carotid catheter must be washed well before SNP injection. The highest dose of ACh can affect SNP response.

References

1. Angus JA, Campbell GR, Cocks TM, Manderson JA (1983) Vasodilatation by acetylcholine is endothelium-dependent: a study by sonomicrometry in canine femoral artery in vivo. J Physiol 344:209–222
2. Vanhoutte PM (2003) Endothelial control of vasomotor function: from health to coronary disease. Circ J 67:572–575
3. Donoghue M, Hsieh F, Baronas E, Godbout K, Gosselin M, Stagliano N, Donovan M,

Woolf B, Robison K, Jeyaseelan R, Breitbart RE, Acton S (2000) A novel angiotensin converting enzyme-related carboxypeptidase (ACE2) converts angiotensin I to angiotensin 1-9. Circ Res 87:E1–9

4. Santos RA, Ferreira AJ, Verano-Braga T, Bader M (2013) Angiotensin-converting enzyme 2, Angiotensin-(1-7) and Mas: new players of the Renin Angiotensin System. J Endocrinol 216(2):R1–R17
5. Santos RA, Simoes-e-Silva AC, Maric C, Silva DM, Machado RP, de Buhr I, Heringer-Walther S, Pinheiro SV, Lopes MT, Bader M, Mendes EP, Lemos VS, Campagnole-Santos MJ, Schultheiss HP, Speth R, Walther T (2003) Angiotensin-(1-7) is an endogenous ligand for the G protein-coupled receptor Mas. Proc Natl Acad Sci U S A 100:8258–8263
6. Faria-Silva R, Duarte FV, Santos RA (2005) Short-term angiotensin(1-7) receptor MAS stimulation improves endothelial function in normotensive rats. Hypertension 46:948–952
7. Sampaio WO, Souza dos Santos RA, Faria-Silva R, da Mata Machado LT, Schiffrin EL, Touyz RM (2007) Angiotensin-(1-7) through receptor Mas mediates endothelial nitric oxide synthase activation via Akt-dependent pathways. Hypertension 49:185–192
8. Xu P, Costa-Goncalves AC, Todiras M, Rabelo LA, Sampaio WO, Moura MM, Santos SS, Luft FC, Bader M, Gross V, Alenina N, Santos RA (2008) Endothelial dysfunction and elevated blood pressure in MAS gene-deleted mice. Hypertension 51:574–580
9. Rabelo LA, Xu P, Todiras M, Sampaio WO, Buttgereit J, Bader M, Santos RA, Alenina N (2008) Ablation of angiotensin (1-7) receptor Mas in C57Bl/6 mice causes endothelial dysfunction. J Am Soc Hypertens 2:418–424
10. Rabelo LA, Alenina N, Bader M (2011) ACE2-angiotensin-(1-7)-Mas axis and oxidative stress in cardiovascular disease. Hypertens Res 34:154–160
11. Langeveld BE, Henning RH, de Smet BJ, Zijlstra F, Driessen A, Tijsma E, van Gilst WH, Roks A (2008) Rescue of arterial function by angiotensin-(1-7): towards improvement of endothelial function by drug-eluting stents. Neth Heart J 16:293–298
12. Scalia R (2007) Evaluation of endothelial function by in vivo microscopy. Methods Mol Med 139:225–235
13. Fitzgerald SM, Bashari H, Cox JA, Parkington HC, Evans RG (2007) Contributions of endothelium-derived relaxing factors to control of hindlimb blood flow in the mouse in vivo. Am J Physiol Heart Circ Physiol 293:H1072–H1082
14. Tamura Y, Naemura A, Inoue A, Ijiri Y, Seki J, Yada T, Goto M, Shinohara M, Kawashima S, Giddings JC, Yamamoto J (2009) Impaired endothelial function may be due to decreased aortic tetrahydrobiopterin, assessed by a new flow-mediated vasodilation in vivo in hypercholesterolemic/atherogenic mice. Blood Coagul Fibrinolysis 20:699–705
15. Wang CH, Chen KT, Mei HF, Lee JF, Cherng WJ, Lin SJ (2011) Assessment of mouse hind limb endothelial function by measuring femoral artery blood flow responses. J Vasc Surg 53:1350–1358
16. Rentzsch B, Todiras M, Iliescu R, Popova E, Campos LA, Oliveira ML, Baltatu OC, Santos RA, Bader M (2008) Transgenic angiotensin-converting enzyme 2 overexpression in vessels of SHRSP rats reduces blood pressure and improves endothelial function. Hypertension 52:967–973

Chapter 29

Vascular Reactivity of Isolated Aorta to Study the Angiotensin-(1-7) Actions

Roberto Q. Lautner, Rodrigo A. Fraga-Silva, Anderson J. Ferreira, and Robson A.S. Santos

Abstract

Since the early 1950s, vascular reactivity using isolated vessel rings has been a useful and efficient model for physiological and pharmacological studies. This experimental model was utilized in the milestone study of Dr. Robert Furchgott to discover the endothelium-derived relaxation factor (EDRF) nitric oxide (NO), opening new avenues and scientific perspectives in the vascular pathophysiology. Moreover, the isolated vessel ring preparation had an important contribution to understand many vasoactive systems. Here, we described the isolated aorta technique and pitfalls about the use of angiotensin-(1-7) peptide in this preparation.

Key words Vascular reactivity, Aortic rings, Endothelium, Vasodilation, Vasoconstriction, Angiotensin-(1-7), A-779, D-Pro^7-Angiotensin-(1-7)

1 Introduction

Historically, the vascular reactivity technique contributed to important discoveries characterizing vascular effects of endogenous substances, such as epinephrine, acetylcholine (Ach), angiotensin (Ang) II, bradykinin, and Ang-(1-7). Indeed, the endothelium-derived relaxation factor (EDRF) nitric oxide (NO) was described using this experimental model culminating with the Nobel Prize 1998 in Physiology and Medicine [1–5].

Ang-(1-7) is a bioactive member of the renin-angiotensin system (RAS) that counter-regulates several Ang II actions, thereby inducing beneficial effects through activation of its own receptor Mas [6]. This peptide is formed mainly by the action of the angiotensin-converting enzyme (ACE) 2 using Ang II as substrate [7]. Based on these observations, a novel concept of the RAS has arisen in which it is formed by two opposite branches, i.e. one deleterious axis composed by ACE/Ang II/AT$_1$, and another protective formed by ACE2/Ang-(1-7)/Mas [8–12].

Rhian M. Touyz and Ernesto L. Schiffrin (eds.), *Hypertension: Methods and Protocols*, Methods in Molecular Biology, vol. 1527, DOI 10.1007/978-1-4939-6625-7_29, © Springer Science+Business Media, LLC 2017

One of the most important effects of Ang-(1-7) is its vasodilatory action in different vascular beds [6, 13–17]. Undoubtedly, the isolated vessel ring preparation was of great importance to describe this Ang-(1-7) action. Nevertheless, because of its biochemical and physiological nature, Ang-(1-7) holds some particularities that might lead to mistakes during the interpretation of the data obtained with the isolated vessel ring technique. Here, we will describe the isolated aorta technique and pitfalls about the use of Ang-(1-7) in this preparation.

2 Materials

2.1 Modified Krebs-Henseleit Buffer

1. To prepare the modified Krebs-Henseleit solution (KHS) just before the use is advisable to avoid microorganism proliferation. This solution needs to be made using pure water (prepared by purifying deionized water to attain a sensitivity of 18 MΩ cm at 25 °C) and analytical grade reagents. Store all reagents at room temperature (unless indicated otherwise). Diligently follow all regulations when disposing of waste materials.
2. The modified KHS consists of 110.8 mmol/L NaCl, 5.9 mmol/L KCl, 25.0 mmol/L $NaHCO_3$, 1.1 mmol/L $MgSO_4$, 2.5 mmol/L $CaCl_2$, 2.3 mmol/L NaH_2PO_4, and 11.5 mmol/L glucose.
3. Modified KHS is gassed with 95% O_2 and 5% CO_2 in order to establish a physiological pH and to provide oxygen source.

2.2 Organ Chamber

1. Due to the large use and applicability of the vascular reactivity model, many commercial isolated organ chamber systems are available. All of these systems are based on the same principle, i.e., they acquire the mechanical activity of the vessel through a force transducer connected to an amplifier. Each system has its own sensibility and precision. Thus, it is important to be aware about these particularities of the systems (e.g., calibration) for a better quality of the acquired data.
2. The organ chamber systems are supplied with an external heating control unit to keep the temperature constant. The desired temperature inside the chamber is about 37.0–37.4 °C. Usually, a thermostat control is located in the water bath and it allows detecting slight changes in the temperature of the water inside the chamber. Thus, required adjustments should be performed measuring the temperature inside the chamber.
3. The mechanical activity (tension) of the vessel is recorded by a force transducer. One end of the vessel ring is connected to the transducer using a holder, while another end is stuck. Therefore, it is important to assure that the vessel holders are properly positioned, without slackness or touching the support.

2.3 Vasoactive Agents

1. Acetylcholine chloride (Sigma-Aldrich, Inc).
2. Phenylephrine hydrochloride (Sigma-Aldrich, Inc).
3. Angiotensin I/II (1-7) [Ang-(1-7), amino acid sequence: H-Asp-Arg-Val-Tyr-Ile-His-Pro-OH] (Bachem, Inc or Phoenix Pharmaceutical, Inc).
4. [D-Ala^7]-Angiotensin I/II (1-7) (A-779, amino acid sequence: H-Asp-Arg-Val-Tyr-Ile-His-D-Ala-OH) (Bachem, Inc or Phoenix Pharmaceutical, Inc) [18].
5. [D-Pro^7]-Angiotensin I/II (1-7) [D-Pro^7-Ang-(1-7), amino acid sequence: H-Asp-Arg-Val-Tyr-Ile-His-D-Pro-OH) (Bachem, Inc or Phoenix Pharmaceutical, Inc) [19].

3 Methods

3.1 Preparing the Krebs-Henseleit Buffer

1. It is indispensable to estimate the total volume of KHS required for the entire experimentation. The total volume will depend on the volume of the chambers, number of samples, duration of the experimentation and protocol design (number of curves, period of incubation, required period of stabilization, etc.). For example, in a simple protocol to evaluate the Ang-(1-7) activity using eight chambers with 10 mL each, it will be necessary 2 L of buffer, as follows:
   - Number of chambers = 8.
   - Volume of the chamber = 10 mL.
   - Changes of buffer during initial stabilization = 4 (total time of stabilization 60 min, buffer replaced every 15 min).
   - Changes of buffer during experimentation = 5.
   - Margin of safety = 20 %.

$$\left(8 \times 10\text{mL} \times 4 \times 5 \times 1.2 = 1920\text{mL}\right)$$

2. Using a 2 L beaker and under agitation, dissolve 6.9 g of NaCl; 0.7 g of KCL; 0.32 g of KH_2PO_4; 0.6 g of $MgSO_4.7\ H_2O$; 4.0 g of glucose; and 4.2 g of $NaHCO_3$ in 1.5 L of pure water. Add the salts one by one and wait until they complete dissolve before adding the next.
3. In other beaker, dissolve 0.74 g of $CaCl_2.2H_2O$ in 300 mL of pure water. After complete dissolution of $CaCl_2$, add it gently to the buffer. This procedure will avoid the precipitation of $CaSO_4$(s) formed in presence of high concentration of $Ca^{+2}_{(aq)}$ and $[SO_4^{-2}]_{(aq)}$. The KHS is completely crystalline and traces of opacity (usually white) indicate precipitation. In this case, the buffer cannot be used and need to be wasted.

4. After dissolving the KHS reagents, adjust the volume for 2 L. Later, warm the buffer to 37 °C and oxygenate it with 95% O_2/5% CO_2. This procedure needs to be performed at least 20 min before setting up the vessels in the chamber.

3.2 Sacrifice of the Animal and Tissue Preparation

1. In order to avoid unnecessary pain and stress to the animal (rat or mouse), as well as interferences due to the use of anesthetics, sacrifice the animals by the decapitation method. Excise the tissues shortly thereafter.
2. Dissect the animal removing the internal organs located in the thoracic and abdominal regions. Be careful to avoid damages to the aorta, which is closely located with the spinal cord. Localize the descending thoracic aorta and remove the excess of adipose and connective tissues around the aorta. Gently, excise the aorta without stretching or pinch the functional area (selected area which will provide the rings) to avoid damages to the endothelium layer. Place it in a petri dish containing modified KHS and remove the remained adipose tissue under a binocular microscope.
3. Cut the aorta in segments (rings), 2 mm for mouse aorta and 4 mm for rat aorta. If desired, identify the rings according to cephalic or distal regions (population of many receptors varies in the regions of the aorta).

3.3 Setting Up the System and Tissue

1. Before sacrifice, the acquisition system needs to be calibrated and the chambers filled with KHS maintained at 37 °C with continuous oxygenation.
2. Gently, place the rings between two L-shaped stainless steel hooks (tissue holders) and immerse them into the chamber. Stretch the vessel to a passive force (e.g., 0.5 g for 2 mm mouse aortic rings and 1.0 g for 4 mm rat aortic rings) to mimic the physiological tonic tension.
3. Allow the vessels to equilibrate for 60 min, replacing the KHS every 15 min. During the stabilization period, the basal tension may decrease due to the adaptation of the vessels. This may occur in the first minutes and it needs to be adjusted to the basal tension.

3.4 Endothelial Function

1. After stabilization, the preparation is ready for stimulation. However, before evaluation of the Ang-(1-7) activity, the endothelium integrity must to be attested. The endothelium functionality is assessed by testing the relaxation produced by Ach in rings pre-contracted with phenylephrine (Fig. 1). Thus, firstly discard the buffer and refill the chamber with fresh buffer (pre-warmed at 37 °C and oxygenated).
2. Add a submaximal dose of phenylephrine to the bath (Fig. 2). The suggested dose is 0.1 μM, e.g., add 10 μL of a stock solution at 0.1 mM into the 10 mL chamber.

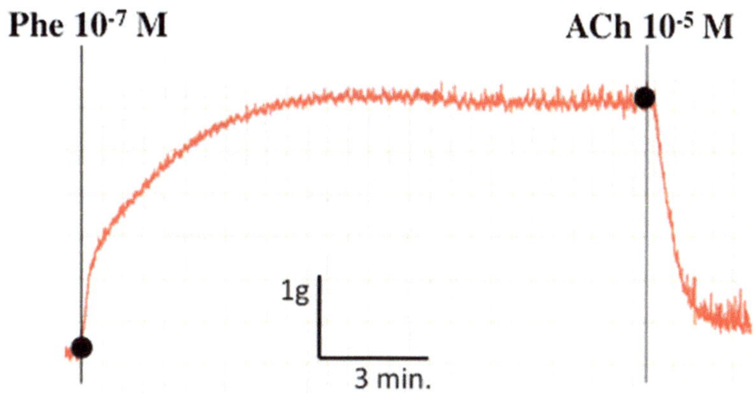

Fig. 1 Typical recording showing rat aortic tension (g) with time. After equilibration at 1.0 g of tension, aortic ring was exposed to phenylephrine and acetylcholine on endothelium-intact ring

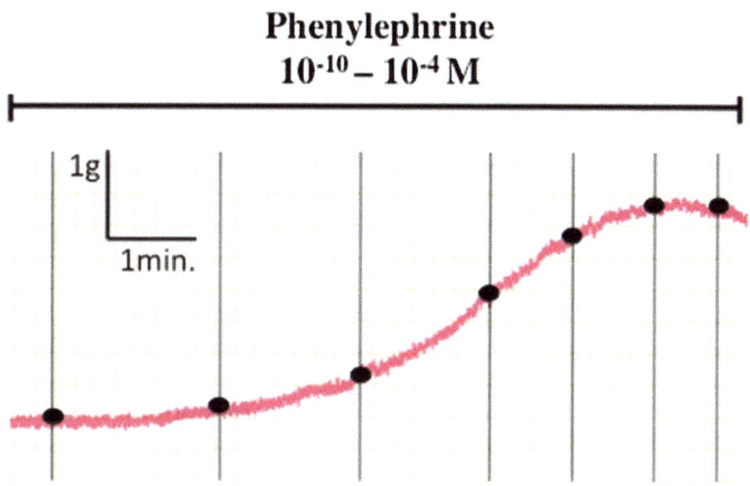

Fig. 2 Typical recording showing rat aortic tension (g) with time. After equilibration at 1.0 g of tension, a cumulative concentration curve was constructed using phenylephrine

3. After the vasoconstriction reaches the stabilization, add Ach at 10 μM, e.g., 10 μL of a stock solution at 10 mM in a chamber with 10 mL of total volume. In the presence of an undamaged endothelium, Ach will cause vasorelaxation (Fig. 1). To consider the endothelium intact, the relaxation produced by Ach needs to reach at least 80% of relaxation in rat aorta and 60% of relaxation in mouse aorta.
4. The percentage of relaxation is calculated considering the delta of the constriction produced by phenylephrine. For instance, considering a preparation with 1.0 g of basal tension in which

the phenylephrine stimulus caused an increase in the tension stabilized at 3.0 g and a relaxation to 1.2 g was reached after Ach incubation, it is possible to conclude that a 90% of relaxation was observed. In other words, the contraction was of 2.0 g and the relaxation was of 1.8 g, giving 90% of relaxation.

5. For endothelium-denuded experiments, prior setting up the ring in the organ chamber system, remove the endothelium by gently rubbing the intimal surface with a wooden stick.
6. To consider a vessel with nonfunctional endothelium, the relaxation produced by Ach should not exceed 5% (Fig. 3).
7. After testing the functionality of the endothelium, wash the preparation three times with fresh buffer (10 min each wash) prior sequential stimulation.

3.5 Ang-(1-7) Activity

1. To assess the vasorelaxant activity of Ang-(1-7) in aorta of rat and mouse, a cumulative concentration curve from 10^{-10} to 10^{-5} M should be performed in pre-constricted vessels. In stabilized preparations, discard the buffer and refill the chamber with fresh buffer (pre-warmed at 37 °C and oxygenated).
2. Add phenylephrine at 0.1 μM, e.g., 10 μL of the stock solution at 0.1 mM in a chamber with 10 mL of total volume.
3. The vessels will contract reaching the stabilization. Sequentially, perform the Ang-(1-7) cumulative concentration curve following the protocol summarized in Table 1.
4. The pharmacological blockade of Ang-(1-7) vasorelaxant activity can be assessed using two different antagonists, A-779 or D-pro^7-Ang-(1-7). Add the antagonist at 10 μM (e.g., 10 μL of the stock solution at 0.1 mM in a chamber with

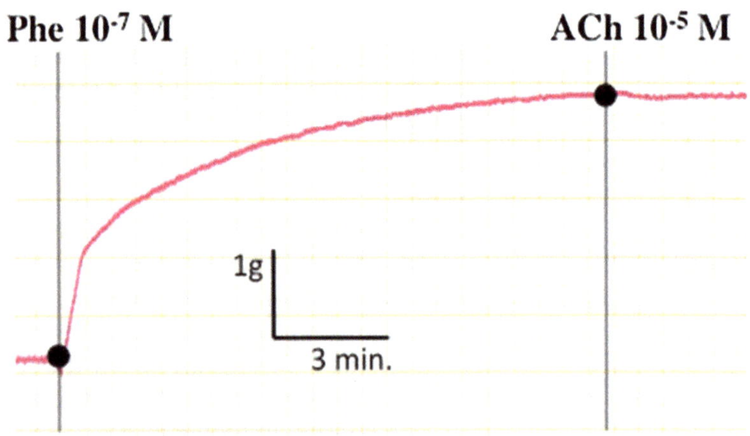

Fig. 3 Typical recording showing rat aortic tension (g) with time. After equilibration at 1.0 g of tension, aortic ring was exposed phenylephrine and acetylcholine on endothelium-denuded ring

Table 1
Protocol pipetting of angiotensin-(1-7) in organ bath containing 10 ml of Krebs-Henseleit solution

Ang-(1-7) concentration (mol/L)	Pipetting volume (μL)	Ang-(1-7) final concentration in organ bath (mol/L)
10^{-7}	10	10^{-10}
	20	3×10^{-10}
	70	10^{-9}
10^{-6}	20	3×10^{-9}
	70	10^{-8}
10^{-5}	20	3×10^{-8}
	70	10^{-7}
10^{-4}	20	3×10^{-7}
	70	10^{-6}

10 mL of total volume) 2–5 min before pre-constriction with phenylephrine. After stabilization of the constriction, proceed with the cumulative curve for Ang-(1-7).

5. The molecular pathways involved in the vasorelaxant effect of Ang-(1-7) may be assessed in this experimental model adding pharmacological tools into the bath before pre-constriction induced by phenylephrine and the cumulative concentration curve of Ang-(1-7). For instance, the aortic preparation may be incubated with N^G-nitro-L-arginine methyl ester (L-NAME), a selective inhibitor of NO synthase (NOS) and/or indomethacin, a nonselective inhibitor of cyclooxygenase (COX), to address the role of NO and prostaglandins, respectively, in the vasorelaxant effect of Ang-(1-7) [15, 20].
6. The analysis of the vasorelaxant effect of Ang-(1-7) in aorta can be performed by the maximal relaxation (E_{max}) and/or by the concentration causing 50% of the maximal response (EC_{50}) expressed as pD_2 ($-\log EC_{50}$).

4 Notes

1. The endothelium is a delicate layer of cells which may be easily damaged during the initial procedures. The removal of the aorta from the animal, its segmentation (rings) and the procedure to place it in the tissue holder are critical. During the removal of the aorta avoid stretching or pinching the selected

area for the rings. Cut the vessel gently when preparing the rings avoiding screw it. When placing the ring in the holders, avoid rubbing the internal surface of the vessel.

2. The vasodilatory effect of Ang-(1-7) is abolished in endothelium-denuded rings [15, 20]. Thus, it is critical the presence of a preserved endothelium in the preparation. The endothelium test with Ach in pre-constricted rings with phenylephrine is fundamental to confirm the endothelium integrity.
3. The vasorelaxant effect of Ang-(1-7) in aortic rings pre-constricted with phenylephrine is rapidly reverted. Therefore, during the cumulative curve of Ang-(1-7), each dose of Ang-(1-7) must be added as soon as the previous dose reaches the plateau. The time for reaching the plateau will depend on the specie and strain and usually occurs about 1 min or even less.
4. Ang-(1-7) does not cause relaxation without pre-constriction of the vessel. Moreover, Ang-(1-7) causes vasorelaxation in aortic rat rings pre-constricted with KCl at 25 mM, but not in rings pre-constricted with KCl at 100 mM (Fig. 4).

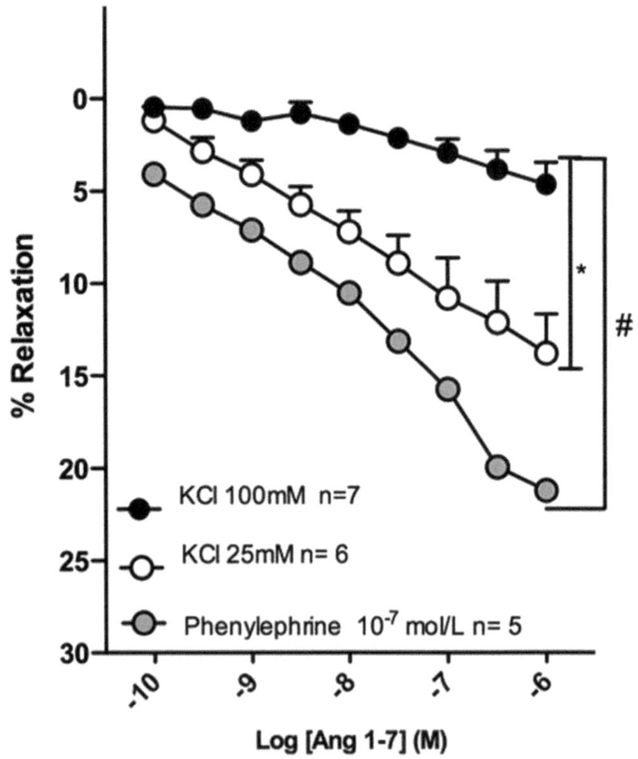

Fig. 4 Ang-(1-7) cause relaxation in vessels pre-constricted with KCl 25 mM, but not with KCL 100 mM. Cumulative concentration curve of Ang-(1-7) caused relaxation in Wistar rat aortic rings pre-constricted with phenylephrine (*gray circle*) and KCl 25 mM (*white circle*), but not in rings pre-constricted with KCl 100 mM (*black circle*). *,#$P<0.05$

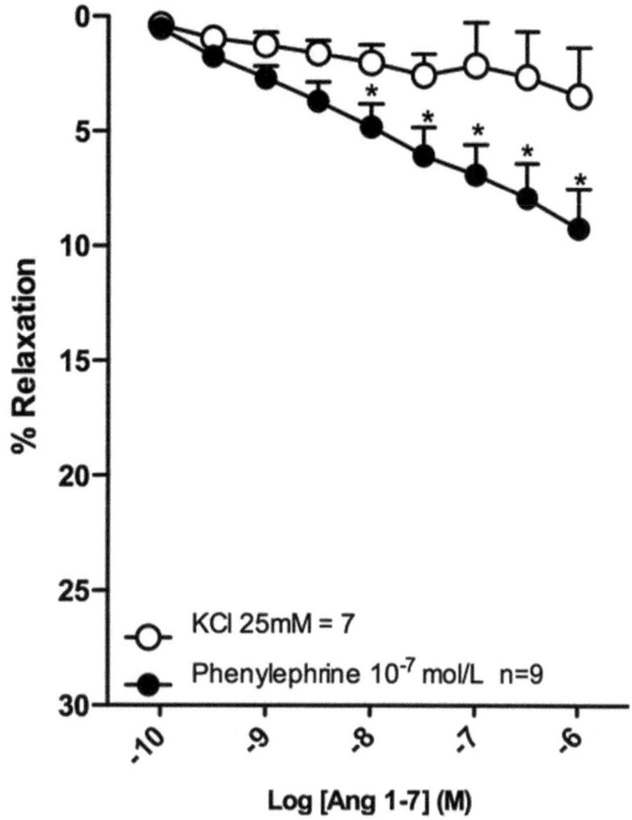

Fig. 5 The vasorelaxant activity of Ang-(1-7) is significantly attenuated in rings kept overnight at 4 °C. Cumulative concentration curve of Ang-(1-7) was performed in Wistar rat aortic rings kept for 24 h in KHR at 4 °C. The vasoactivity of Ang-(1-7) was measured in vessels pre-constricted with phenylephrine (*black circle*) and KCl 25 mM (*white circle*). *$P<0.05$

5. The vasorelaxant activity of Ang-(1-7) is significantly attenuated in rings kept overnight at 4 °C (Fig. 5). Thus, overnight protocols need to be carefully planned and interpreted.
6. Most of the actions of Ang-(1-7) are mediated by Mas [6, 8, 12]. In fact, the vasodilation effect of Ang-(1-7) is absent in two different strains of *Mas*-gene deleted mice [6, 21]. There are two different Mas antagonists, A-779 and D-Pro^7-Ang-(1-7) [18, 19]. However, the use of such blockers needs to be carefully interpreted. Previously, we have shown that the vasodilatory effect of Ang-(1-7) in aortic rings of Sprague–Dawley is blocked by D-pro^7-Ang-(1-7), but not by A-779 [20]. On the other hand, both antagonists abolished the Ang-(1-7) vasodilation in aortic rings of Wistar rats and C57/Bl6 and FVBN mice [6, 21]. These data suggest the existence of different subtypes of Ang-(1-7) receptors, which are sensitive

to distinct antagonists and may be differently expressed in distinct species and strains.

7. Aliquots of Ang-(1-7), A-779, and D-Pro^7-Ang-(1-7) can be stocked at −20 °C, but at high concentration (0.02 μg/10 μL) and not over 3 months.
8. The working solutions of Ang-(1-7), A-779, and D-Pro^7-Ang-(1-7) must be freshly prepared and kept on ice until use.

Acknowledgment

This work was supported by the National Institute of Science and Technology in Nanobiopharmaceutics, Brazil.

References

1. Furchgott RF, Zawadzki JV (1980) The obligatory role of endothelial cells in the relaxation of arterial smooth muscle by acetylcholine. Nature 288:373–376
2. Furchgott RF (1998) Nitric oxide: from basic research on isolated blood vessels to clinical relevance in diabetes. An R Acad Nac Med 115:317–331
3. Furchgott RF (1996) The 1996 Albert Lasker Medical Research Awards. The discovery of endothelium-derived relaxing factor and its importance in the identification of nitric oxide. JAMA 276:1186–1188
4. Vanin AF (1999) 1998 Nobel prize winners for physiology or medicine. Biochemistry 64:98–100
5. Williams N (1998) NO news is good news--but only for three Americans. Science 282:610–611
6. Santos RA, Simoes-e-Silva AC, Maric C, Silva DM, Machado RP, de Buhr I, Heringer-Walther S, Pinheiro SV, Lopes MT, Bader M, Mendes EP, Lemos VS, Campagnole-Santos MJ, Schultheiss HP, Speth R, Walther T (2003) Angiotensin-(1-7) is an endogenous ligand for the G protein-coupled receptor Mas. Proc Natl Acad Sci U S A 100:8258–8263
7. Vickers C, Hales P, Kaushik V, Dick L, Gavin J, Tang J, Godbout K, Parsons T, Baronas E, Hsieh F, Acton S, Patane M, Nichols A, Tummino P (2002) Hydrolysis of biological peptides by human angiotensin-converting enzyme-related carboxypeptidase. J Biol Chem 277:14838–14843
8. Ferreira AJ, Santos RA, Bradford CN, Mecca AP, Sumners C, Katovich MJ, Raizada MK (2010) Therapeutic implications of the vasoprotective axis of the renin-angiotensin system in cardiovascular diseases. Hypertension 55:207–213
9. Ferreira AJ, Santos RA (2005) Cardiovascular actions of angiotensin-(1-7). Braz J Med Biol Res 38:499–507
10. Ferreira AJ, Murca TM, Fraga-Silva RA, Castro CH, Raizada MK, Santos RA (2012) New cardiovascular and pulmonary therapeutic strategies based on the Angiotensin-converting enzyme 2/angiotensin-(1-7)/mas receptor axis. Int J Hypertens 2012:147825
11. Fraga-Silva RA, Da Silva DG, Montecucco F, Mach F, Stergiopulos N, da Silva RF, Santos RA (2012) The angiotensin-converting enzyme 2/angiotensin-(1-7)/Mas receptor axis: a potential target for treating thrombotic diseases. Thromb Haemost 108:1089–1096
12. Fraga-Silva RA, Ferreira AJ, Dos Santos RA (2013) Opportunities for targeting the Angiotensin-converting enzyme 2/angiotensin-(1-7)/mas receptor pathway in hypertension. Curr Hypertens Rep 15:31–38
13. Brosnihan KB, Li P, Ferrario CM (1996) Angiotensin-(1-7) dilates canine coronary arteries through kinins and nitric oxide. Hypertension 27:523–528
14. Porsti I, Bara AT, Busse R, Hecker M (1994) Release of nitric oxide by angiotensin-(1-7) from porcine coronary endothelium: implications for a novel angiotensin receptor. Br J Pharmacol 111:652–654
15. Feterik K, Smith L, Katusic ZS (2000) Angiotensin-(1-7) causes endothelium-dependent relaxation in canine middle cerebral artery. Brain Res 873:75–82
16. Savergnini SQ, Beiman M, Lautner RQ, de Paula-Carvalho V, Allahdadi K, Pessoa DC, Costa-Fraga FP, Fraga-Silva RA, Cojocaru G, Cohen Y, Bader M, de Almeida AP, Rotman G, Santos RA (2010) Vascular relaxation, antihy-

pertensive effect, and cardioprotection of a novel peptide agonist of the MAS receptor. Hypertension 56:112–120

17. Fernandes L, Fortes ZB, Nigro D, Tostes RC, Santos RA, Catelli De Carvalho MH (2001) Potentiation of bradykinin by angiotensin-(1-7) on arterioles of spontaneously hypertensive rats studied in vivo. Hypertension 37:703–709
18. Santos RA, Campagnole-Santos MJ, Baracho NC, Fontes MA, Silva LC, Neves LA, Oliveira DR, Caligiorne SM, Rodrigues AR, Gropen Junior C et al (1994) Characterization of a new angiotensin antagonist selective for angiotensin-(1-7): evidence that the actions of angiotensin-(1-7) are mediated by specific angiotensin receptors. Brain Res Bull 35:293–298
19. Santos RA, Haibara AS, Campagnole-Santos MJ, Simoes e Silva AC, Paula RD, Pinheiro SV, Leite MF, Lemos VS, Silva DM, Guerra MT, Khosla MC (2003) Characterization of a new selective antagonist for angiotensin-(1-7), D-pro7-angiotensin-(1-7).Hypertension41:737–743
20. Silva DM, Vianna HR, Cortes SF, Campagnole-Santos MJ, Santos RA, Lemos VS (2007) Evidence for a new angiotensin-(1-7) receptor subtype in the aorta of Sprague-Dawley rats. Peptides 28:702–707
21. Santos RA, Paula RD, Bader M, Alenina N, Ferreira AJ, Raizada MK, Costa-Fraga FC (2008) Mas-independent vasorelaxant actions of ala1-angiotensin-(1–7), a novel ACE2 product. Hypertension 52:34–131

Chapter 30

Generation of a Mouse Model with Smooth Muscle Cell Specific Loss of the Expression of PPARγ

Yohann Rautureau, Pierre Paradis, and Ernesto L. Schiffrin

Abstract

An inducible tissue-specific knockout (KO) technique has been used to study the role of genes in the adult heart. This KO technique circumvents the developmental effect that could otherwise be observed in a tissue-specific KO. The peroxisome proliferator-activated receptor (PPAR) γ is a transcription factor that when activated has been shown to improve vascular remodeling and endothelial function in hypertensive rodents. Here we describe an inducible tissue specific KO protocol used to study the role of PPARγ in smooth muscle cells (SMC) in angiotensin (Ang) II-induced hypertension in adult mice. Inducible VSMC *Pparγ* KO mice are generated by crossing mice expressing a fusion protein of Cre recombinase with the modified estrogen receptor ligand binding domain (*Cre*ER^{T2}) under the control of the *smooth muscle myosin heavy chain* (*smmhc*, *myh11*) with mice having loxP sites flanking exon 2 of the *Pparγ* gene (*PparγFlox/Flox*). The SMC *Pparγ* KO is induced by treating smMHC-*Cre*ER^{T2}/*PparγFlox/Flox* mice with the estrogen receptor antagonist tamoxifen causing recombination of the two loxP site by CreER^{T2}. SMC KO is confirmed by determining mRNA *Pparγ* levels in aortic media. Presence of the loxP sites is determined by sequencing genomic DNA. Tissue specific expression is assayed using smMHC-*Cre*ER^{T2}/reporter crossed mice.

Key words Hypertension, PPARγ, Arteries, Smooth muscle cell, Cre-LoxP, Tamoxifen, Reporter mice

1 Introduction

Natural ligands of PPARγ are prostaglandins and linolenic acid. Synthetic ligands include the thiazolidinediones (TZDs) such as rosiglitazone and pioglitazone. TZDs have been and are still used as antidiabetic insulin sensitizers. PPARγ is expressed in all the cells of blood vessels including smooth muscle cells (SMC) [1–4]. In hypertension, activation of PPARγ with TZDs decreases blood pressure (BP) and vascular damage. It also improves vascular remodeling and endothelial dysfunction [5, 6]. Studies of the role of PPARγ in SMC using *Sm22α* promoter-driven SMC-specific Cre expression and KO in mice with *Pparγ* floxed gene (*PparγFlox/Flox*) has resulted in paradoxical observations [7, 8]. SMC *Pparγ* inactivation resulted in the perturbation of the blood pressure (BP)

Rhian M. Touyz and Ernesto L. Schiffrin (eds.), *Hypertension: Methods and Protocols*, Methods in Molecular Biology, vol. 1527, DOI 10.1007/978-1-4939-6625-7_30, © Springer Science+Business Media LLC 2017

circadian rhythm and produced an increase [8] or a decrease [9] in BP during the day when transgenic and knockin (KI) *Sm22α*-Cre mice were used respectively with *PparγFlox/Flox* mice. These discrepancies might result from the fact that the expression of *Sm22α* promoter differs between its native genomic and the transgenic environment. For example, transgenic *Sm22α* promoter-driven Cre recombination of LoxP sites could lead to KO in other tissues such as the heart and the kidney [7]. In these KO studies, *Pparγ* disruption occurred in utero, which could causes developmental effects and compensatory mechanisms contributing to the phenotype. It was recently shown that deletion of *Pparγ* in SMC using *Sm22α*-Cre KI mice causing *Pparγ* KO was not restricted to SMC, but also occurred in perivascular fat (PVAT) [10]. The latter prevented the development of PVAT and could contribute to the hypotensive phenotype.

A drug-inducible tissue-specific knockout (KO) technique has been used to circumvent developmental effects *n* order to study the role of genes in the adult heart [11, 12]. Here we describe an inducible tissue-specific KO protocol used to study the role of PPARγ in smooth muscle cells in angiotensin (Ang) II-induced hypertension in adult mice [13]. Inducible SMC *Pparγ* KO mice are generated by crossing mice expressing a fusion protein of Cre recombinase with the modified estrogen receptor ligand binding domain (*Cre*ER^{T2}) under the control of the *smooth muscle myosin heavy chain* (*Smmhc*, *Myh11*) with mice having loxP sites flanking exon 2 of the *Pparγ* gene (*PparγFlox/Flox*) (Fig. 1). CreER^{T2} cannot bind estrogen but can be activated by the estrogen receptor antagonist tamoxifen. SMC *Pparγ* KO is induced by treating *Smmhc-Cre*ER^{T2}/*PparγFlox/Flox* mice with tamoxifen causing recombination of the two loxP sites by CreER^{T2}. SMC KO is confirmed by determining mRNA *Pparγ* levels in aortic media. Presence of the loxP sites is determined by sequencing of genomic DNA. Tissue-specific expression is assayed using smMHC-*Cre*ER^{T2}/reporter crossed mice. The inducible SMC-specific *Pparγ* KO (*Smmhc-Cre*ER^{T2}/*PparγFlox/Flox*) mouse is a useful model to understand the role of SPPARγ in SMC in hypertension induced by different agents.

2 Materials

2.1 Mice

1. Transgenic mice (C57BL/6) expressing a fusion protein of Cre recombinase with the modified estrogen receptor-binding domain (CreER^{T2}) under the control of the *Smooth muscle heavy chain* (*Smmhc, Myh11*) promoter (*Smmhc*-CreER^{T2} mice) [14] can be obtained through collaboration with Dr Stefan Offermanns (Max Planck Institute for Heart and Lung Research, Bad Nauheim, Germany). These mice have been

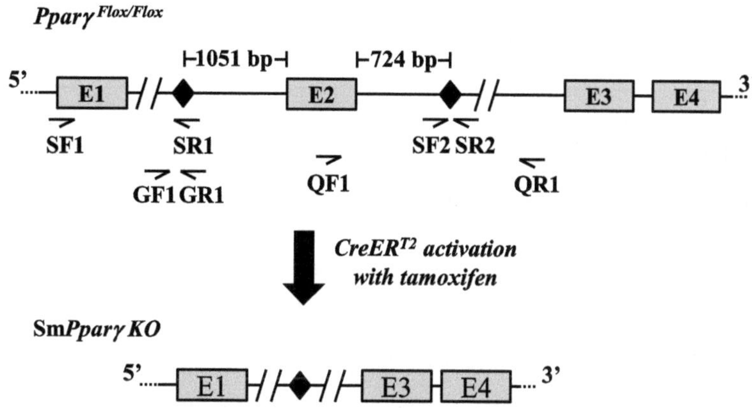

Fig. 1 Strategy for the generation of tamoxifen-inducible SMC *Pparγ* KO mice. Inducible SMC *Pparγ* KO mice were generated by crossing mice expressing a fusion protein of Cre recombinase with the modified estrogen receptor ligand binding domain (*Cre*ER^{T2}) under the control of the *smooth muscle myosin heavy chain* (*Smmhc, Myh11*) with mice having loxP sites flanking exon 2 of the *Pparγ* gene (*PparγFlox/Flox*). CreER^{T2} cannot bind estrogen but can be activated by the estrogen receptor antagonist tamoxifen. SMC *Pparγ* (Sm*Pparγ*) KO is induced by treating *Smmhc-Cre*ER^{T2}/*PparγFlox/Flox* mice with tamoxifen causing recombination of the two loxP sites by CreER^{T2}. *SF#* sequencing forward #, *SR#* sequencing reverse #, *QF1* QPCR forward 1, *QR1* QPCR reverse 1 oligonucleotides are listed in Table 1 have their positions indicated with *half arrows*. *Boxes* represent the exons. *Double arrows* show the number of bases between 5′ and 3′ LoxP sequences and the exon 2

generated using a bacterial artificial chromosome (BAC) containing only the *Myh11* gene, which is integrated as a transgene on the Y chromosome (*see* **Note 1**).

2. *Pparγ* floxed mice (*PparγFlox/Flox*, BALB/c) can be obtained through collaboration with Dr Franck, J. Gonzalez (Laboratory of Metabolism, Division of Basic Sciences, National Cancer Institute, National Institutes of Health, Bethesda, MD, USA) [3]. These mice possess loxP sites on either side of exon 2 of the *Pparγ* gene.
3. Wild-type BALB/c female mice for reproduction (Harlan Laboratories).
4. B6.129S4-*GT(Rosa)26sortm1Sor/*J (*Rosa–lacZ/–lacZ*) reporter mice (The Jackson Laboratory) are in a C57BL/6 background and carry a DNA STOP sequence flanked by two loxP sites that prevent expression of a downstream β-galactosidase (*lacZ*) gene [15]. Upon Cre activation, the STOP sequence is excised and β-galactosidase is expressed in cells where Cre has provoked DNA excision.

Table 1
Oligonucleotides, product sizes, and applications

Gene	Primers	Product size (bp)	Application
PparγFlox/Flox	F: 5′-TCCAATGTTCCCAAACTTACAC-3′ [GF1] R: 5′-cagctatgacttactgaaaagaagc-3′ [GR1]	WT: 209 *Flox*: 244	PCR genotyping
Smmhc-CreER^{T2}	FWT: 5′-TGACCCCATCTCTTCACTCC-3′ RWT: 5′-AACTCCACGACCACCTCATC-3′ RTg:5′-AGTCCCTCACATCCTCAGGTT-3′	WT: 225 CreER^{T2}: 287	PCR genotyping
Rosa–lacZ/+	FWT: 5′-AAAGTCGCTCTGAGTTGTTAT-3′ RWT: 5′-GGAGCGGGAGAAATGGATATG-3′ RTg: 5′-GCGAAGAGTTTGTCCTCAACC-3′	WT:550 *–lacZ*:300	PCR genotyping
RosamT-mG/+	FWT: 5′-CTCTGCTGCCTCCTGGCTTCT-3′ RWT: 5′-CGAGGCGGATCACAAGCAATA-3′ RTg: 5′-TCAATGGGCGGGGGTCGTT-3′	WT: 330 *mT-mG*: 250	PCR genotyping
Pparγ Flox/Flox	F: 5′-ACCATGGTTGACACAGAGA TG-3′[SF1] R: 5′-ACAGCTTAGAAAGAAAGCCTAA CTG-3′[SR1]	753	Sequencing of *PparγFlox/Flox* mouse
Pparγ Flox/Flox	F: 5′-TGACCCATGGACTAATGCTG-3′[SF2] R: 5′-GACCAGGCTTGATGAACTCC-3′[SR2]	630	Sequencing of *PparγFlox/Flox* mouse
Pparγ	F: 5′-AACAGGCCTCATGAAGAACC-3′[QF1] R: 5′-CCAACAGCTTCTCCTTCTCG-3′ [QR1]	298	mRNA quantification by QPCR
Rps16	F: 5′-ATCTCAAAGGCCCTGGTAGC-3′ R: 5′-ACAAAGGTAAACCCCGATCC-3′	211	Housekeeping gene for relative quantification of mRNA by QPCR

Oligonucleotides for PCR genotyping and sequencing quantitative PCR (QPCR) are presented. Oligonucleotides with bracketed abbreviations are depicted in Fig. 1

F forward, *R* reverse, *GF1* genotyping forward 1, *GR1* genotyping reverse 1, *WT* wild-type, *FWT* forward WT, *RWT* reverse WT, *RTg* reverse transgenic referring to CreER^{T2}, *–lacZ* or *mT-mG*, *SF#* sequencing forward #, *SR#* sequencing reverse #, *QF1* QPCR forward 1, *QR1* QPCR reverse 1, *Rps16* 40S ribosomal protein S16

5. B6.129(Cg)-Gt(ROSA)26Sor$^{tm4(}$*Actb-tdtomato,-egfp*$^{)Luo}$/J (*RosamT-mG/mT-mG*) reporter mice [16] (The Jackson Laboratory) are in a C57BL/6 background and possess a membrane-targeted tandem dimer *tomato* (mT) cassette flanked by two loxP sites with a downstream membrane-targeted *enhanced green fluorescent protein* (*egfp*) (mG). These mice express mT prior to Cre-mediated excision in all cell types and mG after excision in cells where Cre has induced DNA excision. The excitation/emission of dtTomato and EGFP are 554/581 and 488/509 nm, respectively.

2.2 Genotyping and Sequencing of Genomic DNA

1. Autoclaved polypropylene tubes, 1.5 mL (Sarstedt).
2. A set of pipettes and disposable tips for volumes of 2, 20, 200 and 1000 μL.
3. Basic digestion buffer for extraction of genomic DNA from mouse tails: 25 mM NaOH, 0.2 mM EDTA, pH 12. Store at room temperature (RT) in a plastic bottle.
4. Heat block: Thermolyne DRI-BATH with three heat blocks.
5. Vortex-Genie 2 (VWR Scientific).
6. Centrifuge 5415D with fixed-angle rotor FA-45-24-11 (Eppendorf).
7. Oligonucleotides (*see* Table 1).
8. Top Taq DNA polymerase (Qiagen).
9. Set of PCR grade 100 mM dNTP (Qiagen). Prepare a 2.5 mM dNTPs working solution and store aliquots at −20 °C until use. Prepare aliquots as small as possible to limit the number of freeze thawing cycle to 3. This is to prevent degradation of dNTPs.
10. Micro-tube opener (Research Product International Corp.)
11. PCR tubes.
12. Centrifuge 5417C with fixed-angle rotor FA-45-28-PCR (Eppendorf) that accommodates six 8-tube strips or 48 individual PCR test tubes.
13. Biometra TGradient Thermocycler (Montreal Biotech).
14. Agarose A, DNase, RNase, and protease free.
15. Diethyl pyrocarbonate (DEPC, Sigma-Aldrich).
16. RNAse-free water. Add 0.01 volume of DEPC to milliQ water contained in an Erlenmeyer flask in a fume hood. Mix until complete dispersion of the DEPC, and continue to mix for at least 10 min and up to overnight. Seal the Erlenmeyer flask with an aluminum foil, and autoclave the water for 45 min. Immediately after autoclaved, place the Erlenmeyer flask upon a heat plate in a fume hood, remove the aluminum foil and boil the water for 30 min or until disappearance of the fruity smell of DEPC. Let the water cool down and store in RNAse-free containers.
17. Ethylenediaminetetraacetic acid (EDTA) 500 mM, pH 8, RNase free. Reserve a bottle of EDTA for RNA applications. Dissolve 14.6 g of EDTA in ~90 mL of RNAse-free water. Adjust the pH to 8 with pellets of NaOH. Adjust the volume to 100 mL. Store in RNAse-free containers.
18. Tris-acetate-EDTA (TAE) electrophoresis buffer, 1× and RNAse-free 50×. A 1× TAE solution is constituted of 2 M Tris-acetate and 50 mM EDTA. Prepare 1× TAE by diluting

RNAse-free 50× stock solution with milliQ water. Prepare 50× TAE RNAse-free stock solution as follows. Dissolve 242 g of Tris base (contained in a bottle reserved for RNA applications) in about 600 mL of RNAse-free water. Add 57.1 mL of glacial acetic acid and 100 mL of RNAse-free 500 mM EDTA pH 8, mix and adjust volume to 1 L with RNAse-free water. Autoclave and store at RT.

19. Ethidium bromide (EtBr) 10 mg/mL, RNAse-free (Sigma-Aldrich).
20. Submerged horizontal electrophoresis system.
21. Agarose gels. Prepare 1 and 2% agarose gel by dissolving agarose in 1× TAE in a microwave. Let the agarose gel solution cool down to 50 °C in a heated water bath. Add 1 μL EtBr solution per 10 mL of gel and mix gently without introducing air bubbles. Pour the gel in a cast and apply a comb to generate the wells.
22. Ficoll type 400 Molecular Biology grade, RNAse-free (Fisher Scientific). Reserve a new bottle for RNA applications.
23. Gel loading solution, RNAse-free. Prepare a RNAse-free and dye-free gel loading by dissolving 7.5 g of Ficoll Type 400 in 50 mL of RNase-free water. Store at room temperature. Imaging system for gel documentation.

2.3 Induction of SMC Specific CreER^{T2} Activation and Pparγ KO or Reporters Activation

1. Peanut oil. Use a bottle that has never been opened.
2. Ultrasonic cleaner B1500A-MTH (VWR).
3. Tamoxifen (Sigma-Aldrich) 15 mg/mL solution. Prepare the stock solution of tamoxifen as follows. Resuspend 100 mg of tamoxifen in 400 μL of 100% ethanol by vortexing. Add 2.5 mL of peanut oil and sonicate in an Ultrasonic Cleaner for 20 min at high sonic power. Add 3.8 mL of peanut oil and mix by vortexing. Sonicate for 10 min. Aliquot the tamoxifen solution and store at −20 °C until use. Each aliquot is thawed once. Prepare the vehicle solution without tamoxifen.
4. Curved feeding and dosing needle 22 G×1 1/2″ (CDMV).
5. One mL Luer-lok™ tip syringe (BD).

2.4 Fixation and Harvesting of Tissues of Reporter Mice

1. Nalgene® polypropylene separatory funnel equipped with Teflon stopcock and polypropylene screw cap, 250 mL (Thermo Scientific).
2. One mL serological pipette.
3. Rubber stoppers.
4. Three-way Luer lock, stopcock.
5. PrecisionGlide needles, 26 G x 5/8 in (BD).
6. Tubing for the perfusion system.

7. Phosphate buffered saline (PBS) 137 mM NaCl, 2.7 mM KCl, 10 mM $Na_2HPO_4 \cdot 2 H_2O$, 2 mM KH_2PO_4, pH 7.4.
8. Paraformaldehyde (PFA) 0.2% fixative solution. Prepare 0.2% PFA fixative solution by diluting 10% PFA aqueous solution (EM grade, Electron Microscopy Sciences) in PBS the day of the experiment.
9. Avertin anesthetic solution. Prepare a stock solution as follows. Prepare first a 100% (1 g/mL) Avertin solution by dissolving 6.25 g of 2,2,2-tribromoethanol (Sigma-Aldrich Canada Co.) in 6.25 mL of tert-amyl alcohol (Sigma-Aldrich) with agitation. Dilute the 100% stock solution to 2.5% (25 mg/mL) by adding 250 mL of milli Q water. Warm up to 50 °C, mix the solution, filter-sterilize, and aliquot and store at −20 °C.
10. Sodium heparin, 10,000 IU/mL. Prepare a working heparin solution by diluting heparin to 1000 IU/mL in PBS. Store aliquots at −20 °C.
11. Styrofoam board to immobilize the mouse for the perfusion.
12. Needles to fix the mouse on the Styrofoam board.
13. Scissors, forceps and hemostatic forceps.
14. Curity Gauze sponges 2″×2″ (Kendall).
15. Fifty mL Falcon tubes.
16. Thirty percentage sucrose dehydration solution. Prepare by dissolving 30 g of sucrose in about 60 mL of PBS. Adjust the volume to 100 mL with PBS.
17. CFSC embedding medium. VWR® Clear Frozen Section Compound (CFSC, VWR International).
18. Cryostat Leica CM3050 S (Leica Microsystems Inc.).
19. Microscope Slides VWR® Superfrost Micro Slides 75×25 mm (VWR international).
20. Foam lined 100-place slide boxes (Fisher Scientific).

2.5 Staining for β-Galactosidase Activity

1. Glutaraldehyde (GTA) 0.5% fixative solution. Prepare 0.5% glutaraldehyde fixative solution by diluting glutaraldehyde 25% solution EM grade distillation purified (Electron Microscopy Sciences) in PBS. The glutaraldehyde 25% solution is stored at −20 °C.
2. IGEPAL CA-630 10% stock solution. Prepare the stock solution by diluting IGEPAL CA-630 nonionic detergent (Sigma-Aldrich Canada Ltd) in water. Store this solution at RT.
3. IGEPAL CA-630 0.02% washing solution. Prepare washing solution by diluting 10% IGEPAL CA-630 stock solution in PBS.

4. $K_3Fe(CN)_6$, 200 mM stock solution. Prepare 50 mL of 200 mM solution by dissolving $K_3Fe(CN)_6$ powder (ACP Chemicals Inc.) in PBS and store at RT in the dark.
5. $K_4Fe(CN)_6•3H_2O$, 200 mM stock solution. Prepare 50 mL of 200 mM solution by dissolving $K_4Fe(CN)_6•3H_2O$ powder (ACP Chemicals Inc.) in PBS and store at RT in the dark.
6. $MgCl_2$ 100 mM stock solution. Prepare this solution by dissolving $MgCl_2$ powder in water. Store at RT.
7. Sodium deoxycholate 10%. Prepare 50 mL of 10% solution by dissolving sodium deoxycholate powder (Sigma-Aldrich Canada Ltd) in water. Store at RT.
8. X-gal (5-bromo-4-chloro-3-indolyl-β-d-galactopyranoside) 20 mg/mL stock solution. Prepare a stock solution by dissolving X-gal (Gold Biotechnology Inc.) in dimethylformamide at a concentration of 20 mg/mL. Store at −20 °C. Avoid repeated freeze thawing.
9. Millex® syringe 0.22 μm filter units, sterile, 25 mm (EMD Millipore).
10. X-gal staining solution. This solution contains 10 mM $K_3Fe(CN)6$, 10 mM $K_4Fe(CN)_6•3H_2O$ 2 mM $MgCl_2$, 0.01% sodium deoxycholate, 0.02% IGEPAL CA-630 and 1 mg/mL of X-gal in PBS. On the day of the experiment, prepare enough X-gal solution using 200 mM $K_3Fe(CN)_6$, 200 mM $K_4Fe(CN)_6•3H_2O$, 10% IGEPAL CA-630, 10% sodium deoxycholate, and 20 mg/mL X-gal stock solutions. Filter the final solution with a Millex® syringe 0.22 μm filter unit to remove undissolved crystals of X-gal.
11. HARLECO® Eosin Y 1% alcoholic solution (EMD Millipore).
12. Anhydrous ethyl alcohol (100% ETOH). Prepare 95% ETOH by diluting 100% ETOH with water.
13. Xylene.
14. EUKITT mounting medium (Electron Microscopy Sciences).
15. Coverslips. Fisherbrand cover glasses no. 1, rectangle 50×24 mm (Fisher Scientific).
16. Upright microscope equipped with a digital camera and acquisition software.

2.6 Determination of Expression of *tdtomato* and *egfp* Reporter Genes

1. Triton X-100 10% solution. Prepare a 10% solution by dilution Triton X-100 (Sigma-Aldrich) in water. Store at RT.
2. Triton X-100 0.1 and 0.5% solutions. Prepare diluted Triton X-100 solutions by diluting 10% Triton X-100 solution in PBS.
3. DAPI (4′,6-diamidino-2-phenylindole, dihydrochloride, Life Technologies). The excitation/emission is 358/461 nm.

Prepare 14.3 mM stock solution by dissolving the DAPI to 5 mg/mL in water. Store aliquots at −20 °C in the dark.

4. DRAQ5® (1,5-bis{[2-(di-methylamino) ethyl]amino}-4, 8-dihydroxyanthracene-9,10-dione) 5 mM in aqueous solution (New England Biolabs). Excitation is possible using a wide range of laser light wave-lengths including 488, 514, 568, 633, or 647 nm. The emission spectrum extends from 670 nm into the low infrared. Store at 4 °C in the dark.

17. Nuclear staining solutions. Prepare DAPI and DRAQ5 working solution on the day of the experiment. Dilute DAPI to 28 μM and DARQ5 to 1 μM in PBS containing 0.1 or 0.5 %Triton X-100 using stock solutions for tissue sections and mesenteric arteries, respectively.
18. Fluoromount™ aqueous mounting medium (Sigma-Aldrich Canada Co.). Store at RT.
19. Confocal microscope. Wave FX spinning disk confocal microscope (Quorum).
20. LSM Pascal confocal scanning microscope (Carl Zeiss Canada Ltd.).

2.7 Quantification of Pparγ mRNA Expression

1. Small animal anesthesia machine.
2. Isoflurane (Baxter Corp.).
3. Oxygen gas (O_2).
4. Cotton tipped applicator (Puritan).
5. Fine tips forceps for microdissection.
6. RNA later® (QIAGEN).
7. Five mL tube, 75 × 12 mm, polypropylene (Sarstedt).
8. RNase AWAY™ Reagent (Life Technologies).
9. AbSolve glassware cleaner (PerkinElmer). Prepare the working solution by diluting Absolve to 2 % in distilled water.
10. RNeasy® MinElute® Cleanup kit (QIAGEN).
11. Dissecting tools cleaned with RNase AWAY™.
12. Polytron PT 1600 E homogenizer (VWR, Mississauga, ON, Canada).
13. Dispersing aggregate PT-DA 1607/2EC.
14. TRIzol® (Life Technologies).
15. Chloroform.
16. RNAse-free submerged horizontal electrophoresis system. Render the electrophoresis RNAse-free by soaking the comb, the gel tray and the electrophoresis chamber in a 2 % solution of AbSolve for 30 min. Rinse all of them with distilled water and dry with Kimwipe.

17. RNAse-free 1% agarose. Prepare 1% agarose RNAse-free gel by using a bottle of agarose reserved for RNA applications and RNAse-free glassware as in Subheading 2.2.
18. RNAse-free 1× TAE electrophoresis buffer. Prepare RNAse-free 1× TAE by diluting RNAse-free 50× stock solution (*see* Subheading 2.2) with milliQ water that was obtained directly from the purification system in a RNAse free Erlenmeyer.
19. Quantitect reverse transcription kit (QIAGEN).
20. Sso Fast Eva Green® Supermix (Bio-Rad).
21. Real-time PCR machine Mx3005P (Agilent).

3 Methods

Use male mice for this study (*see* **Note 1**).

3.1 Generation of Inducible Tissue-Specific KO Mice

1. *Smmhc*-CreER^{T2}/*PparγFlox/Flox* mice are generated by crossing male *Smmhc*-CreER^{T2} (C57BL/6) mice with female *PparγFlox/Flox* (BALB/c) mice using three consecutive matings. The following strategy is designed to ensure that all experimental mice are on equivalent background of third-generation (F3) BALB/c (*see* **Note 2**).
   (a) Cross C57BL/6 male *Smmhc*-CreER^{T2} mice with BALB/c female *PparγFlox/Flox* mice to obtain Fl BALB/c male *Smmhc*-CreER^{T2}/*PparγFlox/+* mice.
   (b) Cross Fl BALB/c male *Smmhc*-CreER^{T2}/*PparγFlox/+* mice with BALB/c female *PparγFlox/Flox* mice to obtain F2 BALB/c male *Smmhc*-CreER^{T2}/ *PparγFlox/Flox* mice.
   (c) Cross male *Smmhc*-CreER^{T2}/Pparγ$^{Flox/Flox}$ mice with Pparγ$^{Flox/Flox}$, BALB/c to obtain the experimental F3 BALB/c male *Smmhc*-CreER^{T2}/Pparγ$^{Flox/Flox}$ mice. Use these mice for induction of KO with tamoxifen (*see* Subheading 3.5).
   (d) Maintain above mating cages to ensure good generation of mice during the study.
2. Use F3 BALB/c control male *Smmhc*-CreER^{T2} mice to control for the effects of CreER^{T2} activation by tamoxifen (*see* **Note 3**). Generate these mice using the above strategy with wild-type BALB/c female for backcrossing.

3.2 Generation of the Reporter

Rosa–lacZ/–lacZ and *RosamT-mG/mT-mG* reporter mice are used to determine the tissue specificity of *Smmhc* driven CreER^{T2} expression and tamoxifen-induced Cre recombinase efficiency.

1. Cross C57BL/6 male *Smmhc*-CreER^{T2} mice with female C57BL/6 *Rosa–lacZ/–lacZ* mice to get C57BL/6 male *Smmhc*-CreER^{T2}/*Rosa–lacZ/+* reporter mice.
2. Cross C57BL/6 male *Smmhc*-CreER^{T2} mice with female C57BL/6 *RosamT-mG/mT-mG* to get C57BL/6 male *Smmhc*-CreER^{T2}/*RosamT-mG/+* mice.

3.3 Genotyping of the Mice

Genomic DNA samples are prepared using a simplified quick DNA extraction method [13, 17] and genotypes are determined by PCR.

3.3.1 Genomic DNA Extraction

1. Collect 3 mm tail biopsies in autoclaved 1.5 mL tubes and store them at −20 °C until use.
2. Add 90 μL of basic digestion buffer to the tubes containing the piece of tail (*see* **Note 4**).
3. Incubate the tubes at 95 °C for 45 min in a heat block.
4. Vortex the tubes to ensure tissue disruption and maximal DNA release.
5. Do a quick centrifugation at 12,000 × *g* at RT to bring down to the bottom of the tube the undigested tissue and lysis solution.
6. Incubate the tubes an additional 15 min at 95 °C. Note that after the last incubation period, the tails might not be completely digested (*see* **Note 5**).
7. Vortex and quickly centrifuge the tube as above.
8. Store DNA samples at −20 °C until used.

3.3.2 PCR Genotyping

Mice are genotype by PCR using conditions that have been determined empirically for each gene (*see* **Note 5**). Take any necessary precaution not to introduce contamination (*see* **Note 6**). Prepare sure to include no template, negative and positive controls in the genotyping. Oligonucleotides used for genotyping are described in Table 1. PCR are performed using Top Taq DNA polymerase using PCR reaction composition described in Table 2.

1. Thaw, vortex, and quick centrifuge at 12,000 × *g* at RT all the controls, samples and reagents.
2. Prepare enough PCR reaction master mix using the composition described in Table 2.
3. Distribute the PCR master mix to the PCR tubes.
4. Pipette the controls and samples to the PCR tubes.
5. Close the lids and centrifuge the PCR tubes at 1000 × *g* for 1 min at RT.
6. All the PCR are run in a thermal cycler as follows. The PCR conditions are denaturation for 3 min at 94 °C, followed by 35

Table 2
Composition of PCR reaction for mouse genotyping

Gene	10× Buffer	10× CoralLoad	2.5 mM dNTPs, μM	Oligonucleotides, μM	Taq (5 U/μL), μL	gDNA, μL
Pparγ Flox/Flox	1×	1×	200	0.40	0.50	1.7
Smmhc-CreER^{T2}	1×	1×	200	0.33	0.25	1.7
Rosa–lacZ/+	1×	1×	200	0.40	0.30	2.5
RosamT-mG/+	1×	1×	200	0.40	0.50	1.5

The final concentration or volume of reagents and volume of genomic DNA (gDNA) for the genotyping of *PparγFlox/Flox*, *Smmhc*-CreER^{T2}, *Rosa–lacZ/+*, and *RosamT-mG/+* mice are presented. The final concentration of $MgCl_2$ is 1.5 mM. Volumes are defined in function of a final reaction volume of 50 μL. Taq, Taq DNA polymerase. The CoralLoad contains gel loading reagent, orange dye, and red dye

cycles of denaturation for 30 s at 94 °C, annealing at 30 s at 60 °C, and elongation for 1 min at 72 °C followed with one final elongation step of 10 min at 72 °C.

7. Centrifuge the PCR tubes at 1000 × *g* for 1 min at RT.
8. Load and migrate PCR products on a 2% agarose gel in 1× TAE electrophoresis buffer (*see* **Note 7**).
9. Take a picture of the gel using an imaging system.

Representative gel pictures for genotyping are shown in Fig. 2.

3.4 Confirmation of LoxP Sequences Flanking the Exon 2 of the Pparγ Gene

The presence of the LoxP sequences in 5′ and 3′ of the exon 2 of *Pparγ* gene is confirmed by sequencing of *PparγFlox/Flox* mouse genomic DNA as follows.

1. Extract genomic DNA from biopsy tails using the simplified quick DNA extraction method described in Subheading 3.3.1.
2. Amplify by PCR two DNA fragments of 753 and 630 bp containing the 5′ and 3′ LoxP sequences using the Platinum *Pfx* DNA polymerase and oligonucleotides presented in Table 1 (*see* **Notes 8** and **9**) as follows.

   (a) Add the *Pfx* Amplification buffer, dNTP, $MgSO_4$, oligonucleotides, Platinum *Pfx* DNA polymerase as recommended by the manufacturer but use a final concentration of 2× for the *Pfx* Amplification buffer. The final volume is 49 μL.

   (b) Add 1 μL genomic DNA per PCR tube.

   (c) Centrifuge the PCR tubes at 1000 × *g* for 1 min at RT.

   (d) Amplify the DNA fragments in a thermal cycler using the following PCR conditions: denaturation at 94 °C for 5 min, followed by 1 cycle of denaturation at 94 °C for

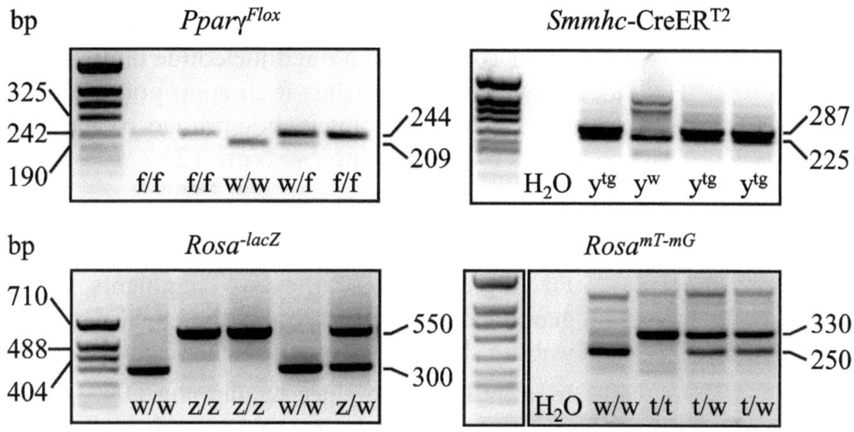

Fig. 2 Genotyping of mice for *PparγFlox*, *Smmhc*-CreER^{T2}, *Rosa–lacZ* and *RosamT-mG* for the presence of LoxP site in *Pparγ* gene, *Smmhc*-CreER^{T2} and presence of *lacZ* or *mT-mG* in *Rosa* locus by PCR are performed as described in the text. The genotype is assigned based on the size of the PCR products determined after agarose gel electrophoresis. Representative images of agarose gel for *PparγFlox*, *Smmhc*-CreER^{T2}, *Rosa–lacZ* and *RosamT-mG* are shown. Pparγ*Flox* genotyping: a PCR product of 209 bp is from a wild-type mouse (w/w), a PCR product of 244 bp is for Pparγ*Flox/Flox* (f/f) and the presence of both PCR products is for *PparγFlox/+* (f/w). *Smmhc*-CreER^{T2} genotyping: a PCR product of 287 bp is from *Smmhc*-CreER^{T2} (the transgene being on the Y chromosome (y^{tg})) and a PCR product of 225 bp is from wild-type (y^{w}). Note that a wild-type PCR product is present also in the *Smmhc*-CreER^{T2} genotype because these mice are heterozygote. *Rosa–lacZ* genotyping: a PCR product of 550 bp is from *Rosa–lacZ/–lacZ* (z/z), a PCR product of 300 bp is from wild-type (w/w), and the presence of both a PCR products corresponds to *Rosa–lacZ/+* (z/w). *RosamT-mG* genotyping: a PCR product of 330 bp is from *RosamT-mG/mT-mG* (t/t), a PCR product of 250 bp is from wild-type (w/w), and the presence of both a PCR products is indicative of *RosamT-mG/+* (t/w). H_2O corresponds to PCR done without tail DNA. Sizes on the left on the gels are for the DNA ladder

15 s, annealing at 55 °C for 30 s, and elongation at 68 °C for 1 min 50 s, and then 35 cycles of denaturation at 94 °C for 15 s, annealing at 58 °C for 30 s, and elongation at 68 °C for 1 min 15 s, and a last step of elongation for 5 min at 68 °C (*see* **Note 9**).

3. PCR products are isolated as follows.
   (a) Add gel loading solution to the PCR tubes and load and run PCR products on a 1 % agarose gel in 1× TAE electrophoresis buffer.
   (b) Visualize on a UV transilluminator, take a picture and cut each band of agarose containing the amplified DNA fragments using a new single edge blade for each DNA fragment (*see* **Note 10**). Collect the bands in sterile 1.5 tubes.
   (c) Extract DNA from the agarose gel bands using the QIAquick gel extraction kit.
      (a) Determine the DNA concentration using a NanoDrop (*see* **Note 11**).

4. Send 100 μL of each DNA fragment diluted to 10 ng/μL in water and 10 μL of each oligonucleotide diluted to 1.6 pmol/μL in water for sequencing at an appropriate facility. Use forward and reverse oligonucleotide primers to amplify the DNA fragments for sequencing (*see* **Note 12**).
5. Analyze the sequences as follows.
   (a) Identify *Pparγ* sequences by aligning forward and reverse DNA sequences of the two fragments to the mouse genome using the Blat tool of the UCSC Genome Browser website (http://www.genome.ucsc.edu) (*see* **Note 13**).
   (b) Identify LoxP sequence by aligning DNA sequences that are conserved on both DNA strands and do not align to the mouse *Pparγ* gene to nonredundant sequences using nucleotide blast tool of NCBI (http://blast.ncbi.nlm.nih.gov). The vector and LoxP sequences integrated in the mouse genome have been previously published [13].

3.5 Induction of SMC Specific CreER^{T2} Activation and KO of Pparγ or Reporter Activation

SMC specific KO is induced by treating *Smmhc*-CreER^{T2}/*PparγFlox/Flox* mice with 1.5 mg tamoxifen per day *per os* for 5 days (*see* **Note 14**). *Smmhc*-CreER^{T2}/*PparγFlox/Flox* are also treated with the vehicle and used as control. *Smmhc*-CreER^{T2} mice are treated with vehicle or tamoxifen to control for the effect of CreER^{T2} activation. *Smmhc*-CreER^{T2}/*Rosa–lacZ/+* and *Smmhc*-CreER^{T2}/*RosamT-mG/+* reporter mice are treated with vehicle or tamoxifen as above to activate the reporter in a SMC-specific fashion. Use the following protocol to treat mice by gavage once a day for 5 days.

1. Thaw enough 15 mg/mL tamoxifen solution and vehicle to treat the mice. Make sure that the solution is at room temperature before administration.
2. Load 1 mL syringe equipped with a curved feeding and dosing needle with tamoxifen solution or vehicle.
3. Eliminate bubbles inside the syringe and adjust volume to 100 μL.
4. Firmly restrain the mouse.
5. Determine the length of tube to insert by measuring the gavage needle externally from the tip of the nose to the last rib.
6. While maintaining the animal in an upright position, insert the gavage needle through the side of the mouth and advance the needle into the esophagus and toward the stomach by following the roof of the mouth (*see* **Note 15**).
7. Inject slowly the tamoxifen solution or vehicle when the correct length of needle has been advanced.
8. Repeat the gavage the four following days.

9. Wait for 7–9 days to give time to eliminate tamoxifen and SMC PPARγ protein (*see* **Note 16**) and then induce an experimental model (for example, hypertension using an angiotensin II infusion for 14 days).

3.6 Study of Inducibility and Tissue-Specificity of Smmhc-CreER^{T2} Transgene in Smmhc-CreERT2/Rosa–lacZ/+ and Smmhc-CreERT2/RosamT-mG/+ Reporter Mice

Determine the inducibility and tissue specifity of *Smmhc*-CreER^{T2} by evaluating the expression of *lacZ* or *tdtomato* and *egfp* reporter gene in *Smmhc*-CreERT2/Rosa–*lacZ*/+ and *tdtomato* and *egfp* reporter genes in *Smmhc*-CreER^{T2}/*RosamT-mG*/+ reporter mice treated or not with tamoxifen as follows. Study mice after waiting for the washout period of 9 days plus the time required by the experimental model induced in the mice.

3.6.1 Determination of Inducibility and Tissue Specificity of Smmhc-CreER^{T2} Transgene in Smmhc-CreER^{T2}/Rosa– lacZ/+

Fixation and Harvesting of Tissues

Perfuse the mice with PBS followed by 0.2 % PFA fixative solution at a constant pressure of 100 mmHg using the principle of Mariotte's bottle (*see* **Note 17** and Fig. 3) and collect tissues for β-galactosidase activity assay as follows.

1. Set up a perfusion system as depicted in Fig. 3 to get a perfusion pressure of 100 mmHg.
2. Fill the funnels with PBS and 0.2 % PFA fixative solution.
3. Prime the perfusion system with PBS and 0.2 % PFA fixative solution.
4. Remove air bubbles from the perfusion lines.
5. Anesthetize *Smmhc*-CreER^{T2}/Rosa–*lacZ*/+ mice by injecting IP 300-375 mg/Kg of Avertin. Wait for 5 min and confirm the depth of anesthesia by rear foot squeezing. Repeat the injection if the depth of anesthesia is not profound enough.
6. Inject mice (ip) with 100 μL of 1000 IU/mL heparin solution.
7. Immobilize the mouse in a dorsal decubitus position on a Styrofoam board by inserting needles through the four limbs in the board.
8. Use scissors to make a "U" shape incision in the abdominal cavity of the animal as follows.
   (a) Pull the abdominal skin close to the genitals of the animal with a forceps.
   (b) Make a hole in the skin and in the muscle in the middle of the abdominal cavity close to the genitals with the scissors.
   (c) Cut the skin and the muscle of the animal from the middle to each side of the animal, then cut the skin and muscle up to the diaphragm with a "U" shape. Make sure not to cut the diaphragm at this point.

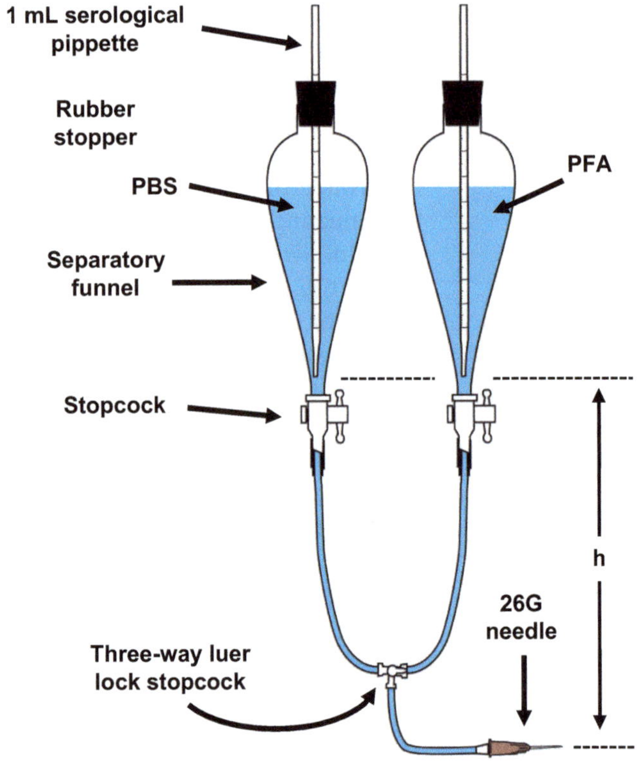

Fig. 3 Perfusion apparatus. Mariotte's bottle is used to perfuse mice at a constant pressure of 100 mmHg. Mariotte's bottle is put together as follows. Replace the screw cap from a polypropylene funnel equipped with Teflon stopcock by a robber stopper with a 1 mL serological pipette inserted through it tightly. Use two funnels, one for phosphate buffered saline (PBS) and one for the paraformaldehyde (PFA) solution. Connect the two bottles to a 26 G needle using tubing, a three-way Luer lock stopcock and necessary adapters. Adjust the pressure of perfusion to 100 mmHg by moving up the funnels so that the height (h) between the tip of the 1 mL pipette and the needle is 135.95 cm

9. Place the skin from the abdominal cavity over the thoracic cage and hold it there with a hemostatic forceps or a long needle pinned to the Styrofoam board.
10. Place wet gauze on one side of the animal.
11. Bring the intestine out of the abdominal cavity on to the wet gauze and place the wet gauze over it.
12. Clean the abdominal cavity with two gauzes to remove the fat tissue over the inferior vena cava.

The next steps should be performed rapidly with no pause as the rupture through the diaphragm abolishes ability of the mouse to breathe.

13. Make a small hole in the diaphragm with the scissors and visualize the heart.
14. Remove the pericardium by turning around the heart with forceps or scissors.
15. Insert the 26 G needle connected to the perfusion line into the left ventricle.
16. While holding with one hand the needle inserted in the left ventricle, punch the vena cava with a needle to create an outflow for the blood and perfusate.
17. Place a corner of a 2″×2″ gauze beside the hole to drain the blood and perfusate out of the peritoneal cavity.
18. Initiate the perfusion with the PBS for 5 min (*see* **Note 18**).
19. Release the needle when the heart stops beating.
20. Switch the perfusion to 0.2% PFA for 12 min (*see* **Note 19**).
21. Stop the perfusion and remove the needle from the animal (*see* **Note 20**).
22. Dissect out the organs to study and store them in ice-cold PBS.
23. Further dissect the organs in PBS to remove unnecessary tissues such as fat around aorta and mesenteric arteries. Use small section of a large organ such as liver for the next step.
24. Transfer the tissues to a 50 mL tube containing 30 mL of 0.2% PFA, and incubate at 4 °C for 24 h with gentle agitation.
25. Transfer the tissues to a 50 mL tube containing 30 mL of 30% sucrose dehydration solution and incubate at 4 °C for 24 h with gentle agitation.
26. Embed tissues in CFSC embedding medium and freeze the blocks on dry ice.
27. Keep embedded tissues frozen at −80 °C until used.

Determination of β-Galactosidase Activity

1. Prepare 10 μm-thick tissue sections as follows.
   (a) Cut 10 μm-thick tissue sections with a cryostat and apply the sections to microscope slides at room temperature to allow attachment of the tissue sections to the slide.
   (b) Store the slides in a slide box in the cryostat until completion of tissue sectioning.
   (c) Use the slides immediately or store them at −80 °C until used.
2. Rinse tissue sections twice in PBS at room temperature.
3. Incubate tissue sections in 0.5% GTA fixative solution for 10 min at 4 °C.
4. Wash tissue sections twice for 10 min in PBS containing 0.02% IGEPAL CA-630 at room temperature.

5. Initiate β-galactosidase reaction by incubating the tissue sections in X-gal staining solution at 37 °C for 16–36 h in the dark. Determine the length of the reaction by monitoring the blue color development under a microscope.
6. Stop the reaction by washing the tissue sections with PBS twice.
7. Counterstain with eosin as follows.
   (a) Incubate the tissue sections in HARLECO® Eosin Y 1 % alcoholic solution for 10 s.
   (b) Wash the tissue sections one time in 95 % ETOH for 1 min.
   (c) Dehydrate the tissue sections by incubating for 1 min in two consecutive baths of 100 % ETOH.
   (d) Incubate for 1 min in two consecutive baths of xylene to remove the ETOH. This step and the following should be done in a fume hood.
   (e) Mount the slide with 120–150 μL of EUKITT mounting medium and cover the slide with a coverslip.
   (f) Let the mounting harden overnight in a fume hood before imaging.
8. Capture the image of the tissue sections using an upright microscope equipped with a digital camera and acquisition software.

Representative images showing tamoxifen induction of *lacZ* expression in SMC of mesenteric artery, aorta, kidney and heart of *Smmhc*-CreER^{T2}/*Rosa–lacZ/+* mice are shown in Figs. 4 and 5.

3.6.2 Study of the Inducibility and Tissue Specificity of Smmhc-CreER^{T2} Transgene in Smmhc-CreERT2/RosamT-mG/+ Mice

1. Anesthetize mice as in Subheading 3.6.1.1.
2. Perfuse the mouse as in Subheading 3.6.1.1.
3. Dissect tissues except mesenteric arteries as in Subheading 3.6.1.1.
4. Collect mesenteric artery segments of 0.5–1 cm long in PBS in 1.5 mL tubes.
5. Embed and cut all tissue, except the mesenteric arteries, in CFSC embedding medium as in Subheading 3.6.1.1.
6. Nuclear stain mesenteric artery segments as follows.
   (a) Incubate mesenteric arteries in PBS 0.5 % Triton X-100 at 4 °C overnight.
   (b) Incubate the mesenteric arteries with DAPI or DRAQ5 working solutions at room temperature for 1 h (*see* **Note 21**).
   (c) Wash two times the mesenteric in PBS at room temperature for 5 min.
   (d) Transfer the mesenteric arteries to a slide.
   (e) Remove excess liquid.

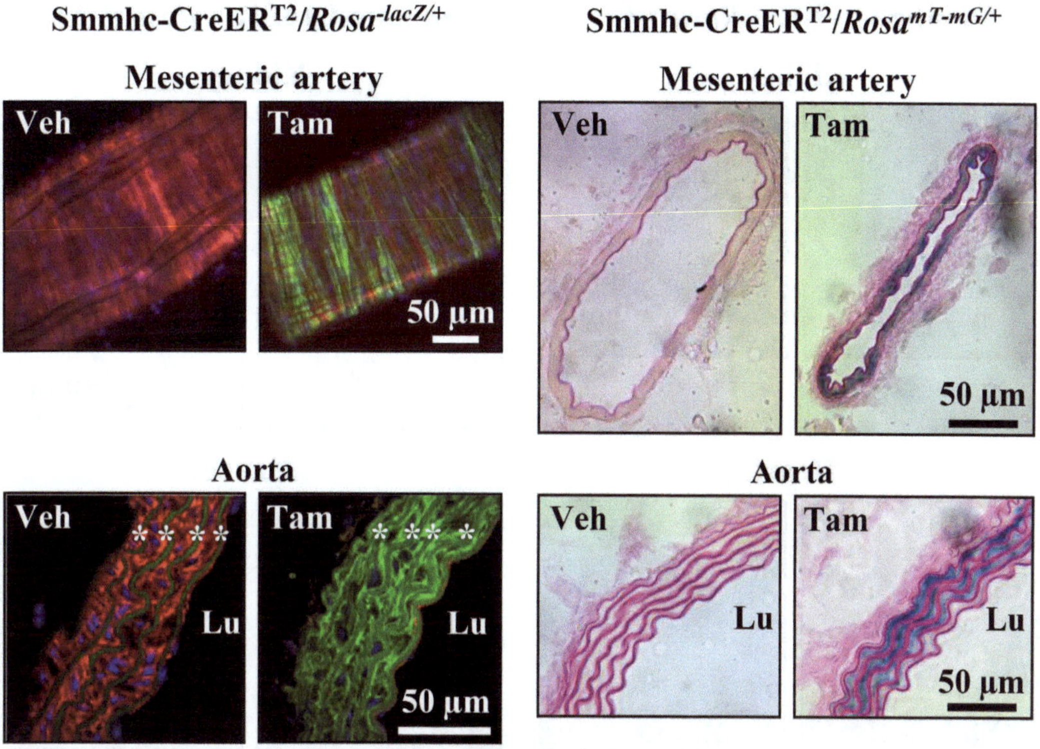

Fig. 4 Activation of Cre recombinase by tamoxifen in mesenteric arteries and aorta of *Smmhc*-CreER^{T2}/*Rosa–lacZ/+* and in *Smmhc*-CreER^{T2}/*RosamT-mG/+* reporter mice. In *Smmhc*-CreER^{T2}/Rosa–*lacZ/+* mice, Cre activation leads to the expression of β-galactosidase. β-galactosidase activity is visualized with blue X-gal staining on tissue sections . In *Smmhc*-CreER^{T2}/ *RosamT-mG/+* mice, Cre activation causex inactivation of the membrane-targeted tandem dimer tomato (mT, red fluorescence) and activation of the membrane-targeted enhanced green fluorescent protein (mG, green fluorescence). Representative immunofluorescence images with nuclei in blue and elastin lamella (*asterisk*) autofluorescence in green are shown in *right panels.* Fluorescence imaging was performed on aorta sections and whole-mounted mesenteric arteries. Representative sections stained in blue for β-galactosidase activity and counterstained with eosin are shown in the *right panels. Veh* vehicle, *Tam* tamoxifen, *Lu* lumen. Reproduced from ref. [13] with permission

(f) Mount the slides with 120–150 μL of Fluoromount™ aqueous mounting medium and cover the slides with a coverslip.

(g) Let the mounting medium harden for 30–45 min before imaging.

7. Nuclear stain tissue sections as follows.

   (a) Wash the tissue sections in PBS for 5 min.

   (b) Incubate the tissue section in Triton X-100 at room temperature for 5 min.

   (c) Incubate the tissue sections with DAPI or DRAQ5 working solutions at room temperature for 20 min

   (d) Wash the tissue sections twice in PBS 5 min.

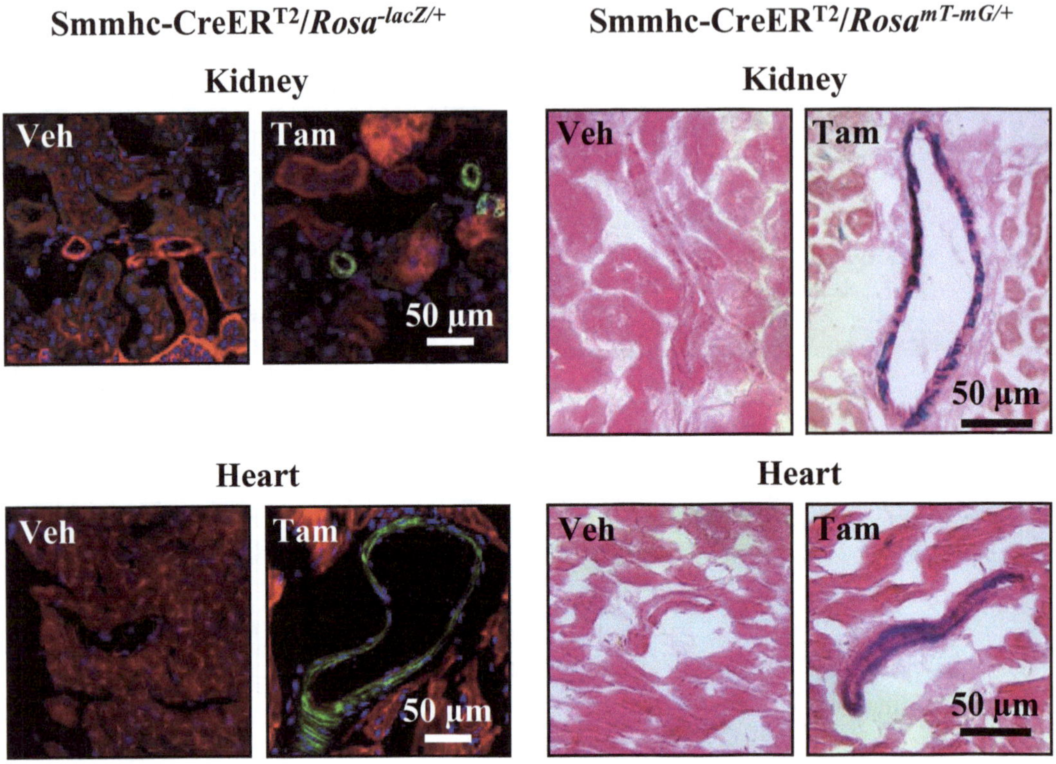

Fig. 5 Activation of Cre recombinase by tamoxifen in the kidney and the heart of *Smmhc*-CreER^{T2}/ Rosa–*lacZ/+* and *Smmhc*-CreER^{T2}/ *RosamT-mG/+* reporter mice. *See* legend of Fig. 2. for details. Reproduced from ref. [13] with permission

(e) Mount the slide with 120–150 μL of Fluoromount™ aqueous mounting medium and cover the slide with a Coverslip.

(f) Let the mounting medium harden for 30–45 min before imaging.

8. Capture the images of the tissue sections and mesenteric artery segments using a confocal microscope.

Representative image sshowing tamoxifen induction of *egfp* expression in SMC of mesenteric artery, aorta, kidney and heart of *Smmhc*-CreER^{T2}/*RosamT-mG/+* mice are shown in Fig. 4 and 5.

3.7 Study of the Efficiency of Induction of PPARγ KO in SMC of Smmhc-CreERT2/PparγFlox/Flox Mice with Tamoxifen

Take all necessary precautions not to introduce RNAses in the sample during the isolation of the RNA. Wear gloves, use disposable RNAse-free plasticware and remove RNAses by cleaning other equipment with RNase AWAY™ or AbSolve reagents. Treat water with DEPC to render it RNAse-free. Make glassware RNAse-free by cooking at 240 °C overnight. Note that RNases are resistant to autoclave.

1. Treat *Smmhc*-CreER^{T2}/*PparγFlox/Flox* mice with tamoxifen or vehicle as described in Subheading 3.5.
2. Twenty-three days later, anesthetize the mice with 3% isoflurane mixed with O_2 at 1 L/mL. Verify depth of anesthesia confirmed by the absence of reaction to rear foot squeezing.
3. Dissect out the thoracic aorta in ice-cold PBS.
4. Remove the fat surrounding the aorta.
5. Open the whole length of the aorta with scissors.
6. Carefully remove the endothelium with a cotton-tipped applicator.
7. Isolate the remaining media from the adventitia (*see* **Note 22**).
8. Place fragments of media in RNA later® on ice until the next step. In general, tissues are processed within 2 h.
9. Place a Polytron PT 1600 E homogenizer equipped with a dispersing aggregate PT-DA 1607/2EC in a fume hood since TRIzol containing phenol and chloroform are used in the following steps.
10. Clean the dispersing aggregate device with RNase AWAY™.
11. Further clean the dispersing aggregate device by homogenizing three times 1 mL of RNAse free water in a 5 mL tube at maximum speed for 10 s.
12. Homogenize media fragments in 1 mL of TRIzol® using the Polytron at maximum speed for 1 min in a 5 mL tube. Clean the dispersing aggregate device between samples by homogenizing sec three times 1 mL of RNAse free water in a 5 mL tube at maximum speed for 10.
13. Incubate the samples at room temperature for 5 min to permit complete dissociation of nucleoprotein complexes.
14. Centrifuge the tubes 5000×*g* at 4 °C for 10 min to remove the insoluble material.
15. Transfer the supernatant to a 1.5 mL tube and add 0.2 mL of chloroform.
16. Shake tubes vigorously by hand for 15 s.
17. Incubate the samples at room temperature for 3 min.
18. Centrifuge the samples at 5000×g at 4 °C for 30 min.
19. Collect 80% of the upper aqueous phase in a 1.5 mL tube without disturbing the interphase and lower organic phase. This is done using a p1000 pipette tip cut with a blade to enlarge the opening in order to decrease the suction force.
20. Add 1 volume of 70% ethanol and mix thoroughly by vortexing.
21. Further purify the RNA with RNeasy MinElute Cleanup Kit according to the manufacturer's instructions. Use 14 μL of RNAse-free water to elute the RNA from the silica-gel membrane.

22. Use 2 μL of RNA solution to measure the RNA concentration and 260 nm/280 nm ratio using a NanoDrop (*see* **Note 23**).
23. Verify the RNA quality by running 100 ng of RNA on RNAse-free 1% agarose gel and 1× TAE electrophoresis buffer (*see* **Note 24**).
24. Capture the image using an Imaging system for gel documentation,
25. Determine the levels of *Pparγ* mRNA by reverse transcription (RT) followed by quantitative PCR (QPCR) as follows.
26. Reverse-transcribe 400 ng of RNA with a Quantitect reverse transcription kit according the manufacturer's instructions.
27. Perform QPCR using oligonucleotides for *Pparγ* and 40S ribosomal protein S16 (*Rps16*, *see* **Note 26**) designed as described in **Note 25** (Table 1) and SsoFast EvaGreen Supermix. The QPCR conditions are 2 min at 96 °C, followed by 40 cycles of 5 s at 96 °C and 30 s at 58 °C.
28. Analyze using the $\Delta\Delta C_t$-method [18].

We previously observed [13] that the treatment of *Smmhc*-CreERT2/*PparγFlox/Flox* mice with tamoxifen treatment caused a 67% reduction of *Pparγ* expression in aortic media (Fig. 6).

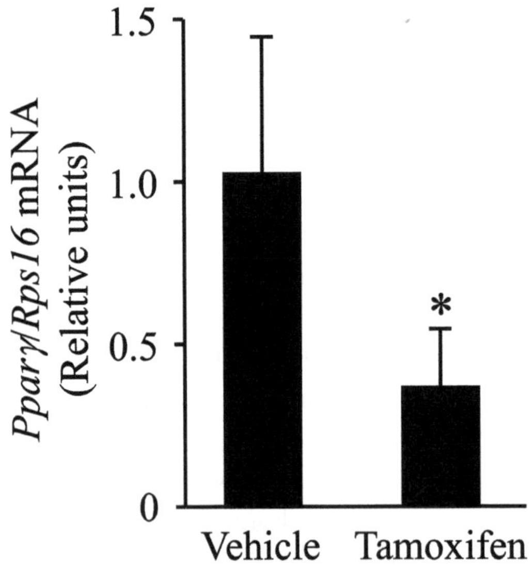

Fig. 6 Tamoxifen treatment results in an efficient reduction in *Pparγ* mRNA expression in *Smmhc*-CreER^{T2}/*PparγFlox/Flox* mice. The *Pparγ* mRNA expression is determined by RT-QPCR in the media of thoracic aorta of *Smmhc*-CreER^{T2}/*PparγFlox/Flox* mice treated with vehicle or tamoxifen. Values are means ± SEM, $n = 4$, *$P < 0.05$ vs. Vehicle. Reproduced from ref. [13] with permission

4 Notes

1. *Smmhc-CreER*^{T2} is a fusion protein of Cre recombinase with a mutated estrogen receptor ligand binding domain under the control of the SMC specific *smooth muscle myosin heavy chain* (*Myh11*) promoter. The modified estrogen receptor ligand binding domain binds tamoxifen, an antagonist of estrogen, but not estrogen. The transgenic construct was designed by knockin of CreER^{T2} into the mouse *Myh11* gene carried by a bacterial artificial chromosome (BAC). This strategy confers a native genomic context to and targets expression of CreER^{T2} only in SMC. Since the transgenic construct is integrated on the Y chromosome, it is impossible to study female mice. Accordingly, only male mice are investigated.
2. The *Smmhc-CreER*^{T2}*/PparγFlox/Flox* mice are in a mixed C57BL/6 and BALB/c background since they are generated by crossing *Smmhc-CreER*^{T2} and *PparγFlox/Flox* mice that are in C57BL/6 and BALB/c backgrounds, respectively. This is a limitation that could have a profound effect on the phenotype. The problem is circumvented by studying mice on equivalent backgrounds. In order to do this, it is important to follow the strategy of mating presented in Subheading 3.1 and always generate the mice the same way so that all the experimental animals, including controls, are Balb/c third-generation backcross. Alternatively, *PparγFlox/Flox* mice in a C57BL/6 background can be obtained from another source or by backcrossing them for 10 generations with C57BL/6 wild-type mice. *PparγFlox/Flox* mice in C57BL/6 background are available from The Jackson Laboratory (B6.129-*Ppargtm2Rev*/J, stock number: 004584). These mice have loxP sites on either side of exons 1 and 2 *Pparγ* gene.
3. It is important to determine whether activation of Cre recombinase produces by itself any effect that could interfere with the study. This is done by treating *Smmhc*-CreER^{T2} mice with tamoxifen or vehicle and looking at an important endpoint of the study. We previously demonstrated that CreER^{T2} activation with tamoxifen had no effect on endothelial function of mesenteric resistance arteries of *Smmhc*-CreER^{T2} mice [13]. After the end of tamoxifen treatment, we waited 2 weeks before sacrifice of the mice and collection of tissues to allow turnover of membrane-targeted tomato proteins in cells that have undergone Cre-mediated excision as previously described [16].
4. The tails might not be digested completely, but this is fine as enough DNA for genotyping by PCR is released.
5. The PCR reaction composition has been optimized empirically for each gene. These conditions should be taken as a starting protocol as they could change between laboratories.

6. The worst problem of genotyping by PCR is cross-contamination. This is revealed by presence of unexpected PCR products in controls such as PCR products in no template controls or unexpected PCR products for the negative or positive controls. The best way to prevent cross-contamination is to change gloves often during the procedure, centrifuge tubes before opening and use a micro-tube opener. A set of pipettes should be reserved for genotyping by PCR. Avoid using the same pipette to prepare the PCR and load the diagnostic agarose gel. Assemble the PCR reaction and run the agarose gel electrophoresis in different rooms.
7. Since the PCR reaction mix contains CoralLoad, the samples are ready to be loaded immediately after the PCR reaction.
8. The strategy of PCR amplification of DNA fragments containing the LoxP sites is designed based on the information provided previously [19].
9. Oligonucleotides are designed to have a melting temperature (Tm) of 60 °C and a 3′ GC clamp using Primer3 [20]. The PCR is performed with an annealing temperature of 58 °C. Sometime, even if the design of the oligonucleotides is right, none or very little DNA is amplified. In this protocol, we are using a trick to improve DNA amplification, which is to do one cycle of DNA amplification with lower stringency (annealing temperature of 55 °C) followed by 35 cycles of DNA amplification with high stringency (annealing temperature of 58 °C).
10. Limit the time of UV exposure to as short as possible as it could cause create nicks in the DNA.
11. Increase the number of PCR reactions if the DNA yield is too low.
12. DNA fragments are sequencing using forward and reverse oligonucleotides to read DNA sequences in both orientations. This ensures elimination of sequencing artifacts.
13. *Pparγ* sequences are confirmed by reading DNA on both strands. The LoxP sequences do not align on the mouse genome. Note that vector sequences could accompany LoxP sequences. Sequences that do not align to the mouse genome may contain the LoxP sites and vector sequences.
14. The *per os* route is used in order to prevent any change induced by the peanut oil on endothelial function and vascular remodeling of mesenteric resistance arteries. It is preferable to avoid the intraperitoneal route and use the oral route to prevent undesirable effects.

15. It is possible that the feeding needle goes in the trachea. This is found when a resistance is encountered while attempting to advance the needle. In this situation, alter the needle position.
16. It is better to wait for 7–9 days before beginning the study. This is to ensure complete elimination of the PPARγ protein and tamoxifen. The half-life of the PPARγ protein is less than 4 h [21], and tamoxifen and metabolites are completely eliminated from serum 4.2 days after oral administration of a single large dose of tamoxifen of 200 mg/mL [22].
17. Mariotte's bottle was invented by the French physicist Edmé Mariotte during the seventeenth century. It permits the delivery of liquid at a constant pressure as long as the liquid remains above the bottom of the tube inserted in the bottle that determines the exit pressure (Fig. 3). The pressure is obtained by adjusting the height of the water column as determined by the bottom of the inlet tube and the exit needle. One hundred mmHg are obtained by having a 135.95 cm water column.
18. If the perfusion is good, the lungs and kidneys should become white and pink, respectively.
19. In this protocol, 2 min is included in the time of perfusion of the PFA to eliminate the PBS contained within the dead volume of the perfusion line. The dead volume should be determined for each new perfusion system.
20. Use a new needle for each animal to perfuse.
21. The proper choice of nuclear stains, DAPI or DRAQ5®, is determined based on the laser and filter availability.
22. PPARγ is expressed in all cell types present in the aorta wall, including endothelial cells and adipocytes. Therefore the effect of $CreER^{T2}$ activation on SMC *Pparγ* mRNA expression could be hidden by mRNA from other types of cells. Remove adventitia and endothelium from the aorta and keep the media rich in SMC for total RNA extraction. Use two fine-tip forceps for microdissection to remove the adventitia from the whole aorta. The color of the media is whiter than the surrounding adventitia.
23. Typically quantity of RNA purified range from 0.5 to 1.5 μg.
24. RNA of good quality is not degraded. It is expected that the electrophoresis profile will present a sharp 28S rRNA band with approximately twice the intensity of the 18S rRNA band with a mRNA smear from high to low size. A decrease in the intensity of 28S band and a shift down in the mRNA smear is indicative of RNA degradation.
25. Oligonucleotides for QPCR are designed using Primer3 [20] to have a melting temperature (T_m) of 60 °C and a 3′ GC clamp

and to generate a PCR product of 250–350 bp. Oligonucleotides are validated for QPCR with a standard curve of cDNA from wild-type mice with a dilution range of 1/10–1/640. The oligonucleotides are good when the PCR efficiency is 100 ± 5 %. This note should be moved down to become Note 26

26. *Rps16* is chosen as a housekeeping gene for relative quantification. This Note should be moved up to become Note 25.

Acknowledgment

We are grateful to André Turgeon, Marie-Eve Deschênes, Véronique Michaud, and Cristina Adriana Ene for excellent technical assistance. The work of the authors was supported by Canadian Institutes of Health Research grants 37917 and 82790, a Canada Research Chair on Hypertension and Vascular Research from Canadian Institutes of Health Research/Government of Canada, the Canada Fund for Innovation, and a Grant from Pfizer Canada Competitive Cardiovascular Grants Program, all to E.L.S.

References

1. Bishop-Bailey D, Hla T (1999) Endothelial cell apoptosis induced by the peroxisome proliferator-activated receptor (PPAR) ligand 15-deoxy-Delta12, 14-prostaglandin J2. J Biol Chem 274:17042–17048
2. Bishop-Bailey D, Warner TD (2003) PPARgamma ligands induce prostaglandin production in vascular smooth muscle cells: indomethacin acts as a peroxisome proliferator-activated receptor-gamma antagonist. FASEB J 17:1925–1927
3. Hevener AL, Olefsky JM, Reichart D, Nguyen MT, Bandyopadyhay G, Leung HY, Watt MJ, Benner C, Febbraio MA, Nguyen AK, Folian B, Subramaniam S, Gonzalez FJ, Glass CK, Ricote M (2007) Macrophage PPAR gamma is required for normal skeletal muscle and hepatic insulin sensitivity and full antidiabetic effects of thiazolidinediones. J Clin Invest 117:1658–1669
4. Zhang J, Fang NY, Gao PJ, Wu LY, Han WQ, Guo SJ, Shen WL, Zhu DL (2008) Peroxisome proliferator-activated receptor-gamma agonists attenuate angiotensin II-induced collagen type I expression in adventitial fibroblasts. Clin Exp Pharmacol Physiol 35:72–77
5. Diep QN, El MM, Cohn JS, Endemann D, Amiri F, Virdis A, Neves MF, Schiffrin EL (2002) Structure, endothelial function, cell growth, and inflammation in blood vessels of angiotensin II-infused rats: role of peroxisome proliferator-activated receptor-gamma. Circulation 105:2296–2302
6. Benkirane K, Viel EC, Amiri F, Schiffrin EL (2006) Peroxisome proliferator-activated receptor gamma regulates angiotensin II-stimulated phosphatidylinositol 3-kinase and mitogen-activated protein kinase in blood vessels in vivo. Hypertension 47:102–108
7. Chang L, Villacorta L, Zhang J, Garcia-Barrio MT, Yang K, Hamblin M, Whitesall SE, D'Alecy LG, Chen YE (2009) Vascular smooth muscle cell-selective peroxisome proliferator-activated receptor-gamma deletion leads to hypotension. Circulation 119:2161–2169
8. Wang N, Yang G, Jia Z, Zhang H, Aoyagi T, Soodvilai S, Symons JD, Schnermann JB, Gonzalez FJ, Litwin SE, Yang T (2008) Vascular PPARgamma controls circadian variation in blood pressure and heart rate through Bmal1. Cell Metab 8:482–491
9. Villacorta L, Schopfer FJ, Zhang J, Freeman BA, Chen YE (2009) PPARgamma and its ligands: therapeutic implications in cardiovascular disease. Clin Sci (Lond) 116:205–218
10. Chang L, Villacorta L, Li R, Hamblin M, Xu W, Dou C, Zhang J, Wu J, Zeng R, Chen YE (2012) Loss of perivascular adipose tissue on peroxisome proliferator-activated receptor-gamma deletion in smooth muscle cells impairs intravascular thermoregulation and enhances atherosclerosis. Circulation 126:1067–1078

11. Davis J, Maillet M, Miano JM, Molkentin JD (2012) Lost in transgenesis: a user's guide for genetically manipulating the mouse in cardiac research. Circ Res 111:761–777
12. Doetschman T, Azhar M (2012) Cardiac-specific inducible and conditional gene targeting in mice. Circ Res 110:1498–1512
13. Marchesi C, Rehman A, Rautureau Y, Kasal DA, Briet M, Leibowitz A, Simeone SM, Ebrahimian T, Neves MF, Offermanns S, Gonzalez FJ, Paradis P, Schiffrin EL (2013) Protective role of vascular smooth muscle cell PPARgamma in angiotensin II-induced vascular disease. Cardiovasc Res 97(3):562–570
14. Wirth A, Benyo Z, Lukasova M, Leutgeb B, Wettschureck N, Gorbey S, Orsy P, Horvath B, Maser-Gluth C, Greiner E, Lemmer B, Schutz G, Gutkind JS, Offermanns S (2008) G12-G13-LARG-mediated signaling in vascular smooth muscle is required for salt-induced hypertension. Nat Med 14:64–68
15. Soriano P (1999) Generalized lacZ expression with the ROSA26 Cre reporter strain. Nat Genet 21:70–71
16. Muzumdar MD, Tasic B, Miyamichi K, Li L, Luo L (2007) A global double-fluorescent Cre reporter mouse. Genesis 45:593–605
17. Truett GE, Heeger P, Mynatt RL, Truett AA, Walker JA, Warman ML (2000) Preparation of PCR-quality mouse genomic DNA with hot sodium hydroxide and tris (HotSHOT). Biotechniques 29(52):54
18. Schefe JH, Lehmann KE, Buschmann IR, Unger T, Funke-Kaiser H (2006) Quantitative real-time RT-PCR data analysis: current concepts and the novel "gene expression's CT difference" formula. J Mol Med (Berl) 84:901–910
19. Akiyama TE, Sakai S, Lambert G, Nicol CJ, Matsusue K, Pimprale S, Lee YH, Ricote M, Glass CK, Brewer HB Jr, Gonzalez FJ (2002) Conditional disruption of the peroxisome proliferator-activated receptor gamma gene in mice results in lowered expression of ABCA1, ABCG1, and apoE in macrophages and reduced cholesterol efflux. Mol Cell Biol 22:2607–2619
20. Rozen S, Skaletsky H (2000) Primer3 on the WWW for general users and for biologist programmers. Methods Mol Biol 132:365–386
21. Waite KJ, Floyd ZE, Arbour-Reily P, Stephens JM (2001) Interferon-gamma-induced regulation of peroxisome proliferator-activated receptor gamma and STATs in adipocytes. J Biol Chem 276:7062–7068
22. Robinson SP, Langan-Fahey SM, Johnson DA, Jordan VC (1991) Metabolites, pharmacodynamics, and pharmacokinetics of tamoxifen in rats and mice compared to the breast cancer patient. Drug Metab Dispos 19:36–43

Chapter 31

Renal Delivery of Anti-microRNA Oligonucleotides in Rats

Kristie S. Usa, Yong Liu, Terry Kurth, Alison J. Kriegel, David L. Mattson, Allen W. Cowley Jr., and Mingyu Liang

Abstract

MicroRNAs are endogenous small, non-protein-coding RNA molecules that play an important role in the regulation of a wide variety of cellular functions and disease processes. A novel role for microRNAs in the development of hypertension and hypertensive tissue injury is emerging in recent studies. Development of hypertension involves multiple organ systems and cannot be modeled in vitro. Therefore, the ability to experimentally alter genes, gene products, or biological pathways, including microRNAs, in an organ-specific manner in intact animal models is particularly valuable to hypertension research. The kidney plays a central role in the long-term regulation of arterial blood pressure. In this chapter, we describe a detailed protocol for using a renal interstitial injection method to deliver anti-miR oligonucleotides to knock down microRNA specifically in the kidney in conscious rats.

Key words MicroRNA, Rat, Kidney, Gene expression, Oligonucleotides

1 Introduction

MicroRNA (miRNA) research has been one of the most exciting and rapidly developing areas of biomedical research over the last decade. MiRNAs are small, non-protein-coding RNA molecules encoded by the genome. MiRNAs participate in the regulation of a wide variety of cellular functions and disease development [1, 2]. A novel role for miRNAs in the development of hypertension and hypertensive tissue injury is emerging in recent studies [3, 4]. Much more remains to be learned about whether and how miRNAs are involved in various mechanistic pathways underlying the development of hypertension and hypertensive tissue injury.

Arterial blood pressure can only be measured and studied in intact animals or human subjects and cannot be modeled in vitro. An implication of this is that animal models of hypertension, such as several widely used rat models of hypertension, and techniques for experimentally altering genes, gene products, or biological pathways in vivo are crucial for hypertension research. Moreover,

Rhian M. Touyz and Ernesto L. Schiffrin (eds.), *Hypertension: Methods and Protocols*, Methods in Molecular Biology, vol. 1527, DOI 10.1007/978-1-4939-6625-7_31, © Springer Science+Business Media LLC 2017

the development of hypertension involves several organ systems, making the ability to experimentally alter genes, gene products, or biological pathways in an organ-specific manner highly valuable to hypertension research.

The kidney plays a central role in long-term regulation of arterial blood pressure [5]. One approach to experimentally altering biological pathways specifically in the kidney is to deliver experimental agents via direct injection or infusion into the kidney interstitium. The approach has been used for various purposes in hypertension research, ranging from experimentally changing renal interstitial hydrostatic pressure to delivering pharmacological agents [6, 7].

Renal interstitial injection can be performed in anesthetized animals. Anesthesia, however, affects arterial blood pressure and its regulation, which complicates the interpretation of blood pressure data. One can carry out renal interstitial injection in conscious animals by implanting an indwelling catheter in the kidney and performing the injection several days after the animal recovered from the surgery and anesthesia [8–10]. The use of chronically implanted renal interstitial catheter avoids acute complications of surgery and anesthesia, which is valuable for studies of blood pressure. The chronically implanted renal interstitial catheter and the continuous saline infusion at a low rate needed to maintain patency of the catheter (see the protocol below) have minimal effect on renal function including glomerular filtration rate, sodium and water excretion, and urinary concentration [10].

Our laboratory has utilized renal interstitial injection to deliver gene expression constructs or gene silencing agents to rat models [11, 12]. For example, we used the approach to deliver plasmid constructs encoding small hairpin RNA targeting 11β-hydroxysteroid dehydrogenase type 1 into the renal interstitium of conscious Dahl salt-sensitive (SS) rats. The treatment resulted in significant knockdown of 11β-hydroxysteroid dehydrogenase type 1 in the renal medulla measured 6 days after the injection and attenuated salt-induced hypertension over 11 days [12].

Delivery of gene expression constructs or silencing agents via renal interstitial injection has unique values compared to using gene knockout or transgenic animals. It allows temporal (timing) and spatial (kidney-specific) control of gene expression or silencing. Temporal control of gene knockout or transgenesis is possible but challenging especially in rats. It is nearly impossible to achieve gene knockout or transgenesis that is restricted to the kidney yet impacts the entire kidney or an entire kidney region, except when global knockout or transgenesis is followed by invasive transplantation of the kidneys to wild-type animals. That is because tissue-specific knockout or transgenesis typically relies on gene promoters that are active in a specific cell type. Yet the kidney contains at least a dozen cell types, and it may not be clear in many cases which specific cell type should be targeted.

In this chapter, we describe a detailed protocol for using the renal interstitial injection method to deliver anti-miR oligonucleotides to knock down miRNA specifically in the kidney in conscious rats. Anti-miR oligonucleotides were designed to suppress the action of miRNAs on their targets. Anti-miR oligonucleotides have a complementary sequence to the miRNA of interest and, when complexed, physically prevent mature miRNAs from interacting with their targets and could induce degradation of miRNAs. Chemical modifications have been introduced to synthesized anti-miR oligonucleotides to provide increased protection and stability in vivo, such as phosphorothioate linkages and locked-nucleic acid (LNA) modifications. Of these, LNA-modified anti-miR oligonucleotides have been reported to provide long lasting, efficient and safe suppression of miRNA in vitro and in vivo [13]. Our laboratory was one of the first to report use of LNA-modified anti-miR in rats [14] and has knocked down miRNAs in the kidney in several studies [14–17].

2 Materials

2.1 Catheter Supplies

- Polyethylene tubing PE 50 (for catheter tip).
- Polyethylene tubing PE 10 (for catheter tip).
- Polyethylene tubing PE 240 (for catheter stopper).
- Tygon Tubing $0.02 \times 0.06 \times 0.02$ (for catheter body).
- 18 G needle.
- 23 G thin wall connector.
- Very thin piece of wire (must fit into the PE10 tubing).
- Flame heater with air.
- Glass pasteur pipette.
- PVC glue.
- 250 ml beaker with water.

2.2 Surgical Supplies

- Standard sharp/blunt scissors.
- Forceps.
- Fine scissors.
- Hemostat.
- Microdissecting forceps.
- Needle holder.
- Fistula and regular needle.
- 25 G needle.
- Vetbond (Midwest Vet).

- Trochar.
- 3.0 silk suture.
- 4.0 braunamid suture.
- 0.9 % NaCl saline.
- Gauze.
- Cotton tip applicator.
- Antibiotic ointment.
- 22 G stopper.
- Stainless steel extension spring (Exacto) with connector.
- Sterile surgical gloves.

2.3 Anti-miR Oligonucleotides

A large quantity (several mg or more) of the LNA-modified anti-miR oligonucleotides (Exiqon) of interest is purchased 4–6 weeks in advance. Purchase anti-miR targeting the miRNA of interest as well as control anti-miR that has scrambled or mutated sequences and chemical modifications similar to the experimental anti-miR. Upon arrival the oligonucleotides is stored in powder form at −20 °C until use.

3 Methods

3.1 Uninephrectomy

Uninephrectomy is necessary for ensuring the remaining kidney, which will receive interstitial injections later, is the sole determinant of the rat's renal function. Uninephrectomy should be performed 7–10 days prior to implantation of the interstitial catheter. This allows for hypertrophy of the remaining kidney and placement of the interstitial catheter tip in the appropriate kidney region.

1. Anesthetize rat with appropriate anesthesia.
2. Shave flank area on the side of the body from the kidney will be removed (*see* **Note 1**).
3. Clean the surgical area with alcohol and Betadine.
4. Make a vertical flank incision through the skin, approximately half inch in length, midway between the ribs and hind leg. Make a cut through the muscle beneath this incision.
5. Using microdissecting forceps, grab the fat attached to the caudal end of the kidney and pull it out (*see* **Note 2**).
6. Carefully dissect the surrounding perirenal fat and connective tissue from the kidney, leaving only the artery, vein, and ureter to be tied off.
7. Tie a knot around these three vessels with 3–0 silk, leaving some space between the kidney and the knot. Cut the vessels here and remove the kidney.

8. Once the kidney is removed, sew up the muscle with 3–0 silk. Use interrupted stitches or a running stitch. Then sew up the skin with 4–0 braunamid, using interrupted stitches.
9. Give antibiotic and analgesia post-op and recover the rat on a warming pad until awake.

3.2 Preparing Renal Interstitial Catheter

1. Cut a piece of PE 50 tubing approximately 1.5 cm long. Hold one end very close to a flame for 5–10 s until the end spreads out, then touch it to a flat surface and press flat (*see* **Note 3**).
2. Cut a piece of PE 10 tubing about 2 cm, slip it over a piece of wire. Insert this into the piece of PE 50 just made.
3. Heat fuse the piece of PE 50 to the PE 10 by holding the place where the PE 50 overlaps the PE 10 and wire over heated air until the tubing becomes clear. This is when the two pieces have melted together. Remove the wire after it cools (*see* **Note 4**).
4. Hold the end of the PE 10 just before it enters the PE 50 over heated air and stretch the tip of the PE 10 to 100 μm diameter tip. Make a 90° bend in the PE 50 tubing by holding the PE 50 tubing just before the PE 10 is covered over the flame. Set this aside (*see* **Note 5**).
5. Measure out 60 cm of the Tygon tubing 0.02×0.06. Wrap one end around a glass pasteur pipette 4–5 times and submerge into boiling water for 20–30 s. Keep holding in place and immediately immerse in cold water for 15–20 s. Remove from glass tube. Tubing should now have a coil curl to provide a flexible spring-like action to minimize the tension (*see* **Note 6**).
6. Push a 23 G thin wall connector half way into the tip set aside earlier. Push the other half into the coiled tygon tubing. Slip a piece of shrink tubing over the connection and use a flame to shrink it. Use a syringe and test for any leaks (*see* **Note** 7).
7. Cut a piece of PE 240 tubing. Cut it into 2–3 cm pieces. Hold an 18 G needle into a flame until hot. Use it to poke a hole in the middle of the tubing. When cooled this piece will slide onto the tygon tubing just before the coiled portion and help prevent the pulling of the catheter from the kidney.
8. Under the hood, apply PVC glue to where the PE 240 is on the tygon tubing. Dry at least 1–2 h. Test the catheter once more for leaks (*see* **Note 8**). A complete renal interstitial catheter is shown in Fig. 1.
9. Sterilize the catheter using methods such as ethylene oxide sterilization.

3.3 Implantation of Renal Interstitial Catheter

1. The interstitial catheter is implanted 7–10 days after the uninephrectomy.
2. Anesthetize rat with appropriate anesthesia.

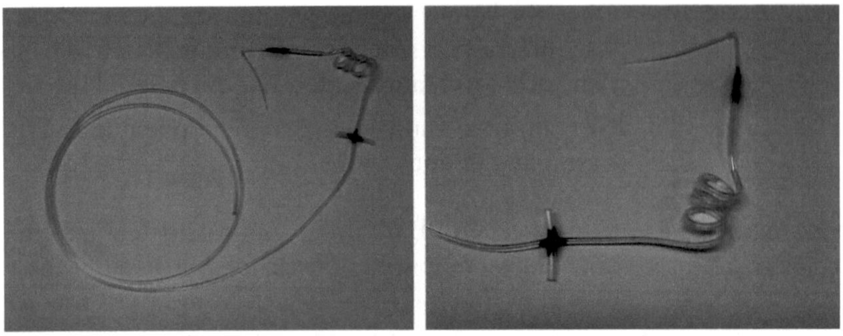

Fig. 1 Renal interstitial catheter. A fully constructed catheter (*left*) and a closer view of the tip of the catheter (*right*) are shown

3. Shave left flank and back (between shoulder blades). Apply alcohol and Betadine to surgical sites.
4. Fill the catheter with 0.9% NaCl saline and insert a 22 G plug in the end.
5. Make a 2–3 cm transverse incision in the left flank. Blunt dissect through fascia and connective tissue with sharp/blunt scissors down to muscle (*see* **Note 9**).
6. Make a 2–3 cm transverse incision in the muscle directly below skin incision.
7. Blunt dissect up towards the shoulder blades on the back where the incision will be made for the catheter to exteriorize and the spring to be attached.
8. Make a 1.5 cm incision in the back between the shoulder blades. Blunt dissect around incision and down toward interstitial flank incision to create a track for trochar.
9. Insert trochar under the skin in flank incision and push up and out spring incision.
10. Thread interstitial catheter into trochar and out the scapula end. Remove trochar. Carefully pull catheter about half way out the scapular incision.
11. Pull out the kidney by grabbing the fat close to the distal end of the kidney with small forceps. Insert a cotton tip in the incision so that the kidney does not slip back into the cavity.
12. Measure catheter tip length by placing it against the kidney and approximating the length to the junction between the outer and inner medulla (this is *usually* where interstitial catheters are placed). Cut the catheter tip to this length with the fine scissors (*see* **Note 10**).
13. Using a 25 G needle to puncture a hole on the top center of the kidney through the capsule and insert the needle approximately 1–2 mm deep (*see* **Note 11**).

14. Remove needle and stop bleeding by putting pressure on the hole with a cotton tip. The bleeding should stop in 1–2 min.
15. Have Vetbond glue ready to apply. Insert catheter into hole with fine forceps, making sure it goes straight down into the medulla.
16. Secure the catheter in place with a small amount of Vetbond at flanged PE50 on top of kidney. Continue to hold the catheter in place until glue is dry (about 1–2 min) (*see* **Note 12**). A schematic of a kidney with an implanted interstitial catheter of which the tip is situated at the boundary between the outer and inner medulla is shown in Fig. 2.
17. Grab a piece of fat from around kidney and place over glue and extending onto kidney. Apply a small amount of Vetbond onto the fat and let dry (*see* **Note 13**).
18. Paint kidney with antibiotic ointment, being careful not to touch the glue. Slide kidney back into cavity by picking up muscle and skin around incision.
19. Grab coils of catheter and place in cavity as well (*see* **Note 14**).
20. Pull spring end of catheter until cross bar of catheter is just above incision under skin (*see* **Note 15**).
21. Sew up muscle with interrupted stitches or a running stitch using 3–0 suture.
22. Sew up skin with interrupted stitches using 4–0 suture. Apply antibiotic ointment to incision.

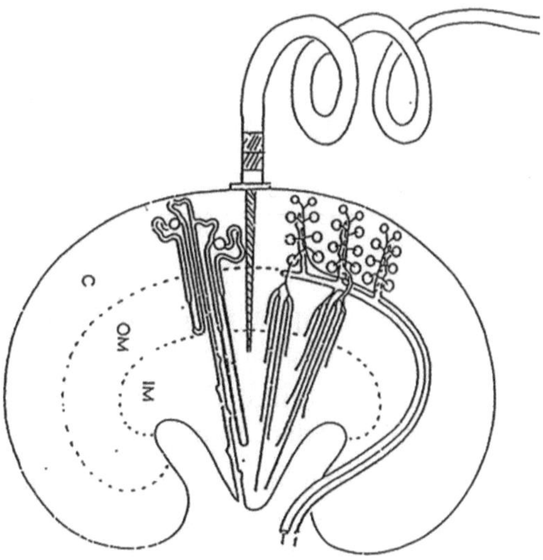

Fig. 2 A schematic of a kidney with an implanted interstitial catheter. *C* cortex, *OM* outer medulla, *IM* inner medulla

23. Turn animal over to dorsal side up and feed the catheter line through the spring. Attach the spring to the scapula muscle using 3–0 silk, and then sew up skin as before with 4–0 suture.
24. Give antibiotic and analgesia post-operatively and recover the animal on a warming pad until awake.
25. After recovery from anesthesia, animal is housed individually in metabolic cages and the spring protecting the catheter is attached to a swivel to allow freedom of movement.

3.4 Maintaining Interstitial Catheter

1. Following post-surgery the interstitial catheter will need to be maintained with a continuous infusion using a Harvard-style syringe pump at a rate of 8 μl/min with 0.9% NaCl saline throughout the study to maintain catheter patency.
2. The saline infusion is accomplished by attaching the interstitial catheter to a swivel which is connected to an infusion pump (*see* **Note 16**).
3. Allow animal to recover at least 7 days before administering anti-miR oligonucleotides.

3.5 Injection of Anti-miR Oligonucleotides into the Renal Interstitium in Conscious Rats

1. Dissolve LNA anti-miR oligonucleotides with 0.9% NaCl saline to make stock solution at desired concentration (*see* **Note 17**).
2. Dilute the stock solution with 0.9% NaCl saline to desired concentration (*see* **Note 18**).
3. Inject 1 mg/kg body weight into the interstitial catheter at a rate of 100 μl over 3 min (*see* **Notes 19** and **20**).
4. After injection; return to normal infusion rate with 0.9% NaCl saline at 8 μl/min.
5. Efficiency of miRNA knockdown and the effect on blood pressure and other phenotypes can be analysed between several hours and several weeks after the anti-miR administration (*see* **Note 21**).

4 Notes

1. Typically the right kidney is removed, and the left kidney is left to be studied.
2. A cotton tip applicator can also be used. Place it under the kidney to help lift it out.
3. Holding the end to the flame for too long will cause it to melt. A round flat surface should be created if done correctly. Also make sure a hole can still be seen in the middle so that the catheter is not plugged.

4. Ensure the catheter does not get to too close over the flame, which will cause it to melt, leading to leakage.
5. The PE 10 can be stretched before being inserted into the PE 50 end. This helps to ensure if it stretches too far and breaks, one would not have to redo the catheter. The easiest way to stretch the PE10 is slow heat with slight tension. The PE 50 bends easily and does not require much heat to bend into a 90 angle.
6. Keeping tension on the tubing and holding it in place will ensure tight coils. Ice can also be added to the cold water beaker to set the coils faster.
7. Place the catheter close to the flame to shrink the tubing, but avoid getting the tip of the catheter too close otherwise it will melt. PVC glue can also be applied around the edge of the shrink tubing after it has shrunk to ensure the catheter is sealed. To test for leaks, fill a 1 cc syringe with milliQ water and fill the catheter, then using a hemostat, clamp the tip of the catheter and slightly press on the syringe to apply pressure. Check the tip where the PE10 and PE 50 connect and then the connection to the tygon.
8. Ensure the PVC glue is applied all the way around the PE240 connector. Allowing the glue to dry overnight and testing it the next day is the best method.
9. Incision should be no more than 1–2 cm. Blunt dissection to the muscle is recommended so there is less irritation to the tissue which allows quicker recovery.
10. Catheter placement is verified at the end of the study. For rats up to about 9 weeks of age, a depth of 2–3 mm usually allows the catheter tip to be situated at the inner and outer medulla junction.
11. Creating a puncture just short of your catheter depth will minimize kidney damage. Insertion of the catheter should show little resistance and slide readily in place.
12. Apply 1–2 drops of the glue. Hold the catheter steady until it dries otherwise it can slip out.
13. Apply one drop.
14. Be careful not to pull on the catheter otherwise the catheter tip can slip out of the kidney. If one grabs the coil with one forceps and stretches the muscle wall with another forceps, the coils should fall right into the body cavity.
15. The cross bar should fit comfortably under the skin. If it presses into the muscle or skin, cut each end of the PE240 shorter so it does not irritate the area.
16. 0.02×0.06 tygon tubing works the best for connecting the swivel from the animal to the syringe on the pump. Use a 16 G needle with a blunt tip to connect the tubing to the syringe.

17. Place the needed amount of oligonucleotide powder into a tube and add saline. Vortex gently. Place the remaining powder back in the freezer.
18. The concentration depends on the dose of anti-miR. The total volume for injection into one kidney should be approximately 100–150 μl.
19. The dose of specific anti-miR will have to be empirically determined.
20. Minimize any air entering the interstitial catheter by ensuring there are no air bubbles in the syringe. Injection should be slow and steady.
21. A single administration of anti-miR could be effective for several weeks. However, repeated administrations may be necessary in some cases. The frequency of repeated administrations may be between daily and weekly and should be determined empirically.

Acknowledgment

This work was supported by NIH grants HL111580 to M.L., HL082798 to A.W.C. and M.L., and HL029587 to A.W.C. and D.L.M.

References

1. Ambros V (2004) The functions of animal microRNAs. Nature 431(7006):350–355
2. Krol J, Loedige I, Filipowicz W (2010) The widespread regulation of microRNA biogenesis, function and decay. Nat Rev Genet 11(9):597–610
3. Kriegel AJ, Mladinov D, Liang M (2012) Translational study of microRNAs and its application in kidney disease and hypertension research. Clin Sci (Lond) 122(10):439–447
4. Liang M, Liu Y, Mladinov D, Cowley AW Jr, Trivedi H, Fang Y, Xu X, Ding X, Tian Z (2009) MicroRNA: a new frontier in kidney and blood pressure research. Am J Physiol Renal Physiol 297(3):F553–F558
5. Cowley AW Jr (1992) Long-term control of arterial blood pressure. Physiol Rev 72(1):231–300
6. Granger JP, Haas JA, Pawlowska D, Knox FG (1988) Effect of direct increases in renal interstitial hydrostatic pressure on sodium excretion. Am J Physiol 254(4 Pt 2):F527–F532
7. Lu S, Roman RJ, Mattson DL, Cowley AW Jr (1992) Renal medullary interstitial infusion of diltiazem alters sodium and water excretion in rats. Am J Physiol 263(5 Pt 2):R1064–R1070
8. Cowley AW Jr, Mattson DL, Lu S, Roman RJ (1995) The renal medulla and hypertension. Hypertension 25(4 Pt 2):663–673
9. Lu S, Mattson DL, Cowley AW Jr (1994) Renal medullary captopril delivery lowers blood pressure in spontaneously hypertensive rats. Hypertension 23(3):337–345
10. Mattson DL, Lu S, Nakanishi K, Papanek PE, Cowley AW Jr (1994) Effect of chronic renal medullary nitric oxide inhibition on blood pressure. Am J Physiol 266(5 Pt 2):H1918–H1926
11. Liang M, Kretschmer P, Kauser K, Perryman M, Kurth T, Tadisch G, Taylor N, Skelton M, Rubanyi GM, Cowley AW Jr (2003) Ultrasound-enhanced gene delivery and siRNA-induced gene silencing in the rat renal medulla. J Am Soc Nephrol 14:28A
12. Liu Y, Singh RJ, Usa K, Netzel B, Liang M (2008) Renal medullary 11β-hydroxysteroid dehydrogenase type 1 in Dahl salt-sensitive hypertension. Physiol Genomics 36(1):52–58
13. Elmén J, Lindow M, Schütz S, Lawrence M, Petri A, Obad S, Lindholm M, Hedtjärn M,

Hansen HF, Berger U, Gullans S, Kearney P, Sarnow P, Straarup EM, Kauppinen S (2008) LNA-mediated microRNA silencing in non-human primates. Nature 452(7189):896–899

14. Liu Y, Taylor NE, Lu L, Cowley AW Jr, Ferreri NR, Yeo NC, Liang M (2010) Renal medullary microRNAs in Dahl salt-sensitive rats: miR-29b regulates several collagens and related genes. Hypertension 55(4):974–982

15. Kriegel AJ, Liu Y, Cohen B, Usa K, Liu Y, Liang M (2012) MiR-382 targeting of kallikrein 5 contributes to renal inner medullary interstitial fibrosis. Physiol Genomics 44(4):259–267

16. Mladinov D, Liu Y, Mattson DL, Liang M (2013) MicroRNAs contribute to the maintenance of cell type-specific physiological characteristics: miR-192 Targets Na^+/K^+-ATPase β1. Nucleic Acids Res 41(2):1273–1283

17. Xu X, Kriegel AJ, Liu Y, Usa K, Mladinov D, Liu H, Fang Y, Ding X, Liang M (2012) Delayed ischemic preconditioning contributes to renal protection by upregulation of miR-21. Kidney Int 82(11):1167–1175

Chapter 32

In Vivo Analysis of Hypertension: Induction of Hypertension, In Vivo Kinase Manipulation, and Assessment of Physiologic Outputs

Satoru Eguchi and Katherine Elliott

Abstract

Using an in vivo model system to study signal transduction will include several steps: (1) induce hypertension in the animal, (2) manipulate kinase activation and signal transduction pathways as desired, and (3) observe physiologic outputs. This chapter provides the reader with overviews of the techniques our lab uses to manipulate signal transduction pathways and determine the effects on hypertension.

Key words Angiotensin II, EGF receptor, Hypertension, End organ damage, Hypertrophy, Fibrosis

1 Introduction

This chapter provides the reader with instructions on how to induce hypertension in mice by infusion of angiotensin II (Ang II), suggestions for various methods to manipulate specific signal transduction components in vivo, and finally how to assess physiologic outputs. The focus is on Epidermal Growth Factor Receptor (EGFR) as an example of a tyrosine kinase and ERK as an example of MAP kinase (MAPK). Both tyrosine kinases and MAP kinases initiate signal transduction cascades that start with an autophosphorylation event [1].

Although there are many animal model systems useful for studying hypertension [2] chronic Ang II infusion is an easy, reliable and relatively inexpensive method. An osmotic minipump is inserted under the skin of the mouse and delivers a steady dose of AngII for 2–4 weeks, resulting in hypertension and eventually end-organ damage [3].

In order to study the signal transduction pathways involved in hypertension in vivo, the kinases will need to be manipulated. The two main ways to inhibit kinases in vivo are through pharmacologic methods and gene knockout. Pharmacologic inhibition of

Rhian M. Touyz and Ernesto L. Schiffrin (eds.), *Hypertension: Methods and Protocols*, Methods in Molecular Biology, vol. 1527, DOI 10.1007/978-1-4939-6625-7_32, © Springer Science+Business Media LLC 2017

EGFR or ERK is relatively quick and inexpensive but often, non-specific effects make data difficult to interpret. Animal knockout systems are more specific but are costly and time consuming. Additionally, systemic knockouts can often be lethal and have unexpected results. A more refined system to use is the cre-lox mice with cre under the control of the sm22α promoter to create a vascular smooth muscle cell specific knockout. Alternatively, an inducible cre system could be used. This chapter does not have space to detail the breeding of transgenic mice, but we can explain the PCR based genotyping protocol used to determine pups that can be used for experiments.

It is important to determine the expression and phosphorylation levels of the kinases in question. This is accomplished by immunohistochemistry or western blotting. Finally, signal transduction events are best studied when physiologic outputs are monitored. This chapter will provide guidance for evaluating hypertension by radiotelemetry [4], which is considered the "gold standard" for measuring blood pressure in laboratory animals, as well as methodologies to assess end organ damage in the mice. Specifically, analysis of fibrosis using Sirius red staining of aortic sections and Masson's trichrome staining of heart and kidney sections will be detailed.

2 Materials

2.1 Osmotic Minipump Implantation

1. Micro-osmotic minipump, Alzet model 1002.
2. 1.0 ml syringe.
3. Anesthesia.
4. Straight hemostat.
5. Suture.

2.2 Genotyping of Sm22a cre-lox Mice

1. 2 week old pups.
2. 50 mM NaOH.
3. 1 M Tris–HCl pH 8.0.
4. PCR kit containing polymerase, buffers, dNTPs.
5. Cre primers.

2.3 Western Blot

1. 1× SDS loading buffer: 0.05 M Tris–HCl pH 6.8, 2% (w/v) SDS, 6% (v/v) β-mercaptoethanol, 1% (w/v) bromophenol blue.
2. Sonicator.
3. 7.5% or 10% SDS PAGE gel, either preformed or make your own.
4. Nitrocellulose membrane.

5. Overnight transfer buffer: 4.5 g tris base, 21.6 g glycine, 1200 ml H_2O, 330 ml methanol.
6. 10× TBS: 60.57 g tris base, pH 7.5, 116.88 g NaCl, H20 up to 1000 ml.
7. TBS-Tween: 100 ml 10× TBS, 1 ml Tween 20, 900 ml dH_2O.
8. Nonfat dry milk.
9. Primary antibody.
10. HRP-conjugated secondary antibody, usually anti-mouse or anti-rabbit.
11. ECL reagents.
12. X-ray film.
13. Autoradiography cassette and developer.

2.4 Immunohisto chemistry

1. Xylene.
2. Ethanol.
3. Citrate buffer: 10 mM Citrate, pH 6.0.
4. H_2O_2.
5. Methanol.
6. Phosphate buffered saline (PBS).
7. PBS-T: PBS with 0.1 % Tween 20.
8. Goat serum.
9. Bovine serum albumin (BSA).
10. Avidin.
11. Biotin.
12. Primary antibody.
13. Biotinylated goat anti-rabbit or biotinylated horse anti-mouse for secondary antibody.
14. Vectastain ABC kit for ABC complex: 1.2 ml 0.1 % BSA PBS-T, 20 μl A, 20 μl B, stand at room temperature for 30 min before using.
15. DAB substrate kit for DAB reaction buffer: 1.2 ml distilled water, 20 μl buffer, 40 μl DAB, 20 μl H_2O_2
16. Hematoxylin.
17. Acid alcohol: 498 ml 95 % ethanol, 2 ml concentrated HCl.
18. Blueing agent.

2.5 Telemetry

1. Anesthesia.
2. Suture.
3. Telemetry unit.

2.6 Sirius Red Staining

1. Paraffin-embedded tissue sections mounted on slides.
2. Xylene.
3. Ethanol.
4. Weigert's iron hematoxylin A solution.
5. Weigart's iron hematoxylin B solution.
6. 0.1 % Sirius Red in saturated picric acid.
7. 0.01 N HCl.

2.7 Masson's Trichrome Staining

1. Paraffin-embedded tissue sections mounted on slides.
2. Xylene.
3. Ethanol.
4. Weigert's iron hematoxylin A solution.
5. Weigart's iron hematoxylin B solution.
6. Bouin's solution.
7. Biebrich scarlet-acid fuchsin solution.
8. Phosphotungstic-phosphomolybdic acid solution.
9. Aniline blue solution.
10. 1 % acetic acid.

3 Methods

3.1 Osmotic Minipump Implantation

Fill micro-osmotic pump

1. Weigh the empty pump and flow moderator, together (*see* **Note 1**).
2. Prepare stock solution of AngII (*see* **Note 2**). Taking into account the animal's weight, calculate dilution of stock solution so that 1000 ng/kg/min is delivered to the animal for 2 weeks.
   (a) $140\{[10/(1000 \times \text{body weight}/1 \times 10^6/0.25 \times 60)] - 1\}$.
3. Draw the solution of Ang II into a 1 ml syringe. Attach the 27 G filling tube (*see* **Note 3**).
4. Remove the flow moderator from the pump and hold the pump upright. Insert the filling tube as far as possible into the opening at the top of the pump.
5. Inject drug slowly into pump. Remove tube when solution reaches the outlet.
6. Wipe excess solution and insert flow moderator until the white flange is flush with the top of the pump.
7. Weigh the filled pump to determine the weight of the solution loaded (*see* **Note 4**).

8. Place filled pumps in eppendorf tubes and cover with 0.9% sterile saline. Incubate at 37 °C overnight (*see* **Note 5**).

Implantation

1. Anesthetize animal.
2. Shave and disinfect the skin on the right shoulder where the implantation site will be.
3. Make a midline skin incision, 0.5 cm long, perpendicular to the tail. Carefully tent up the incision and use straight hemostats to make a subcutaneous tunnel underneath the skin to create a pocket for the mini-pump.
4. Insert the filled pump into the cavity with the flow moderator pointing away from the incision (*see* **Note 6**).
5. Close the wound with three or four interrupted sutures.

3.2 Genotyping of Sm22α cre-lox Mice

1. Through standard breeding practices, breed experimental mice that are cre/+;lox/lox.
2. Use a freshly cut mouse toe from a 2 week old pup (*see* **Note 7**).
3. With tissue in an eppendorf tube, add 180 μl of 50 mM NaOH, then vortex for 30 s.
4. Boil sample for 10 min then vortex for 30 s.
5. Add 20 μl of 1 M Tris–HCl pH 8.0, then vortex for 30 s.
6. Spin at 10,000 × *g* for 5 min.
7. Use 0.5 μl of supernatant for PCR.
8. Perform PCR with Cre primers to identify cre positive mice. Perform PCR with primers flanking lox site to identify +/+, +/lox, and lox/lox mice.
9. Experimental animals are cre positive; lox/lox mice. Control mice can be cre positive; +/+ mice or cre positive; +/lox depending on the gene to be knocked out.

3.3 Western Blot to Quantitate Kinases

Prepare samples of mouse tissue

1. Homogenize tissue in RIPA buffer.
2. Quantitate protein by standard methods.
3. Dilute sample for western using RIPA buffer so that each sample has equivalent protein amount and volume in final 1× SDS Sample buffer (*see* **Note 8**).

Run western blot

1. Run sample on 7.5% or 10% SDS PAGE with stacking gel at 50 V until sample through stacking gel. Increase voltage to 100 V.
2. Transfer the protein to nitrocellulose membrane by overnight transfer at 30 V in 4 °C using Overnight Transfer Buffer.

3. Wash membrane three times for 10 min in TBS-Tween, with slight rocking.
4. Block membrane with 5% (w/v) nonfat dry milk in TBS-Tween for 1 h at room temperature, with slight rocking.
5. Incubate blot with primary antibody in TBS-Tween overnight at 4 °C, with slight rocking.
6. Wash membrane three times for 10 min in TBS-Tween, with slight rocking.
7. Incubate blot with secondary antibody (HRP-conjugated anti-mouse or anti-rabbit) in TBS-Tween for 1 h at room temperature, with slight rocking.
8. Wash membrane three times for 10 min in TBS-Tween, with slight rocking.
9. Add ECL reagents, incubate at room temperature for 1 min, expose to X-ray film.

3.4 Immunohisto chemistry to Evaluate Phosphorylation of Kinase

Deparaffinize and hydrate slides

1. Incubate slide in Xylene, twice for 5 min.
2. Incubate slide in 100% ethanol, twice for 3 min.
3. Incubate slide in 90% ethanol, once for 2 min.
4. Incubate slide in 70% ethanol, once for 2 min.
5. Incubate slide in distilled water, once for 2 min.

Unmasking

1. Incubate slide in boiling citrate buffer, 10 min.
2. Incubate slide at room temperature, 20 min.
3. Wash slide with distilled water, three times for 3 min.

Deactivation of endogenous peroxidase

1. Incubate slide in 0.3% H_2O_2 in MeOH, 20 min.
2. Wash slide with distilled water, three times for 2 min.
3. Wash slide with PBS, three times for 1 min.

Blocking (*see* **Note 9**)

1. Incubate slide in PBS-T with 5% Normal Goat Serum and 1% BSA for 60 min at room temperature.
2. Wash slide with 0.1% BSA PBS-T, two times for 1 min.
3. Incubate slide with one drop of Avidin for 10 min.
4. Wash slide with 0.1% BSA PBS-T, two times for 1 min.
5. Incubate slide with one drop Biotin for 10 min.
6. Wash slide with 0.1% BSA PBS-T, two times for 1 min.

Primary antibody

1. Incubate slide with primary antibody (diluted in 1 % BSA PBS-T) overnight at 4 °C.
2. Wash slide with 0.1 % BSA PBS-T four times for 5 min.

Secondary antibody

1. Incubate slide with Biotinylated Goat anti-rabbit IgG or Biotinylated Horse anti-mouse IgG in 1 % BSA PBS-T for 90–120 min at room temperature.
2. Wash slide with 0.1 % BSA in PBS-T, four times for 5 min.

Amplification

1. Incubate slide with ABC complex for 30 min.
2. Wash slide with PBS, three times for 5 min.

Development

1. Perform DAB reaction for 1–10 min depending on antibody.
2. Wash slide with distilled water, three times for 3 min.

Counter stain

1. Wash slide with hematoxylin for 30 s.
2. Wash slide with distilled water for 15 s.
3. Wash slide with acid alcohol for 20 s.
4. Wash slide with distilled water for 15 s.
5. Wash slide with blueing agent for 20 s.
6. Wash slide with distilled water for 1 min.

Dehydration and penetration (Fig. 1)

1. Wash slide with 70 % EtOH for 1 min.
2. Wash slide with 100 % EtOH three times for 1 min.
3. Wash slide with CitriSolv three times for 1 min.
4. Wash slide with Xylene one time for 5 min.

3.5 Telemetry to Evaluate Hypertension (See Note 10)

1. Create a subcutaneous pocket in left shoulder by cutting a 1 cm linear incision.
2. Make a midline incision from the sternum to the jaw, approximately 2 cm. Retract the salivary glands to expose the muscles of the trachea.
3. Insert the transmitter into the subcutaneous pocket on the left shoulder (Fig. 2) and guide the catheter subcutaneously to the neck.
4. Loosely tape the animal's forelimbs to the table.

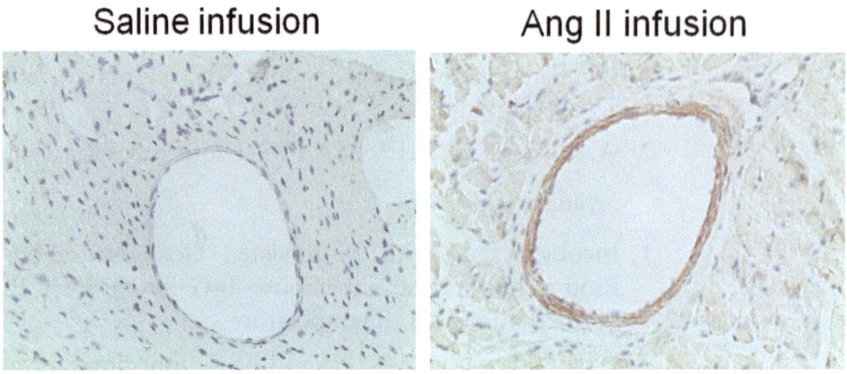

Fig. 1 IHC data using anti-EGFR-pY1068 with heart samples with coronary arteries

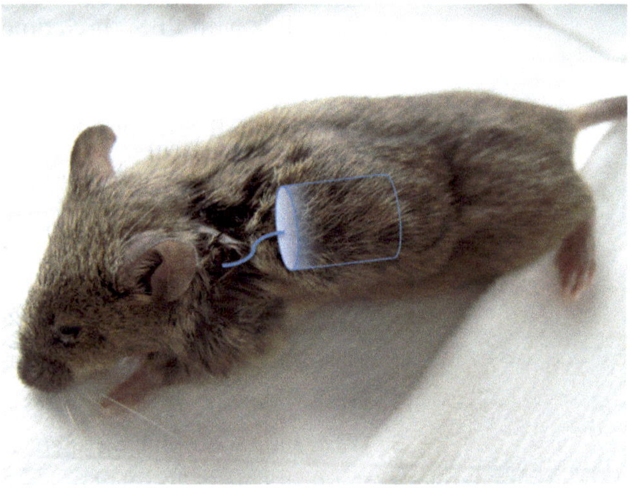

Fig. 2 Location of the transmitter

5. Locate the carotid artery along the left side of the trachea and carefully isolate the vessel from the connective tissue and vagus nerve (*see* **Note 11**).
6. Pass two lengths of nonabsorbable suture (6-0) underneath the isolated section of artery.
7. Position one suture just proximal to the bifurcation of the external and internal carotid arteries and ligate the vessel.
8. Position the other suture close to the clavicle and apply tension to elevate the artery and occlude blood flow.
9. Cut the vessel just below the point of ligation with fine micro scissors and insert the catheter. Alternatively, a bent-tipped syringe needle can be used to incise the vessel wall and introduce the catheter into the artery (Fig. 3) [5]. Advance the tip so that the catheter notch is a few millimeters above the clavicle. Tie in the catheter using the two sutures.

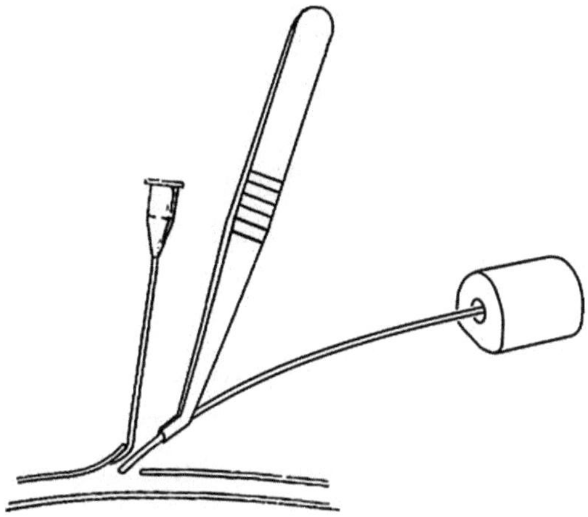

Fig. 3 Bent tip syringe to help introduce telemetry catheter

10. Confirm that the radiotelemetry is transmitting. If not working well, change the position of the catheter tip and retry.
11. Close the catheter skin incision with nonabsorbable sutures (5-0 or 6-0).
12. Close the telemetry skin incision with nonabsorbable sutures (5-0 05 6-0).
13. Allow animal to recover at least 10 min on warming pad.
14. Starting the next day, measure blood pressure continuously.

3.6 Sirius Red Staining to Evaluate End Organ Damage (See Note 12)

Deparaffinize and hydrate slides

1. Incubate slide in xylene, twice for 5 min.
2. Incubate slide in 100% ethanol, twice for 3 min.
3. Incubate slide in 90% ethanol, once for 2 min.
4. Incubate slide in 70% ethanol, once for 2 min.
5. Incubate slide in distilled water, once for 2 min.

Staining

1. Make iron hematoxylin working solution by mixing a 1:1 ratio of Weigert's iron hematoxylin A and Weigart's iron hematoxylin B solutions.
2. Stain slide with hematoxylin working solution for 10 min at room temperature.
3. Wash slide, twice for 3 min.
4. Stain slide with Sirius Red (0.1% in saturated picric acid) for 1 h at room temperature.
5. Wash slide with 0.01 N HCl, twice for 3 min.

Dehydration and penetration

1. Incubate slide in 70% ethanol for 3 min.
2. Incubate slide in 100% ethanol for 3 min.
3. Incubate slide in xylene, twice for 5 min.
4. Mount slides (Fig. 4).

3.7 Masson's Trichrome Staining to Evaluate End Organ Damage (See Note 13)

Deparaffinize and hydrate slides

1. Incubate slide in xylene, twice for 5 min.
2. Incubate slide in 100% ethanol, twice for 3 min.
3. Incubate slide in 90% ethanol, once for 2 min.
4. Incubate slide in 70% ethanol, once for 2 min.
5. Incubate slide in distilled water, once for 2 min.

Staining

1. Stain slide with Bouin's solution for 1 h at 56 °C.
2. Rinse slide in tap water, three times for 3 min.
3. Make hematoxylin working solution by mixing a 1:1 ratio of Weigert's iron hematoxylin A and Weigart's iron hematoxylin B solutions.
4. Stain slide with hematoxylin working solution for 7.5 min at room temperature.
5. Rinse slide in distilled water for 30 s.
6. Stain slide in Biebrich scarlet-acid fuchsin solution for 7.5 min.
7. Rinse slide in distilled water for 30 s.
8. Differentiate slide in phosphotungstic-phosphomolybdic acid solution for 5 min (*see* **Note 14**).
9. Stain slides in aniline blue solution for 5 min.
10. Differentiate slide in 1% acetic acid solution for 1 min.

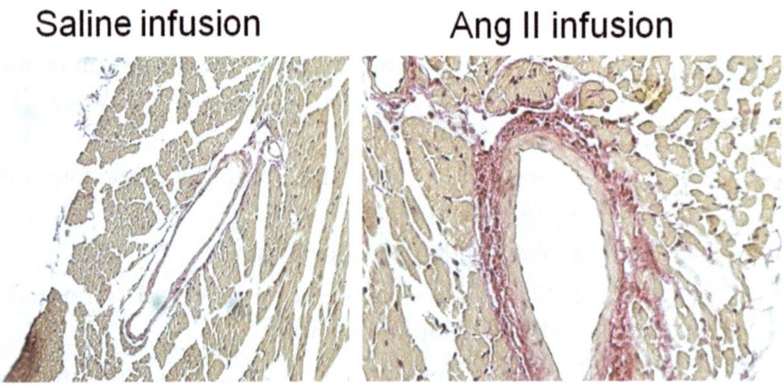

Fig. 4 Sirius Red staining data in heart samples with coronary arteries

11. Rinse slide in distilled water for 30 s.
12. Nuclei will stain black; collagen will stain blue; muscle, cytoplasm, and keratin will stain red.

Dehydration and penetration

1. Incubate slide in 70% ethanol for 3 min.
2. Incubate slide in 100% ethanol for 3 min.
3. Incubate slide in xylene, twice for 5 min.
4. Mount slides.

4 Notes

1. Use sterile technique including filter sterilization of drug.
2. Store as filter sterilized solution of 10 mM Ang II in saline.
3. Avoid air bubbles.
4. Weight of pump in milligrams is equivalent to volume in milliliters.
5. Incubate overnight for a 2 week pump and 48 h for a 4 week pump.
6. If the pocket is not large enough to hold the implant comfortably, remove the implant and enlarge the pocket as described above.
7. Do not freeze tissue sample.
8. Make a 5× sample buffer to use for final sample dilution.
9. Starting at this step, work with slides in a moisturizing box.
10. Potential adverse effects from this procedure may include: anesthetic related respiratory distress, infection of the subcutaneous pocket, catheter insertion site, dehiscence of the surgical site, seroma formation around the transmitter, hind limb paresis or paralysis related to ischemia or nerve damage, hemorrhage due to leaking of the vessel around the catheter insertion site.
11. Do not disturb the vagus nerve.
12. This procedure works best on paraffin-embedded sections.
13. This procedure works well on both paraffin-embedded sections and frozen tissue samples.
14. Immerse until collagen is no longer red.

References

1. Shirai H, Autieri M, Eguchi S (2007) Small gtp-binding proteins and mitogen-activated protein kinases as promising therapeutic targets of vascular remodeling. Curr Opin Nephrol Hypertens 16:111–115
2. Sarikonda KV, Watson RE, Opara OC, Dipette DJ (2009) Experimental animal models of hypertension. J Am Soc Hypertens 3:158–165
3. Qin Z (2008) Newly developed angiotensin ii-infused experimental models in vascular biology. Regul Pept 150:1–6
4. Kurtz TW, Griffin KA, Bidani AK, Davisson RL, Hall JE, Subcommittee of P, Public Education of the American Heart A (2005) Recommendations for blood pressure measurement in humans and experimental animals. Part 2: blood pressure measurement in experimental animals: a statement for professionals from the subcommittee of professional and public education of the American heart association council on high blood pressure research. Hypertension 45:299–310
5. Takayanagi T, Kawai T, Forrester SJ, Obama T, Tsuji T, Fukuda Y, Elliott KJ, Tilley DG, Davisson RL, Park JY, Eguchi S. (2015) Role of epidermal growth factor receptor and endoplasmic reticulum stress in vascular remodeling induced by angiotensin II. Hypertension 65(6): 1349–55
6. Huetteman DA, Bogie H (2009) Direct blood pressure monitoring in laboratory rodents via implantable radio telemetry. Methods Mol Biol 573:57–73

INDEX

Rhian M. Touyz and Ernesto L. Schiffrin (eds.), *Hypertension: Methods and Protocols*, Methods in Molecular Biology, vol. 1527, DOI 10.1007/978-1-4939-6625-7, © Springer Science+Business Media LLC 2017

D

E

F

H

T

U

V

W

MIX
Papier aus verantwortungsvollen Quellen
Paper from responsible sources
FSC® C105338

If you have any concerns about our products,
you can contact us on
ProductSafety@springernature.com

In case Publisher is established outside the EU,
the EU authorized representative is:
Springer Nature Customer Service Center GmbH
Europaplatz 3, 69115 Heidelberg, Germany

Printed by Libri Plureos GmbH
in Hamburg, Germany